T0257565

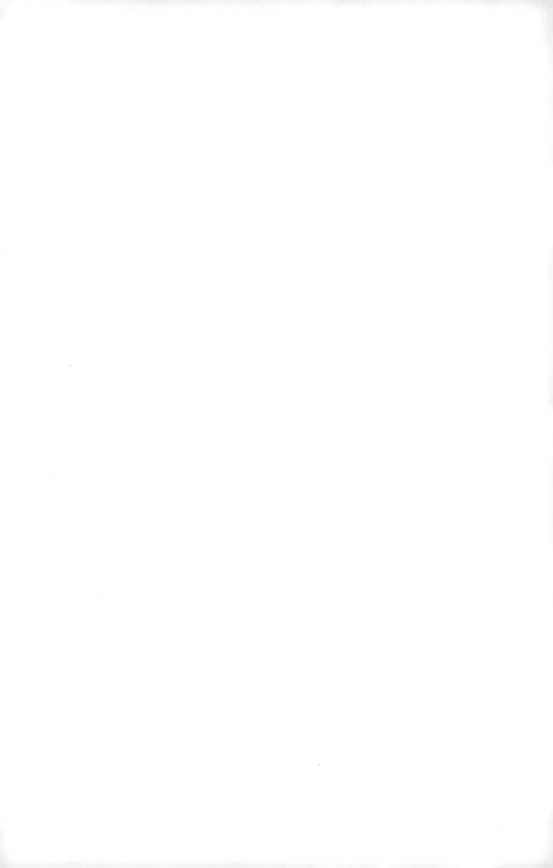

Diverse Applications of Gene Therapy

Diverse Applications of Gene Therapy

Edited by **Harvey Summers**

New Jersey

Published by Foster Academics,
61 Van Reypen Street,
Jersey City, NJ 07306, USA
www.fosteracademics.com

Diverse Applications of Gene Therapy
Edited by Harvey Summers

International Standard Book Number: 978-1-63242-117-3 (Hardback)

Printed in the United States of America.

Contents

Preface   VII

Section 1   Applications: Inherited Diseases   1

Chapter 1   Gene Therapy for Retinitis Pigmentosa   3
             Hiroshi Tomita, Eriko Sugano, Hitomi Isago,
             Namie Murayama and Makoto Tamai

Chapter 2   Gene Therapy for Primary Immunodeficiencies   21
             Francisco Martin, Alejandra Gutierrez-Guerrero and Karim
             Benabdellah

Chapter 3   Gene Therapy for Diabetic Retinopathy – Targeting the
             Renin-Angiotensin System   34
             Qiuhong Li, Amrisha Verma, Ping Zhu, Bo Lei, Yiguo Qiu,
             Takahiko Nakagawa, Mohan K Raizada and William W Hauswirth

Chapter 4   Gene Therapy for the *COL7A1* Gene   59
             E. Mayr, U. Koller and J.W. Bauer

Chapter 5   Gene Therapy for Erythroid Metabolic Inherited Diseases   88
             Maria Garcia-Gomez, Oscar Quintana-Bustamante, Maria Garcia-
             Bravo, S. Navarro, Zita Garate and Jose C. Segovia

Chapter 6   Targeting the Lung: Challenges in Gene Therapy for
             Cystic Fibrosis   116
             George Kotzamanis, Athanassios Kotsinas,
             Apostolos Papalois and Vassilis G. Gorgoulis

Chapter 7   Molecular Therapy for Lysosomal Storage Diseases   138
             Daisuke Tsuji and Kohji Itoh

Section 2   **Applications: Others**   **155**

Chapter 8   **Gene Therapy in Critical Care Medicine**   **157**
             Gabriel J. Moreno-González and Angel Zarain-Herzberg

Chapter 9   **Gene Therapy for Chronic Pain Management**   **177**
             Isaura Tavares and Isabel Martins

Chapter 10   **Insulin Trafficking in a Glucose Responsive Engineered**
             Human Liver Cell Line is Regulated by the Interaction
             of ATP-Sensitive Potassium Channels and
             Voltage-Gated Calcium Channels   **194**
             Ann M. Simpson, M. Anne Swan, Guo Jun Liu,
             Chang Tao, Bronwyn A O'Brien, Edwin Ch'ng, Leticia M. Castro,
             Julia Ting, Zehra Elgundi, Tony An, Mark Lutherborrow,
             Fraser Torpy, Donald K. Martin, Bernard E. Tuch
             and Graham M. Nicholson

Chapter 11   **Clinical and Translational Challenges in Gene Therapy of**
             Cardiovascular Diseases   **218**
             Divya Pankajakshan and Devendra K. Agrawal

Chapter 12   **Feasibility of Gene Therapy for Tooth Regeneration by**
             Stimulation of a Third Dentition   **251**
             Katsu Takahashi, Honoka Kiso, Kazuyuki Saito, Yumiko Togo,
             Hiroko Tsukamoto, Boyen Huang and Kazuhisa Bessho

Chapter 13   **Gene Therapy Perspectives Against Diseases of the**
             Respiratory System   **269**
             Dimosthenis Lykouras, Kiriakos Karkoulias, Christos
             Tourmousoglou, Efstratios Koletsis, Kostas Spiropoulos and
             Dimitrios Dougenis

             Permissions

             List of Contributors

Preface

This book has been a concerted effort by a group of academicians, researchers and scientists, who have contributed their research works for the realization of the book. This book has materialized in the wake of emerging advancements and innovations in this field. Therefore, the need of the hour was to compile all the required researches and disseminate the knowledge to a broad spectrum of people comprising of students, researchers and specialists of the field.

Gene therapy has been extensively researched in this all-inclusive book. Gene therapy as a field has gained its due regard after all these years of poor outcomes. Issues in the past which were troubling scientists and practitioners are now being easily resolved. The growth of secure and effective gene transfer and development in the field of cell therapy has now brought new ways to deal with varied diseases. The book aims at compiling information from different resources about various gene therapy tools, practical achievements of gene therapy and its future usage. Some of the important chapters discuss non-viral delivery systems in gene therapy, transgene expression, plasmid transgene expression in vivo - promoter and tissue variables, DNA electrotransfer as an effective tool for gene therapy, siRNA and gene formulation.

At the end of the preface, I would like to thank the authors for their brilliant chapters and the publisher for guiding us all-through the making of the book till its final stage. Also, I would like to thank my family for providing the support and encouragement throughout my academic career and research projects.

Editor

Applications: Inherited Diseases

Gene Therapy for Retinitis Pigmentosa

Hiroshi Tomita, Eriko Sugano, Hitomi Isago,
Namie Murayama and Makoto Tamai

Additional information is available at the end of the chapter

1. Introduction

The retina comprises diverse differentiated neurons that have specific functions. Photoreceptor cells, the first-order neurons in the retina, have photopigments (rhodopsin and opsin) that absorb photons. Signals produced by the photoreceptor cells are transmitted to second-order neurons. Finally, visual signals are transmitted to the brain from the third-order neurons, the retinal ganglion cells (RGCs). Major diseases that cause blindness in advanced countries include glaucoma, diabetic retinopathy, retinitis pigmentosa (RP), and age-related retinopathy. Loss of vision due to these diseases is irreversible. However, with regard to glaucoma, eye drops that have the effect of reducing intraocular pressure have been developed. In diabetic retinopathy, effective surgical treatments such as vitrectomy and photocoagulation have been established. Blindness due to glaucoma and diabetic retinopathy can be prevented by administering these treatments in the early phase. On the other hand, in diseases caused by gene mutations, such as RP, effective treatments for delaying photoreceptor degeneration have not yet been established. Degeneration of photoreceptor cells results in loss of vision, even if other retinal neurons are intact [1-3].

RP is a disease that causes blindness due to photoreceptor degeneration. Symptoms include night blindness and loss of peripheral and central vision. Approximately 1 in 4,000 people are affected by this disease [4]. In 1990, Dryja et al. [5] first identified a point mutation in the rhodopsin gene from RP patients. A number of gene mutations responsible for RP has subsequently been identified. Most of these genes are associated with the phototransduction pathway in the retina. In some cases, the mutated gene exists not only in photoreceptor cells but also in retinal pigment epithelial cells. To date, 53 causative genes and 7 loci of RP have been identified (http://www.sph.uth.tmc.edu/Retnet/). Leber's congenital amaurosis (LCA) is another retinal degenerative disease predicted to affect approximately 1/81000 individuals [6]. Most LCA patients have severe visual defects in childhood. Histological analysis of the retinas of LCA patients shows marked retinal atrophy in the outer retinal layer, vascular thickening and sclerosis, and atrophy of the retinal pigment epithelium (RPE) [7]. Leber classified the disease as a type of RP on the basis of these characteristics. Later, Franceschetti and Dieterle differentiated it from retinal dystrophy based on the features of electroretinograms (ERGs) in these patients. Many gene mutations involved in LCA have been identified and the disease has been classified into 15 subtypes based on the affected gene [8-13]. Among these, LCA2, accounting for 10% of LCA cases [14], is due to a mutation in the RPE65 gene, which encodes all-*trans* retinyl ester isomerase. Deficiency in RPE65, leads to severe loss of visual function. Thus, in the case of LCA2, the cause of the disease is clearly identified as the biochemical blockade of the visual cycle caused by RPE65 deficiency [11,12]. Replacement therapy using the RPE65 gene is a candidate therapeutic strategy for LCA2. Indeed, successful results have been reported in RPE65 replacement therapy with the LCA2 animal model, Briard dogs [15]. After proof-of-principle studies [16], phase I trials using adeno-associated virus vector type 2 were conducted in 3 independent groups [17]. The results showed no adverse effects such as systemic dissemination of vector or immunological responses to the vector or transgene. Importantly, improvement of visual function as evaluated by microperimetry was observed in 1 subject [18,19]. Two other groups also reported improvement in visual function [20,21]. Continuous follow-ups for 1.5 years [22] have confirmed the safety and tolerability of replacement gene therapy [23]. The various hereditary forms of RP are as follows: autosomal dominant, recessive, and X-linked recessive. The Pro23 -> His gene mutation in the rhodopsin gene [24,25] occurs in 20–30% of all RP patients in Europe and the U.S. In contrast, the occurrence in Japan is only a few percent. Thus, in addition to the diversity of the gene mutations, their frequencies vary characteristically among different races. Differences in the progression, clinical findings, and development of the disease are also observed among different patients, even in those with the same mutation. A common feature of photoreceptor cell death caused by various gene mutations is eventual apoptosis via a common pathway [26]. Based on this rationale, various kinds of methods to prevent apoptosis, such as chemical treatment [27,28] and gene therapy, including gene replacement and neurotrophic factor supplementation [29-31], have been investigated. However, these strategies have not been successful in the complete prevention of cell death, although they have been shown to delay degeneration. The diversity of clinical features and gene mutations makes it difficult to develop effective treatments for RP.

A retinal prosthesis, comprising electrodes, an image processor, and a camera, is the only method to restore vision that has been studied [32-36]. Recently, a new strategy involving gene therapy for restoring vision has been developed using bacteriorhodopsin family genes [37,38]. The channelrhodopsin-2 (ChR2) gene derived from the green alga *Chlamydomonas* functions as a photoreceptor and cation-selective channel [39]. After the absorption of photons by photopigments, photon acquisition is completed by a chain reaction involving certain photoreceptor-specific proteins. Thus, the phototransduction pathway in photoreceptor cells requires not only photopigments but also certain photoreceptor-specific proteins, which complicates the reaction. Due to the inherent characteristics of ChR2, photosensitive neurons can be produced by the transfer of the ChR2 gene into neurons [40-42]. Here, we introduce new strategies for restoring vision by using channelrhodopsins.

2. Materials and methods

All the experiments performed for this report were approved by the Tohoku University Animal Care Committee, which is accredited by the Ministry of Education, Culture, Sports, Science, and Technology of Japan. Every effort was made to minimize the number and suffering of animals used in the following experiments.

Animals

We used 2 types of photoreceptor degeneration models: a genetically blind rat model and a light-induced photoreceptor degeneration model. The experimental design for each of these models is shown in Fig. 1.

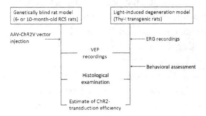

Figure 1. Experimental design. Two types of photoreceptor degeneration models were used in this study. The photo-receptor cells of RCS rats degenerate by 3 months after birth due to the Mertk gene mutation. On the other hand, Thy-TG rats have native photoreceptors. Therefore, we subjected TG rats to continuous light exposure to induce pho-toreceptor degeneration. To confirm photoreceptor degeneration, ERGs were recorded before performing behavioral assessments. Finally, the eyes from all animals were subjected to histological examination.

Genetically blind rats

Royal College of Surgeons (RCS; rdy/rdy) rats [43,44] were used as model animals for photorecep-tor degeneration in our experiments. The RCS rat, an animal model of recessively inherited retinal degeneration, is widely used in the study of photoreceptor degeneration. The gene responsible is the receptor tyrosine kinase gene Mertk [45], and mutations in MERTK, the human ortholog of the RCS rat retinal dystrophy gene, cause RP [46]. Photoreceptor degeneration is almost complete by 3 months after birth. We intravitreously injected the AAV-ChR2V vector into 6-month- or 10-month-old RCS rats. The rats were obtained from CLEA Japan, Inc. (Tokyo, Japan).

Thy-I ChR2 transgenic rats

We established transgenic (TG) rats harboring the ChR2 gene regulated by the Thy-1.2 promoter to investigate contrast sensitivity at each spatial frequency [47]. The rat Thy-1.2 antigen has been found to be abundant in the brain and thymus [48,49]. In the retina, the Thy-1.2 antigen is recognized as a marker specific to RGCs [50,51]. It is necessary to induce the degeneration of native photoreceptor cells in order to investigate the visual function conferred by ChR2-expressing RGCs, because the Thy-I TG rat has native photoreceptor cells. For this purpose, Thy-I TG rats were subjected to light-induced photoreceptor degeneration. Briefly, Thy-I TG rats were kept in cyclic light (12 hours ON/OFF: 5–10 lux/dark) for at least 2 weeks prior to light exposure. The rats were then exposed to a 3000-lux intensity of fluorescent light for 7 days [28]. We used a light exposure box (NK Systems, Tokyo, Japan) to control the timing and light intensity for the induction of photoreceptor degeneration. After induction, we recorded ERGs to confirm photoreceptor degeneration.

Preparation of the adeno-associated virus vector

The adeno-associated virus (AAV) vector with the ChR2 gene was constructed as described previously [38]. Following this, the AAV Helper-Free System (Stratagene, La Jolla, CA) was used to produce infectious AAV-Venus (control) and AAV-ChR2V virions, which were purified by a single-step column purification method as previously described [52].

Recording of ERGs and visual electrophysiology (VEP)

ERGs and VEP readings were recorded using a Neuropack (MEB-9102; Nihon Kohden, Tokyo, Japan) according to methods previously described [38,53]. Briefly, rats were dark-adapted overnight, and the pupils were dilated with 1% atropine and 2.5% phenylephrine hydrochloride. Small contact lenses with gold wire loops were placed on both corneas, and a silver wire reference electrode was inserted subcutaneously between the eyes. Eyes were stimulated with flash light stimuli of 10-ms duration using a blue LED. Full-field scotopic ERGs were recorded, band-pass filtered at 0.3–500 Hz, and averaged for 5 responses at each light intensity. For VEP recordings, recording electrodes (silver-silver chloride) were placed epidurally on each side, 7 mm behind the bregma and 3 mm lateral of the midline, and a reference electrode was placed epidurally on the midline 12 mm behind the bregma, at least 7 days before the experiments [54,55]. Under ketamine-xylazine anesthesia, the pupils were dilated with 1% atropine and 2.5% phenylephrine hydrochloride. The ground electrode clip was placed on the tail. Photic stimuli of 20-ms duration were generated under various intensities by pulse activation of a blue LED. The high- and low-pass filters were set to 50 kHz and 0.05 kHz, respectively. One hundred consecutive response waveforms were averaged for each VEP measurement.

Determination of transduction efficiency

At the end of the experiment, RCS and Thy-TG rats were sacrificed, and their eyes were resected and fixed in 4% paraformaldehyde and 0.1 M phosphate buffer, pH 7.4 [56]. The eye of each rat was flat-mounted on a slide and covered with Vectashield medium (Vector Laboratories, Burlingame, CA) to prevent the degradation of fluorescence. Then, the number of positive cells was counted.

3. Behavioral assessment

The spatial vision of each animal was quantified by its optomotor response. We used a virtual optomotor system to evaluate the contrast sensitivities of each spatial frequency. The original virtual optomotor system described by Prusky et al. [57] was modified for rats [47]. When a drum is rotated around an animal with printed visual stimuli on the inside wall, the animal tracks the stimulus by turning its head. A light-dark grating pattern was displayed on computer monitors (ProLite E1902WS; Iiyama, Tokyo, Japan) arranged in a square around a platform. The software controlled the speed of virtual optomotor rotation, which was set at 12 degrees per second (2 rpm) in all experiments. The spatial frequency and the contrast of the grating pattern were varied but the average brightness was kept constant.

The animal was allowed to move freely on the platform in the virtual optomotor system. The grating session was started at a low spatial frequency (0.06 cycles/degree) with maximal contrast. An experimenter assessed whether the animals tracked the rotation, by monitoring the head movement and the presented rotating stimulus simultaneously on another display connected to the video camera. If head movement simultaneous with the rotation was evident, the experimenter judged that the animal could discriminate the grating, and proceeded to the next grating session. If the movement was ambiguous, the same grating session was presented again. All behavioral tests were double-blinded and performed during the first few hours of the animals' light cycle (light on at 8 AM).

4. Results

4.1. Recording of VEP measurements in RCS rats

VEP measurements in 6- or 10-month-old RCS rats are expected to be abolished due to loss of photoreceptor cells. Generally, in RCS rats, photoreceptor degeneration is almost complete by 3 months after birth. Indeed, VEP measurements were not evoked even by the maximal LED flash in any of the aged RCS (rdy/rdy) rats (Fig. 2A). On the other hand, robust VEPs were evoked by the blue LED flash in RCS rats injected with the AAV-ChR2V vector (Fig. 2A). Initially, small VEP responses were observed at 2 weeks after AAV injection (data not shown), and the maximum amplitudes of VEP were observed 8 weeks later [58]. There were notable differences in sample waveforms from 6- and 10-month-old rats injected with AAV-ChR2V. Amplitudes and latencies of VEPs from 6-month-old rats were larger and shorter, respectively, than those from 10-month-old rats (Fig. 2B).

4.2. Transduction efficiencies of ChR2 in retinas of RCS rats

The expression of the ChR2 gene was evaluated by measuring Venus fluorescence in RCS rat retinas (Fig. 3A). The number of positive cells in rats injected at 10 months of age was significantly less than that injected at 6 months of age (Fig. 3B). The number of RGCs decreased linearly with age, following photoreceptor degeneration in the RCS rats (Fig. 3C). We have previously shown [56] that the ChR2 gene is mainly expressed in RGCs upon intravitreous injection of the AAV-ChR2V vector. Therefore, the observed decrease in the number of RGCs with age suggests that the transduction efficiencies at both ages are very similar.

4.3. Photoreceptor degeneration in Thy-I TG rats

There were 11–12 rows of photoreceptor nuclei in the outer nuclear layer (ONL) of the Thy-1 TG rats; this is a number usually observed in rodents without retinal degeneration [59].

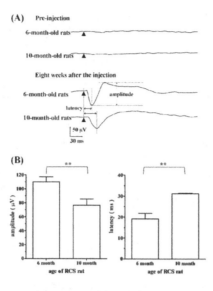

Figure 2. VEP recordings before and after the injection of AAV-ChR2V. (A) VEP recordings from both 6-month- and 10-month-old RCS rats showed no responses. However, VEPs responses were clearly elicited 8 weeks after injection. (B) The amplitudes and latencies from rats injected with AAV-ChR2 at 6 months of age (n = 8) were significantly larger and shorter than those injected at 10 months of age (n = 4).

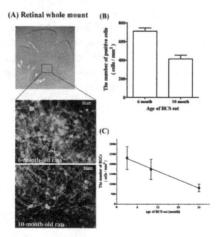

Figure 3. Transduction efficiencies of ChR2 in retinas of RCS rats. (A) Retinal whole-mount specimens obtained from rats injected with AAV-ChR2 at 6 and 10 months of age. (B) Venus-positive cells expressing the ChR2 gene were observed in whole-mount specimens. (C) The number of RGCs decreased with age.

Following continuous light exposure, photoreceptor cells disappeared (Fig. 4A). ERGs showed no response, indicating that the photoreceptor cells degenerated in the whole retina (Fig. 4B).

However, robust VEP measurements could be recorded, even though the photoreceptor cells had completely degenerated (Fig. 4B). Intense expression of the ChR2 gene was observed in the entire retina, with about 45% of RGCs positive for ChR2 (Fig. 4C).

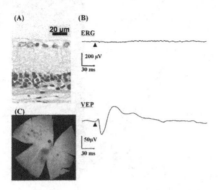

Figure 4. Electrophysiological response of Thy-I TG rats after photoreceptor degeneration. (A) Hematoxylin-eosin staining of the retina showed the degeneration of the native photoreceptor cells after continuous light exposure. (B) Extensive expression of the ChR2 gene was observed throughout the retina. (C) The ERG response was completely abolished following continuous light exposure, indicating that native photoreceptor cells had degenerated throughout the retina. VEP measurements could still be recorded after photoreceptor degeneration.

4.4. Behavioral assessment in photoreceptor degenerated-Thy-I TG rat

In our virtual optomotor system, a stimulus of blue stripes over a black background was produced according to a sine wave function with variable amplitude and frequency (Fig. 5A). All the photoreceptor-degenerated Thy-I TG and wild-type (normal) rats tracked the virtual rotating blue/black gratings (Fig. 5B). However, tracking stopped when the contrast was reduced below a specific threshold. We observed that contrast sensitivity was small at the minimal spatial frequency of 0.06 cycles per degree (CPD), increased with an increase in spatial frequency, and was negligible at spatial frequencies over 0.52 CPD. Therefore, the relationship followed an inverted U-shaped curve, as noted in previous reports [57]. In photoreceptor-degenerated Thy-I TG rats, no reduction of contrast sensitivity was observed at any spatial frequency. Unexpectedly, the contrast sensitivity was instead somewhat enhanced at low spatial frequencies such as 0.09 or 0.18 CPD (Fig. 5C).

5. Discussion

The photo-acquisition system of mammalian photoreceptor cells, which mediates various photoreceptor-specific proteins, is very complicated. In contrast, the corresponding system in green algae such as *Chlamydomonas* and *Volvox* is simpler. ChR2 contains a 13-*cis* retinal that absorbs a photon, inducing a conformational change. The ChR2 functions as a cation-selective ion channel. For this reason, the transfer of a single gene, ChR2, to RGCs allows the generation

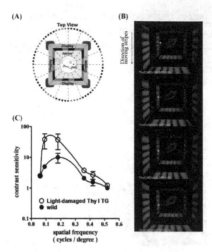

Figure 5. Behavioral assessment using a digital optomotor. (A) The digital optomotor consisted of 4 displays sur-rounding a platform. The number of stripes and the contrast were controlled by software. (B) Superimposed images from movies showed that the rats were able to discriminate the moving stripes. The arrow indicates the direction of the moving stripes. The asterisk indicates the point of the rat's nose. (C) The contrast sensitivities of photoreceptor-degenerated Thy-I TG rats were higher at low spatial frequencies compared to those of wild-type (normal) rats (n = 8).

of photosensitive RGCs. In the normal visual pathway, the light incident upon the eyes is first received by photoreceptor cells located at the end of the retinal layers. The photoreceptor cells control neurotransmitter release, and second-order neurons located in the inner nuclear layer respond to the neurotransmitter. Finally, RGCs produce action potentials and transmit to the lateral geniculate nucleus (LGN) via the optic nerve (Fig. 6). In RP, the photo-acquisition system is damaged due to the degeneration of photoreceptor cells, even if the other retinal layers remain intact. RGCs that are rendered photosensitive by the transfer of the ChR2 gene can directly respond to light and transmit signals to the brain. In this newly organized photo-acquisition system, the other retinal neurons besides the RGCs are not required for the perception of light.

Although VEP responses recovered after ChR2 gene transfer, the amplitudes and waveforms were different between rats injected with AAV-ChR2V at 6 and 10 months of age. One possibility is that RGC activity decayed after photoreceptor degeneration. However, our data show that the number of RGCs decreased after photoreceptor degeneration (Fig. 3C). The calculated RGC transduction efficiencies in 6-month-old rats were the same as those in 10-month-old rats. The differences in the recorded amplitudes and latencies shown in Fig. 2 appear to be due to differences in the number of photosensitive RGCs. We previously reported that the RGC transduction efficiency in 10-month-old rats was about 28% [38]. Subsequently, Isago et al. showed that the RGC transduction efficiencies in 6- and 10-month-old rats were 28.3 and 27.7%, respectively [56]. The data clearly indicates that the transduction efficiency is the same, although the number of ChR2-expressing cells was lower, corresponding to the decrease in the number of RGCs.

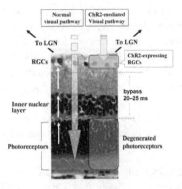

Figure 6. Summary of the visual pathway in ChR2-expressing RGCs. In the normal visual pathway, light (visual signals) is received by photoreceptor cells located at the end of the retinal layer. Photoreceptor cells produce signals that are transmitted to the inner nuclear layer. Finally, RGCs generate action potentials and thereby transmit signals to the LGN. RGCs play a role in transferring the visual signal to the brain. On the other hand, ChR2-expressing retinal ganglion cells directly receive light, produce action potentials, and transmit them to the LGN. Therefore, there is no need for mediation by other retinal cells.

To investigate visual acuity resulting from ChR2-expressing RGCs, we established a TG rat model expressing the ChR2 gene in RGCs. Photoreceptor-degenerated TG rats clearly tracked the rotation of blue-black stripes in a virtual optomotor. However, RCS rats that received the ChR2 gene in the AAV vector did not track the rotation of the virtual optomotor at any spatial frequency. Recently, we tested the behavior of RCS rats using a mechanical optomotor system and showed that the intensity of luminosity the rat received was the most important factor influencing their tracking of the rotation of the column [53]. A luminosity of over 500 lux was needed to induce head tracking in ChR2-expressing RCS rats. However, the maximum luminosity of the virtual optomotor was about 100 lux. It was therefore too low to induce head tracking in RCS rats. The question then arises: what is the difference between the TG and RCS rats? We do not have a reasonable explanation for this. One possibility is that the number of ChR2-expressing RGCs in the TG rat is greater than that in the RCS rat. About 45% of the RGCs expressed ChR2 in the TG rat. Compared to the TG rat, the transduction efficiency in the RCS rat is about 28% independent of the age of the animal. This may affect the light sensitivity. As the another explanation, in the case of TG rats, ChR2 is expressed after birth; therefore, there is a possibility that retinal organization and function might be altered, that cannot be ruled out.

RGCs are merely one of the candidate cell types that could receive the ChR2 gene. Lagali et al. [60] succeeded in transferring the ChR2 gene into ON-bipolar cells in the retina and confirmed the restoration of visual and behavioral responses. ON- and OFF-bipolar cells receive synaptic input from photoreceptors. Considering that ChR2 can elicit light-on responses, ON-bipolar cells seem to be the most appropriate cells for the transfer of the ChR2 gene. However, 2 questions arise in this regard. First, how can we deliver the ChR2 gene into ON-bipolar cells for human gene therapy? Lagali et al. [60] transferred the ChR2 gene into neonatal mice by electroporation of the plasmid vector. It is generally difficult to transfer a gene into the depths of the retina via intravitreous injection of AAV vectors, in spite of the development of various serotypes of AAV vectors for retinal gene therapy [61-65]. Second, does synaptic transmission remain intact after photoreceptor degeneration? Some studies have reported that retinal remodeling is triggered in bipolar cells and horizontal cells following photoreceptor degeneration [66-70]. Recently, Doroudchi et al. [71] succeeded in transferring the ChR2 gene into ON-bipolar cells by the subretinal injection of a modified AAV vector (AAV8-Y733F) [72] that included a specific promoter for ON-bipolar cells (mGRM6-SV40), and demonstrated the behavioral recovery of the light response. These 2 questions could be resolved by these attractive methods used the specific promoter and the modified AAV vectors if the recovered visual acuity is investigated using a behavioral approach.

Since the discovery of ChR2, bacteriorhodopsins that have similar functions as that of ChR2 derived from *Chlamydomonas* have been identified. Channelrhodopsin-1 from the green alga *Volvox* [73] is a light-activated cation channel that has a different wavelength sensitivity from that of *Chlamydomonas*-derived ChR2. Halorhodopsin, which functions as a light-activated chloride channel, has been identified in *Halobacterium salinarum* [74,75]. Researchers have attempted to discover new light-activated ion channel genes, or to artificially design more functional ones [76-78]. In the future, more effective gene therapy strategies for restoring vision in RP might be developed using newly developed genes and vectors.

6. Conclusion

Target diseases for gene therapy were previously restricted to lethal and severe diseases that lead to death. In our country (Japan), the gene therapy guidelines were updated in 2002, whereby diseases in which bodily functions are severely impaired, such as loss of arms or legs, blindness, and deafness, were added to the list of target diseases for gene therapy. Based on these guidelines, people suffering from impaired vision caused by RP are eligible for gene therapy. However, gene therapy using genes derived from living organisms other than humans has not previously been tested in clinical trials. Safety studies, especially immunological reactions, using appropriate animal models in ChR2-based gene therapy is important before proceeding to clinical trials.

Acknowledgements

This work was partly supported by Grants-in-Aid for Scientific Research from the Ministry of Education, Culture, Sports, Science and Technology of Japan (No. 24390393 and 23659804) and the Program for the Promotion of Fundamental Studies in Health Sciences of the National Institute of Biomedical Innovation (NIBIO). We express our heartfelt appreciation to Dr. Ichiro Hagimori in Narita Animal Science Laboratory Co. Ltd., whose enormous support and insightful comments were invaluable during the course of this study.

Author details

Hiroshi Tomita[1,2*], Eriko Sugano[1], Hitomi Isago[1], Namie Murayama[1] and Makoto Tamai[2]

*Address all correspondence to: htomita@iwate-u.ac.jp

1 Department of Chemistry and Bioengineering, Iwate University, Morioka, Iwate, Japan

2 Tohoku University Hospital, Sendai, Miyagi, Japan

References

[1] Humayun, M. S, Prince, M, & De Juan, E. Jr., Barron Y, Moskowitz M, Klock IB, Milam AH. Morphometric analysis of the extramacular retina from postmortem eyes with retinitis pigmentosa. Invest Ophthalmol Vis Sci (1999). , 40(1), 143-148.

[2] Santos, A, Humayun, M. S, & De Juan, E. Jr., Greenburg RJ, Marsh MJ, Klock IB, Milam AH. Preservation of the inner retina in retinitis pigmentosa. A morphometric analysis. Arch Ophthalmol (1997). , 115(4), 511-515.

[3] Stone, J. L, Barlow, W. E, Humayun, M. S, & De Juan, E. Jr., Milam AH. Morphometric analysis of macular photoreceptors and ganglion cells in retinas with retinitis pigmentosa. Arch Ophthalmol (1992). , 110(11), 1634-1639.

[4] Hartong, D. T, Berson, E. L, & Dryja, T. P. Retinitis pigmentosa. Lancet (2006). , 368(9549), 1795-1809.

[5] Dryja, T. P, Mcgee, T. L, Reichel, E, Hahn, L. B, Cowley, G. S, Yandell, D. W, Sandberg, M. A, & Berson, E. L. A point mutation of the rhodopsin gene in one form of retinitis pigmentosa. Nature (1990). , 343(6256), 364-366.

[6] Stone, E. M. Leber congenital amaurosis- a model for efficient genetic testing of heterogeneous disorders: LXIV Edward Jackson Memorial Lecture. Am J Ophthalmol (2007). , 144(6), 791-811.

[7] Blum, M, Hykin, P. G, Sanders, M, & Volcker, H. E. Theodor Leber: a founder of ophthalmic research. Surv Ophthalmol (1992). , 37(1), 63-68.

[8] Dharmaraj, S, Leroy, B. P, Sohocki, M. M, Koenekoop, R. K, Perrault, I, Anwar, K, Khaliq, S, Devi, R. S, Birch, D. G, De Pool, E, Izquierdo, N, Van Maldergem, L, Ismail, M, Payne, A. M, Holder, G. E, Bhattacharya, S. S, Bird, A. C, Kaplan, J, & Maumenee, I. H. The phenotype of Leber congenital amaurosis in patients with AIPL1 mutations. Arch Ophthalmol (2004). , 122(7), 1029-1037.

[9]   Dryja, T. P, Adams, S. M, Grimsby, J. L, Mcgee, T. L, Hong, D. H, Li, T, Andreasson, S, & Berson, E. L. Null RPGRIP1 alleles in patients with Leber congenital amaurosis. Am J Hum Genet (2001). , 68(5), 1295-1298.

[10] Lotery, A. J, Jacobson, S. G, Fishman, G. A, Weleber, R. G, Fulton, A. B, Namperumalsamy, P, Heon, E, Levin, A. V, Grover, S, Rosenow, J. R, Kopp, K. K, Sheffield, V. C, & Stone, E. M. Mutations in the CRB1 gene cause Leber congenital amaurosis. Arch Ophthalmol (2001). , 119(3), 415-420.

[11] Marlhens, F, Bareil, C, Griffoin, J. M, Zrenner, E, Amalric, P, Eliaou, C, Liu, S. Y, Harris, E, Redmond, T. M, Arnaud, B, Claustres, M, & Hamel, C. P. Mutations in RPE65 cause Leber's congenital amaurosis. Nat Genet (1997). , 17(2), 139-141.

[12] Perrault, I, Rozet, J. M, Calvas, P, Gerber, S, Camuzat, A, Dollfus, H, Chatelin, S, Souied, E, Ghazi, I, Leowski, C, & Bonnemaison, M. Le Paslier D, Frezal J, Dufier JL, Pittler S, Munnich A, Kaplan J. Retinal-specific guanylate cyclase gene mutations in Leber's congenital amaurosis. Nat Genet (1996). , 14(4), 461-464.

[13] Perrault, I, Hanein, S, Zanlonghi, X, Serre, V, Nicouleau, M, Defoort-delhemmes, S, Delphin, N, Fares-taie, L, Gerber, S, Xerri, O, Edelson, C, Goldenberg, A, & Duncombe, A. Le Meur G, Hamel C, Silva E, Nitschke P, Calvas P, Munnich A, Roche O, Dollfus H, Kaplan J, Rozet JM. Mutations in NMNAT1 cause Leber congenital amaurosis with early-onset severe macular and optic atrophy. Nat Genet (2012). in press.

[14] Cremers, F. P. van den Hurk JA, den Hollander AI. Molecular genetics of Leber congenital amaurosis. Hum Mol Genet (2002). , 11(10), 1169-1176.

[15] Acland, G. M, Aguirre, G. D, Ray, J, Zhang, Q, Aleman, T. S, Cideciyan, A. V, Pearce-kelling, S. E, Anand, V, Zeng, Y, Maguire, A. M, Jacobson, S. G, Hauswirth, W. W, & Bennett, J. Gene therapy restores vision in a canine model of childhood blindness. Nat Genet (2001). , 28(1), 92-95.

[16] Acland, G. M, Aguirre, G. D, Bennett, J, Aleman, T. S, Cideciyan, A. V, Bennicelli, J, Dejneka, N. S, Pearce-kelling, S. E, Maguire, A. M, Palczewski, K, Hauswirth, W. W, & Jacobson, S. G. Long-term restoration of rod and cone vision by single dose rAAV-mediated gene transfer to the retina in a canine model of childhood blindness. Mol Ther (2005). , 12(6), 1072-1082.

[17] Simonelli, F, Ziviello, C, Testa, F, Rossi, S, Fazzi, E, Bianchi, P. E, Fossarello, M, Signorini, S, Bertone, C, Galantuomo, S, Brancati, F, Valente, E. M, Ciccodicola, A, Rinaldi, E, Auricchio, A, & Banfi, S. Clinical and molecular genetics of Leber's congenital amaurosis: a multicenter study of Italian patients. Invest Ophthalmol Vis Sci (2007). , 48(9), 4284-4290.

[18] Cideciyan, A. V, Hauswirth, W. W, Aleman, T. S, Kaushal, S, Schwartz, S. B, Boye, S. L, Windsor, E. A, Conlon, T. J, Sumaroka, A, Roman, A. J, Byrne, B. J, & Jacobson, S. G. Vision 1 year after gene therapy for Leber's congenital amaurosis. N Engl J Med (2009). , 361(7), 725-727.

[19] Maguire, A. M, Simonelli, F, Pierce, E. A, & Pugh, E. N. Jr., Mingozzi F, Bennicelli J, Banfi S, Marshall KA, Testa F, Surace EM, Rossi S, Lyubarsky A, Arruda VR, Konkle B, Stone E, Sun J, Jacobs J, Dell'Osso L, Hertle R, Ma JX, Redmond TM, Zhu X, Hauck B, Zelenaia O, Shindler KS, Maguire MG, Wright JF, Volpe NJ, McDonnell JW, Auricchio A, High KA, Bennett J. Safety and efficacy of gene transfer for Leber's congenital amaurosis. N Engl J Med (2008). , 358(21), 2240-2248.

[20] Bainbridge, J. W, Smith, A. J, Barker, S. S, Robbie, S, Henderson, R, Balaggan, K, Viswanathan, A, Holder, G. E, Stockman, A, Tyler, N, Petersen-jones, S, Bhattacharya, S. S, Thrasher, A. J, Fitzke, F. W, Carter, B. J, Rubin, G. S, Moore, A. T, & Ali, R. R. Effect of gene therapy on visual function in Leber's congenital amaurosis. N Engl J Med (2008). , 358(21), 2231-2239.

[21] Maguire, A. M, High, K. A, Auricchio, A, Wright, J. F, Pierce, E. A, Testa, F, Mingozzi, F, Bennicelli, J. L, Ying, G. S, Rossi, S, Fulton, A, Marshall, K. A, Banfi, S, Chung, D. C, Morgan, J. I, Hauck, B, Zelenaia, O, Zhu, X, Raffini, L, Coppieters, F, De Baere, E, Shindler, K. S, Volpe, N. J, Surace, E. M, Acerra, C, Lyubarsky, A, Redmond, T. M, Stone, E, Sun, J, Mcdonnell, J. W, Leroy, B. P, Simonelli, F, & Bennett, J. Age-dependent effects of RPE65 gene therapy for Leber's congenital amaurosis: a phase 1 dose-escalation trial. Lancet (2009). , 374(9701), 1597-1605.

[22] Simonelli, F, Maguire, A. M, Testa, F, Pierce, E. A, Mingozzi, F, Bennicelli, J. L, Rossi, S, Marshall, K, Banfi, S, Surace, E. M, Sun, J, Redmond, T. M, Zhu, X, Shindler, K. S, Ying, G. S, Ziviello, C, Acerra, C, Wright, J. F, Mcdonnell, J. W, High, K. A, Bennett, J, & Auricchio, A. Gene therapy for Leber's congenital amaurosis is safe and effective through 1.5 years after vector administration. Mol Ther (2010). , 18(3), 643-650.

[23] Colella, P, & Auricchio, A. Gene Therapy of Inherited Retinopathies: A Long and Successful Road from Viral Vectors to Patients. Hum Gene Ther (2012). , 23(8), 796-807.

[24] Berson, E. L, Sandberg, M. A, & Dryja, T. P. Autosomal dominant retinitis pigmentosa with rhodopsin, valine-345-methionine. Trans Am Ophthalmol Soc (1991). discussion 128-130., 89, 117-128.

[25] Olsson, J. E, Gordon, J. W, Pawlyk, B. S, Roof, D, Hayes, A, Molday, R. S, Mukai, S, Cowley, G. S, Berson, E. L, & Dryja, T. P. Transgenic mice with a rhodopsin mutation (Pro23His): a mouse model of autosomal dominant retinitis pigmentosa. Neuron (1992). , 9(5), 815-830.

[26] Chang, G. Q, Hao, Y, & Wong, F. Apoptosis: final common pathway of photoreceptor death in rd, rds, and rhodopsin mutant mice. Neuron (1993). , 11(4), 595-605.

[27] Ranchon, I. LaVail MM, Kotake Y, Anderson RE. Free radical trap phenyl-N-tert-butylnitrone protects against light damage but does not rescue and S334ter rhodopsin transgenic rats from inherited retinal degeneration. J Neurosci (2003). , 23H.

[28] Tomita, H, Kotake, Y, & Anderson, R. E. Mechanism of protection from light-induced retinal degeneration by the synthetic antioxidant phenyl-N-tert-butylnitrone. Invest Ophthalmol Vis Sci (2005). , 46(2), 427-434.

[29] Cayouette, M, & Gravel, C. Adenovirus-mediated gene transfer of ciliary neurotrophic factor can prevent photoreceptor degeneration in the retinal degeneration (rd) mouse. Hum Gene Ther (1997). , 8(4), 423-430.

[30] Jomary, C, Vincent, K. A, Grist, J, Neal, M. J, & Jones, S. E. Rescue of photoreceptor function by AAV-mediated gene transfer in a mouse model of inherited retinal degeneration. Gene Ther (1997). , 4(7), 683-690.

[31] Bennett, J, Zeng, Y, Bajwa, R, Klatt, L, Li, Y, & Maguire, A. M. Adenovirus-mediated delivery of rhodopsin-promoted bcl-2 results in a delay in photoreceptor cell death in the rd/rd mouse. Gene Ther (1998). , 5(9), 1156-1164.

[32] Chow, A. Y, & Peachey, N. The subretinal microphotodiode array retinal prosthesis II. Ophthalmic Res (1999).

[33] Dobelle, W. H. Artificial vision for the blind by connecting a television camera to the visual cortex. ASAIO J (2000). , 46(1), 3-9.

[34] Rizzo, J. F. rd, Wyatt J, Loewenstein J, Kelly S, Shire D. Perceptual efficacy of electrical stimulation of human retina with a microelectrode array during short-term surgical trials. Invest Ophthalmol Vis Sci (2003). , 44(12), 5362-5369.

[35] Gekeler, F, Kobuch, K, Schwahn, H. N, Stett, A, Shinoda, K, & Zrenner, E. Subretinal electrical stimulation of the rabbit retina with acutely implanted electrode arrays. Graefes Arch Clin Exp Ophthalmol (2004). , 242(7), 587-596.

[36] Weiland, J. D, Cho, A. K, & Humayun, M. S. Retinal prostheses: current clinical results and future needs. Ophthalmology (2011). , 118(11), 2227-2237.

[37] Bi, A, Cui, J, Ma, Y. P, Olshevskaya, E, Pu, M, Dizhoor, A. M, & Pan, Z. H. Ectopic expression of a microbial-type rhodopsin restores visual responses in mice with photoreceptor degeneration. Neuron (2006). , 50(1), 23-33.

[38] Tomita, H, Sugano, E, Yawo, H, Ishizuka, T, Isago, H, Narikawa, S, Kugler, S, & Tamai, M. Restoration of visual response in aged dystrophic RCS rats using AAV-mediated channelopsin-2 gene transfer. Invest Ophthalmol Vis Sci (2007). , 48(8), 3821-3826.

[39] Nagel, G, Szellas, T, Huhn, W, Kateriya, S, Adeishvili, N, Berthold, P, Ollig, D, Hegemann, P, & Bamberg, E. Channelrhodopsin-2, a directly light-gated cation-selective membrane channel. Proc Natl Acad Sci U S A (2003). , 100(24), 13940-13945.

[40] Boyden, E. S, Zhang, F, Bamberg, E, Nagel, G, & Deisseroth, K. Millisecond-time-scale, genetically targeted optical control of neural activity. Nat Neurosci (2005). , 8(9), 1263-1268.

[41] Ishizuka, T, Kakuda, M, Araki, R, & Yawo, H. Kinetic evaluation of photosensitivity in genetically engineered neurons expressing green algae light-gated channels. Neurosci Res (2006). , 54(2), 85-94.

[42] Li, X, Gutierrez, D. V, Hanson, M. G, Han, J, Mark, M. D, Chiel, H, Hegemann, P, Landmesser, L. T, & Herlitze, S. Fast noninvasive activation and inhibition of neural and network activity by vertebrate rhodopsin and green algae channelrhodopsin. Proc Natl Acad Sci U S A (2005). , 102(49), 17816-17821.

[43] LaVail MM, Sidman RL, O'Neil D.Photoreceptor-pigment epithelial cell relationships in rats with inherited retinal degeneration. Radioautographic and electron microscope evidence for a dual source of extra lamellar material. J Cell Biol (1972). , 53(1), 185-209.

[44] Mullen, R. J. LaVail MM. Inherited retinal dystrophy: primary defect in pigment epithelium determined with experimental rat chimeras. Science (1976). , 192(4241), 799-801.

[45] Cruz, D, Yasumura, PM, Weir, D, Matthes, J, Abderrahim, MT, & La, H. , Vollrath D. Mutation of the receptor tyrosine kinase gene Mertk in the retinal dystrophic RCS rat. Hum Mol Genet 2000;9(4):645-651.

[46] Gal, A, Li, Y, Thompson, D. A, Weir, J, Orth, U, Jacobson, S. G, Apfelstedt-sylla, E, & Vollrath, D. Mutations in MERTK, the human orthologue of the RCS rat retinal dystrophy gene, cause retinitis pigmentosa. Nat Genet (2000). , 26(3), 270-271.

[47] Tomita, H, Sugano, E, Fukazawa, Y, Isago, H, Sugiyama, Y, Hiroi, T, Ishizuka, T, Mushiake, H, Kato, M, Hirabayashi, M, Shigemoto, R, Yawo, H, & Tamai, M. Visual properties of transgenic rats harboring the channelrhodopsin-2 gene regulated by the thy-1.2 promoter. PLoS One (2009). e7679.

[48] Barclay, A. N, & Hyden, H. Localizatin of the Thy-1 antigen in rat brain and spinal cord by immunofluorescence. J Neurochem (1978). , 31(6), 1375-1391.

[49] Mason, D. W, & Williams, A. F. The kinetics of antibody binding to membrane antigens in solution and at the cell surface. Biochem J (1980). , 187(1), 1-20.

[50] Barnstable, C. J, & Drager, U. C. Thy-1 antigen: a ganglion cell specific marker in rodent retina. Neuroscience (1984). , 11(4), 847-855.

[51] Perry, V. H, Morris, R. J, & Raisman, G. Is Thy-1 expressed only by ganglion cells and their axons in the retina and optic nerve? J Neurocytol (1984). , 13(5), 809-824.

[52] Sugano, E, Tomita, H, Ishiguro, S, Abe, T, & Tamai, M. Establishment of effective methods for transducing genes into iris pigment epithelial cells by using adeno-associated virus type 2. Invest Ophthalmol Vis Sci (2005). , 46(9), 3341-3348.

[53] Tomita, H, Sugano, E, Isago, H, Hiroi, T, Wang, Z, Ohta, E, & Tamai, M. Channelrho-dopsin-2 gene transduced into retinal ganglion cells restores functional vision in ge-netically blind rats. Exp Eye Res (2010). , 90(3), 429-436.

[54] Iwamura, Y, Fujii, Y, & Kamei, C. The effects of certain H(1)-antagonists on visual evoked potential in rats. Brain Res Bull (2003). , 61(4), 393-398.

[55] Papathanasiou, E. S, Peachey, N. S, Goto, Y, Neafsey, E. J, Castro, A. J, & Kartje, G. L. Visual cortical plasticity following unilateral sensorimotor cortical lesions in the neo-natal rat. Exp Neurol (2006). , 199(1), 122-129.

[56] Isago, H, Sugano, E, Wang, Z, Murayama, N, Koyanagi, E, Tamai, M, & Tomita, H. Age-dependent differences in recovered visual responses in Royal College of Sur-geons rats transduced with the Channelrhodopsin-2 gene. J Mol Neurosci (2012). , 46(2), 393-400.

[57] Prusky, G. T, Alam, N. M, Beekman, S, & Douglas, R. M. Rapid quantification of adult and developing mouse spatial vision using a virtual optomotor system. Invest Ophthalmol Vis Sci (2004). , 45(12), 4611-4616.

[58] Sugano, E, Isago, H, Wang, Z, Murayama, N, Tamai, M, & Tomita, H. Immune re-sponses to adeno-associated virus type 2 encoding channelrhodopsin-2 in a geneti-cally blind rat model for gene therapy. Gene Ther (2011). , 18(3), 266-274.

[59] Rapp, L. M, & Smith, S. C. Morphologic comparisons between rhodopsin-mediated and short-wavelength classes of retinal light damage. Invest Ophthalmol Vis Sci (1992). , 33(12), 3367-3377.

[60] Lagali, P. S, Balya, D, Awatramani, G. B, Munch, T. A, Kim, D. S, Busskamp, V, Cep-ko, C. L, & Roska, B. Light-activated channels targeted to ON bipolar cells restore visual function in retinal degeneration. Nat Neurosci (2008). , 11(6), 667-675.

[61] Auricchio, A, Kobinger, G, Anand, V, Hildinger, M, Connor, O, Maguire, E, Wilson, A. M, & Bennett, J. M. J. Exchange of surface proteins impacts on viral vector cellular specificity and transduction characteristics: the retina as a model. Hum Mol Genet (2001). , 10(26), 3075-3081.

[62] Yang, P, Seiler, M. J, Aramant, R. B, & Whittemore, S. R. Differential lineage restric-tion of rat retinal progenitor cells in vitro and in vivo. J Neurosci Res (2002). , 69(4), 466-476.

[63] Weber, M, Rabinowitz, J, Provost, N, Conrath, H, Folliot, S, Briot, D, Cherel, Y, Che-nuaud, P, Samulski, J, Moullier, P, & Rolling, F. Recombinant adeno-associated virus serotype 4 mediates unique and exclusive long-term transduction of retinal pigment-ed epithelium in rat, dog, and nonhuman primate after subretinal delivery. Mol Ther (2003). , 7(6), 774-781.

[64] Lotery, A. J, Derksen, T. A, Russell, S. R, Mullins, R. F, Sauter, S, Affatigato, L. M, Stone, E. M, & Davidson, B. L. Gene transfer to the nonhuman primate retina with

recombinant feline immunodeficiency virus vectors. Hum Gene Ther (2002). , 13(6), 689-696.

[65] Allocca, M, Mussolino, C, Garcia-hoyos, M, Sanges, D, Iodice, C, Petrillo, M, Vandenberghe, L. H, Wilson, J. M, Marigo, V, Surace, E. M, & Auricchio, A. Novel adeno-associated virus serotypes efficiently transduce murine photoreceptors. J Virol (2007). , 81(20), 11372-11380.

[66] Marc, R. E, Jones, B. W, Anderson, J. R, Kinard, K, Marshak, D. W, Wilson, J. H, Wensel, T, & Lucas, R. J. Neural reprogramming in retinal degeneration. Invest Ophthalmol Vis Sci (2007). , 48(7), 3364-3371.

[67] Marc, R. E, Jones, B. W, Watt, C. B, & Strettoi, E. Neural remodeling in retinal degeneration. Prog Retin Eye Res (2003). , 22(5), 607-655.

[68] Strettoi, E, & Pignatelli, V. Modifications of retinal neurons in a mouse model of retinitis pigmentosa. Proc Natl Acad Sci U S A (2000). , 97(20), 11020-11025.

[69] Strettoi, E, Pignatelli, V, Rossi, C, Porciatti, V, & Falsini, B. Remodeling of second-order neurons in the retina of rd/rd mutant mice. Vision Res (2003). , 43(8), 867-877.

[70] Strettoi, E, Porciatti, V, Falsini, B, Pignatelli, V, & Rossi, C. Morphological and functional abnormalities in the inner retina of the rd/rd mouse. J Neurosci (2002). , 22(13), 5492-5504.

[71] Doroudchi, M. M, Greenberg, K. P, Liu, J, Silka, K. A, Boyden, E. S, Lockridge, J. A, Arman, A. C, Janani, R, Boye, S. E, Boye, S. L, Gordon, G. M, Matteo, B. C, Sampath, A. P, Hauswirth, W. W, & Horsager, A. Virally delivered channelrhodopsin-2 safely and effectively restores visual function in multiple mouse models of blindness. Mol Ther (2011). , 19(7), 1220-1229.

[72] Pang, J. J, Dai, X, Boye, S. E, Barone, I, Boye, S. L, Mao, S, Everhart, D, Dinculescu, A, Liu, L, Umino, Y, Lei, B, Chang, B, Barlow, R, Strettoi, E, & Hauswirth, W. W. Long-term retinal function and structure rescue using capsid mutant AAV8 vector in the rd10 mouse, a model of recessive retinitis pigmentosa. Mol Ther (2011). , 19(2), 234-242.

[73] Zhang, F, Prigge, M, Beyriere, F, Tsunoda, S. P, Mattis, J, Yizhar, O, Hegemann, P, & Deisseroth, K. Red-shifted optogenetic excitation: a tool for fast neural control derived from Volvox carteri. Nat Neurosci (2008). , 11(6), 631-633.

[74] Zhang, Y, Ivanova, E, Bi, A, & Pan, Z. H. Ectopic expression of multiple microbial rhodopsins restores ON and OFF light responses in retinas with photoreceptor degeneration. J Neurosci (2009). , 29(29), 9186-9196.

[75] Kolbe, M, Besir, H, Essen, L. O, & Oesterhelt, D. Structure of the light-driven chloride pump halorhodopsin at 1.8 A resolution. Science (2000). , 288(5470), 1390-1396.

[76] Govorunova, E. G, Spudich, E. N, Lane, C. E, Sineshchekov, O. A, & Spudich, J. L. New channelrhodopsin with a red-shifted spectrum and rapid kinetics from Mesostigma viride. MBio (2011). ee00111., 00115.

[77] Prigge, M, Schneider, F, Tsunoda, S. P, Shilyansky, C, Wietek, J, Deisseroth, K, & Hegemann, P. Color-tuned Channelrhodopsins for Multiwavelength Optogenetics. J Biol Chem (2012). in press.

[78] Wang, H, Sugiyama, Y, Hikima, T, Sugano, E, Tomita, H, Takahashi, T, Ishizuka, T, & Yawo, H. Molecular determinants differentiating photocurrent properties of two channelrhodopsins from chlamydomonas. J Biol Chem (2009). , 284(9), 5685-5696.

Chapter 2

Gene Therapy for Primary Immunodeficiencies

Francisco Martin, Alejandra Gutierrez-Guerrero and
Karim Benabdellah

Additional information is available at the end of the chapter

1. Introduction

Primary immunodeficiencies (PID) are caused by mutations in genes involved in the normal development or activity of the immune system [1, 2]. PIDs include B- and T-cell defects, phagocytic disorders, and complement deficiencies with the common feature of frequent life-threatening infections. The phenotypes vary from asymptomatic (IgA deficiency) to severe PIDs (such as Severe combined immunodeficiencies). Treatment of patients with severe PIDs relies in intravenous injection of immunoglobulins, bone marrow transplantation (BMT) and antibiotics. Identical and haploidentical BMT are the only curative treatment, however, the lack of a HLA-matched donor in over 70% of the patients make necessary the development of new therapeutic strategies [3, 4]. Gene therapy (GT) could be the best alternative for the treatment of patients with severe PID that lack a HLA-matched donor [5]. The aim of GT strategies is the stable correction of the mutated gene on the patient's own haematopoietic stem cells (HSCs).

The first successful gene therapy clinical trial used gamma-retroviral derived vectors expressing common cytokine-receptor gamma chain (γc) cDNA in HSCs from X-linked severe combined immunodeficiency (SCID-X1) patients [6]. So far, using a very similar vector platform, over 50 PID patients treated with GT can been considered "cured" from SCID-X1, adenosine deaminase deficiency (ADA) and Wiskott-Aldrich syndrome (WAS) PID [7-13]. However, in six children, GT treatment resulted in clonal T-cell proliferation (leukaemia-like disease) [9].

The results obtained in the SCID-X1, ADA and WAS clinical trials clearly showed the importance to improve vector's safety and efficiency [8,14, 15]. Lentiviral-based vectors have been the vector of choice to enhance efficiency and, at the same time, reduce the side effects of gammaretroviral vectors (see below). Several GT clinical trials for SCID-X1, chronic granulomatous disease (CGD) and WAS PID using lentiviral vectors (LVs) have started in the last few years.

This chapter intend to illustrate the past, present and near future of GT for the treatment of severe PIDs

2. Gamma-retroviral vector based gene therapy clinical trials for primary immunodeficiencies

2.1. Gammaretrovirus-based vectors

Gammaretrovirus, also named oncoretrovirus, are efficient, integrative, easy to manipulate and poorly immunogenic. Vector derived for these retroviruses are often named "retroviral vectors" and "oncoretroviral vectors". All the clinical data that will be presented in this section was obtained using a similar gammaretroviral backbone: **LTR---ψ-----transgene------LTR**. As consequence the therapeutic gene is expressed through the promoter and enhancer sequences present at the viral LTR. Another common aspect of all the GT strategies presented in this section is the modification of the patient's hematopoietic stem cells (HSCs). However HSCs are quiescent or very slowly dividing cells and gammaretroviral-based vectors require active cell division for transduction [16]. Therefore HSCs transduction protocols require cytokine "pre-stimulation" to induce cell proliferation [17], a process that can modify the characteristics of the haematopoietic precursors [18]. However, since LTR-driven gammaretroviral vectors were the only integrative vectors available at the time, several clinical trials started on SCID-X1, ADA CGD and WAS. An overall conclusion of these clinical trials was that GT is as efficient and safe as haploidentical BMT. However it was also evident the necessity of improving the vector system before GT of PID could be of general use in clinic.

2.2. X-linked Severe Combined Immunodeficiency (SCID-X1)

SCID-X1 is a monogenic disease caused by mutations in the interleukin-2 receptor gamma chain gene (γc). Patients with SCID-X1 deficiency do not have T nor NK cells, consequently B-lymphocyte function is also intrinsically compromised [19]. SCID-X1 has been an attractive GT target because patient's cells expressing the transgene have a growth advantage over non-expressing cells [20, 21]. Therefore, GT could, in theory, achieved complete immune reconstitution with a relatively low number of gene-corrected cells. The Fischer group at the "Unité d'Immunologie et d'Hématologie Pédiatriques, Hôpital Necker" in France achieved the first unequivocal success of gene therapy in the two patients treated [6]. The authors transduced patients HSCs (CD34+) with a Murine Leukaemia Virus (MLV) based vector expressing the γc cDNA following pre-activation with stem cell factor (SCF), polyethylene glycol-megakaryo-cyte differentiation factor (PG-MDF), IL-3 and Flt3-L. The continuation of this work and other clinical trials in other countries enrolled a total of 20 SCID-X1 patients [7, 8, 22, 23]. Between 5 and 12 years after GT, 17 of the 20 treated patients are alive and display full or nearly full correction of the T cell deficiency [24, 25]. The GT treatment led to clear benefits since patients recover from ongoing infections with poor prognosis (disseminated infections) and live in a normal environment without evidence of increased susceptibility to infection.

However, 5 of the 20 patients with SCID-X1 on GT trials developed leukaemia 3-6 years after treatment. Four patients were successfully treated with chemotherapy and they are alive and doing well. However the other patient died from chemotherapy-refractory leukemia [26]. This leukaemia-like disease was a result of vector-mediated up-regulation of host cellular onco-genes (i.e. LMO2) [8, 27]. Several studies have demonstrated that MLV-derived vectors integration favour transcriptionally active genes near transcription start sites (TSSs) [28-30]. Leukemogenesis could also be the result of insertional mutagenesis (activation of the LMO2 oncogene) combined with the acquisition of genetic abnormalities unrelated to vector inser-tion, such as the increase activity of NOTCH1 or the deletion of CDKN2A gene [8].

However, in spite of the secondary effects observed, the results obtained with GT using first generation MLV-based vectors are comparable to those obtained with HLA-identical HSC transplant (HSCT). It is expected that next generation vectors will certainly improve these results as it will discussed later.

2.3. Adenosine Deaminase (ADA) Severe Combined Immunodeficiency (ADA-SCID)

ADA-deficiency has been also considered an important target for GT. The ADA gene codify for an enzyme that is expressed in all tissues and catalyses the deamination of 2'-deoxyade-nosine and adenosine to 2'deoxyinosine and inosine. Its absence or malfunction cause the accumulation of purine metabolites that are toxic to the cells. Although the ADA gene is expressed in all tissues, the accumulation of purine metabolites in the immune cells is the main problem. As consequence, ADA patients suffer from lymphopenia, reduced (or absent) cellular and humoral immunity, failure to thrive and recurrent infections. Additionally, the accumu-lation of purine metabolites in other tissues also produces skeletal, hepatic, renal, lung, and neurologic abnormalities [31, 32]. Like for SCID-X1, bone marrow transplantation (BMT) is the best therapeutic alternative. However, contrary to SCID-X1, there are other treatment options that allow ADA patients to have near-normal lives: Enzyme replacement therapy (ERT) with polyethylene-glycol-conjugated bovine ADA (PEG-ADA). However, although ERT treatment is well tolerated and can partially restore immune function, its effect decline over time and, in addition, lifelong treatment is very expensive[33].

ADA deficiency has been successfully treated by GT using a similar approach to that for SCID-X1, but requiring mild bone-marrow chemoablation [34]. The authors showed immunological and metabolic reconstitution after transplantation of gene-modified CD34+ using ADA-expressing-MLV based vectors. The selective growth advantage of ADA-expressing lympho-cytes played an important role in the success of this trial. Similar findings have been reported by Gaspar et. al. [23] and again by Aiuti et al[10]. In total, over 40 patients with ADA have been treated in Italy, UK and USA. At present all patients are alive and 29 of them do not require ERT [9, 10, 23, 25, 34-36].

It is important to remark that no leukaemia-like disease have been observed in the ADA-SCID GT trial. The author propose that the differences between SCID-X1 and ADA might be related with SCID-X1 genetic background or the role of the therapeutic transgene (*ADA* is a house-keeping enzyme whereas γc is a potential oncogene growth factor receptor). However, in the last clinical trial some non-life threatening adverse effects have been reported such as neutro-penia (2 patients), treatment-related infections (2 patients), Epstein-Barr virus reactivations (1 patient) and autoimmune hepatitis (1 patient).

2.4. X-linked Chronic Granulomatous Disease (X-CGD)

Chronic granulomatous disease (CGD) is a rare PID characterized by severe, life threatening bacterial and fungal infections. Patients with CGD have also defective degradation of inflam-matory mediators leading to granuloma formation. All of these defects are caused by muta-tions in the nicotinamide adenine dinucleotide phosphate (NADPH) oxidase subunits in phagocytic cells [37]. gp91[phox] mutations occur in up to 70% of the CGD cases and represent the X-linked form of this disorder (X-CGD). Neutrophils, monocytes, macrophages, and eosinophils from CGD patients cannot generate superoxide and other reactive oxygen intermediates to destroy invading bacteria and fungi.

Contrary to SCID-X1 and ADA, CGD is a difficult target for GT, since the expression of the correct form of the gene does not provide selective advantage to hematopoietic progenitors. In addition, myeloid cells have a short life span and therefore a large amount of HSC must be corrected to achieve clinical benefits. Myeloablative conditioning is therefore required to increase the amount of gene-modified cells that engraft into the patients. Several GT clinical trials for CGD have been conducted since 1997. Initial studies using retroviral vector to express p47-phox into CD34+ cells, resulted in low and short-term engraftment of CGD-corrected cells [38]. More recent GT clinical trials on X-CGD conducted in Franckfurt, Zurinch, London, USA and Seoul resulted in higher correction and clinical benefit in several patients. Dr Grez´s group showed the most dramatic effects in two children (5 and 8 years old) showing recovery from severe pulmonary and spinal aspergillosis. GT treatment also achieved recovery from paraparesis of both legs in one of the children [39]. However, the efficacy was only partial due to a progressive lost of gene-corrected cells over time [39-41]. The lost of transgene expression was, at least in part, due to inactivation of the vector promoter. However, there are other hypothesis that point to the potential toxicity of ectopic expression of gp91 gene on HSCs as a potential cause of the lost of gene-corrected cells [42]. In addition, three patients developed a myelodisplastic syndrome (MDS) due to transactivation of the MDS/EVI oncogene by the retroviral enhancer [40]. The MDS was fatal for two of the patients while the third was treated with HSCTs. These results revealed the importance of developing new, safer and more efficient vectors for GT in CGD.

2.5. Wiskott-Aldrich Syndrome (WAS)

Wiskott–Aldrich syndrome (WAS) is a X-linked PID caused by mutation in the WAS gene coding for the Wiskott-Aldrich syndrome protein (WASP), a hematopoietic-specific member of regulators of the actin cytoskeleton [43, 44]. The most severe form of WAS (where the mutation cause total absence of protein or function) is characterized by recurrent infections, microtrombocytopenia, eczema and higher susceptibility to autoimmune diseases and lymphoid malignancies [45].

As for other PID, HLA-identical sibling HSC donor transplantation is considered the treatment of choice (over 80% survival rate). Allogeneic HSCTs is offering nowadays good outcomes due to improvements in HLA-typing and new alternative donor sources and myeloablative conditioning regimens [46]. However, patients lacking a HLA-matched donor still require alternative therapeutic approaches. In this direction GT could be an alternative in the near future for these patients. In fact WAS is an attractive target for GT since expression of WASP confer selective growth advantage [47-52].

Dr Klein group (Hannover Medical School, Hannover, Germany) performed the first clinical trial for WAS GT [53]. 10 patients were enrolled in this trial and they received autologous CD34$^+$ cells transduced with LTR-driven gammaretroviral vectors expressing WASP. All patients received reduced intensity conditioning with Busulfan. Most of the patients treated gain WASP expression in multiple lineages. Platelet counts increased and clinical condition improved with resolution of eczema and bleeding disorder [54, 55]. However, as occurred in the SCID-X1 clinical trials, four out of 10 of the treated patients developed leukaemia [55, 56]. The presence of the strong LTR enhancer and the patient's predisposition to develop lymphomas could favour the high frequency of leukaemia in this trial.

3. Lentiviral-vector based gene therapy clinical trials for primary immunodeficiencies

As soon as the first cases of leukaemia appeared in the SCID-X1 GT trial, it was clear that LTR-driven gammaretroviral vectors were not the vector of choice to go further into clinic. Improvements in the gammaretroviral vectors and the design of new integrative vectors became the main goal in the GT field. Several groups have dedicated considerable effort to understand the mechanism of leukomogenesis upon gammaretroviral transduction. The LMO2 oncogene was found in 4/5 cases in the SCID-X1 trial and it is now clear that retrovirus-mediated gene transfer can deregulate proto-oncogene expression through the LTR enhancer activity. With this in mind, Dr. Naldini's group have developed self-inactivated (LTR mutated) lentiviral vectors (based in HIV-1) which have one of the best efficiency/safety ratio [57-59]. LVs, contrary to gammaretroviral vectors are able to achieve efficient transduction of HSCs with minimal activation [60]. They are also safer than gammaretroviral vectors due to their less genotoxic integration site [61-63]. Several clinical trials for PID have started using HIV-1-based vectors and some promising results have already been shown on international meetings. In most cases, the general structure of the vectors is as follow: **LTRΔU3-- ψ ----human promoter ------ transgene------- LTRΔU3**

There are at the moment two GT clinical trials on going for SCID-X1 using lentiviral vectors (http://www.wiley.com/legacy/wileychi/genmed/clinical/). One is designed for newly diagnose children (St Jude Children's Research Hospital) and other is a Phase I/II non-randomized clinical trial designed to treat 13 patients with SCID-X1 who are between 2 and 30 years of age and who have clinically significant impairment of immunity. Both cases are based on mice experiments showing a better profile of lentiviral vectors both in term of reconstitution and safety [64].

Dr Gaspar and Dr Kohn have launched two other clinical trials using lentiviral vectors to treat ADA patients in UK and USA respectively. Both groups use EF1 promoter driven lentiviral vectors produced at the same site (Indiana University Vector Production Facility) through a Transatlantic Gene Therapy Consortium. The primary objective of the trial is to examine the safety of the protocol in 10 patients transplanted with LV gene-modified CD34+ cells. The protocol will involve non-myeloablative conditioning with busulfan and withholding of PEG-ADA ERT. As secondary objectives the trial will aim for the expression of ADA in peripheral blood leucocytes and immune reconstitution.

CGD is probably the PID where the necessity to improve vector efficiency and safety has been more obvious. The absence of the selective advantage of the gene-modified cells and the short life span of myeloid cells reduce the clinical benefits of gammaretroviral vectors but kept all the secondary effects. In addition, the potential toxicity of ectopic expression of gp91^{phox} on HSCs required the use of physiologically regulated vectors [65] expressing the transgene specifically in granulocytes. Very encouraging results have been obtained in animal models using transcriptionally regulated LV [66, 67]. The first clinical trial for CGD using LV started on November 2011 directed by Adrian Thrasher at Great Ormond Street Hospital for Children (UK). The primary outcome measures will be overall survival but the trial will also study reduction in frequency of infections and long-term immune reconstitution (http://clinicaltrials.gov/ct2/show/NCT01381003].

As SCID-X1 and CGD, GT for WAS has also good reasons to change the therapeutic vectors (see above). There are four clinical trials on going for WAS using LV (FR-0047, UK-0168 and US-1052: journal of gene medicine GT clinical trials data base; NCT01515462: Clincaltrial.gov). All trials will use a similar construct which drive the expression of the WASP cDNA through its own promoter. The WASp-promoter-driven LVs are haematopoietic-specific [47, 49, 68], physiological [49, 69] and avoid deleterious effects of over-expression in non-target cells[70]. Preliminary data presented at the 20th European Society of Gene and Cell Therapy by the Italian and French groups showed impressive results both, in terms of immune reconstitution and safety profile. It is important to note that integration site analysis in these patients did not show any preference for the proto-oncongens LMO2 or EVI1. In addition they didn't observe, at the time of analysis, any evidence of clonal dominance (usually indicative of proto-oncogenes activation).

4. Future directions

Based on the data shown, it does appear that new generation LVs driving the expression of the transgene through physiological promoters could be a big step toward GT clinical translation. Exciting results are expected on the clinical trials undergoing at the moment. Still, LV integrates randomly at active sites in the cell genome and can therefore alter its normal expression pattern. New, undesired side effects could appear in the future. New vectors must still consider improving two safety aspects: 1- genotoxicity (genomic alteration due to vector integrations) and 2- ectopic/unregulated expression of the transgene. Strategies to minimize or eliminate genotoxicity problems can be grouped in those based in improving retroviral vectors and those based in the development of non-viral technologies such as gene editing (revised in [14, 65]).

Acknowledgements

This work has been financed by Fondo de Investigaciones Sanitarias ISCIII (Spain) and Fondo Europeo de Desarrollo Regional (FEDER) from the European Union, through the research grant Nº PS09/00340, by the Consejería de Innovación Ciencia y Empresa (grants Nº P09-CTS-04532 and PAIDI-Bio-326) and Consejería de Salud (grant Nº PI0001/2009) from the Junta de Andalucía and FEDER/ Fondo de Cohesion Europeo (FSE) de Andalucía 2007-2013 to F.M.

Author details

Francisco Martin*, Alejandra Gutierrez-Guerrero and Karim Benabdellah

*Address all correspondence to: francisco.martin@genyo.es

Gene and Cell Therapy Group. Human DNA variability department. GENYO. Centre for Genomics and Oncological Research: Pfizer, University of Granada, Andalusian Regional Government. Parque Tecnológico Ciencias de la Salud (PTCS), Granada, Spain

References

[1] Marodi L, Notarangelo LD. Immunological and genetic bases of new primary immunodeficiencies. Nat Rev Immunol. 2007 Nov;7(11):851-61.

[2] Pessach I, Walter J, Notarangelo LD. Recent advances in Primary Immunodeficiencies: identification of novel genetic defects and unanticipated phenotypes. Pediatric research. 2009 Jan 28.

[3] Filipovich A. Hematopoietic cell transplantation for correction of primary immunodeficiencies. Bone Marrow Transplant. 2008 Aug;42 Suppl 1:S49-S52.

[4] Neven B, Leroy S, Decaluwe H, Le Deist F, Picard C, Moshous D, et al. Long-term outcome after hematopoietic stem cell transplantation of a single-center cohort of 90 patients with severe combined immunodeficiency. Blood. 2009 Apr 23;113(17): 4114-24.

[5]   Kildebeck E, Checketts J, Porteus M. Gene therapy for primary immunodeficiencies. Curr Opin Pediatr. 2012 Dec;24(6):731-8.

[6]   Cavazzana-Calvo M, Hacein-Bey S, de Saint Basile G, Gross F, Yvon E, Nusbaum P, et al. Gene therapy of human severe combined immunodeficiency (SCID)-X1 disease. Science. 2000;288(5466):669-72.

[7]   Cavazzana-Calvo M, Lagresle C, Hacein-Bey-Abina S, Fischer A. Gene therapy for severe combined immunodeficiency. Annu Rev Med. 2005;56:585-602.

[8]   Howe SJ, Mansour MR, Schwarzwaelder K, Bartholomae C, Hubank M, Kempski H, et al. Insertional mutagenesis combined with acquired somatic mutations causes leukemogenesis following gene therapy of SCID-X1 patients. J Clin Invest. 2008 Sep 2;118(9):3143-50.

[9]   Fischer A, Cavazzana-Calvo M. Gene therapy of inherited diseases. Lancet. 2008 Jun 14;371(9629):2044-7.

[10] Aiuti A, Cattaneo F, Galimberti S, Benninghoff U, Cassani B, Callegaro L, et al. Gene therapy for immunodeficiency due to adenosine deaminase deficiency. N Engl J Med. 2009 Jan 29;360(5):447-58.

[11] Ott MG, Schmidt M, Schwarzwaelder K, Stein S, Siler U, Koehl U, et al. Correction of X-linked chronic granulomatous disease by gene therapy, augmented by insertional activation of MDS1-EVI1, PRDM16 or SETBP1. Nat Med. 2006 Apr;12(4):401-9.

[12] Boztug K, Schmidt M, Schwarzer A, Banerjee PP, Diez IA, Dewey RA, et al. Stem-cell gene therapy for the Wiskott-Aldrich syndrome. N Engl J Med. 2010 Nov 11;363(20): 1918-27.

[13] Galy A, Thrasher AJ. Gene therapy for the Wiskott-Aldrich syndrome. Curr Opin Allergy Clin Immunol. 2011 Dec;11(6):545-50.

[14] Romero Z, Toscano MG, Unciti JD, Molina I, Martin F. Safer Vectors For Gene Therapy Of Primary Immunodeficiencies. Curr Gene Ther. 2009 Aug 1.

[15] Toscano MG, Romero Z, Munoz P, Cobo M, Benabdellah K, Martin F. Physiological and tissue-specific vectors for treatment of inherited diseases. Gene Ther. 2011 Feb; 18(2):117-27.

[16] Miller DG, Adam MA, Miller AD. Gene transfer by retrovirus vectors occurs only in cells that are actively replicating at the time of infection. Mol Cell Biol. 1990 Aug; 10(8):4239-42.

[17] Demaison C, Brouns G, Blundell MP, Goldman JP, Levinsky RJ, Grez M, et al. A defined window for efficient gene marking of severe combined immunodeficient-repopulating cells using a gibbon ape leukemia virus-pseudotyped retroviral vector. Hum Gene Ther. 2000;11(1):91-100.

[18] Baum C, Dullmann J, Li Z, Fehse B, Meyer J, Williams DA, et al. Side effects of retroviral gene transfer into hematopoietic stem cells. Blood. 2003 Mar 15;101(6):2099-114.

[19] Noguchi M, Yi H, Rosenblatt HM, Filipovich AH, Adelstein S, Modi WS, et al. Interleukin-2 receptor gamma chain mutation results in X-linked severe combined immunodeficiency in humans. Cell. 1993 Apr 9;73(1):147-57.

[20] Stephan V, Wahn V, Le Deist F, Dirksen U, Broker B, Muller-Fleckenstein I, et al. Atypical X-linked severe combined immunodeficiency due to possible spontaneous reversion of the genetic defect in T cells. N Engl J Med. 1996 Nov 21;335(21):1563-7.

[21] Hacein-Bey-Abina S, Fischer A, Cavazzana-Calvo M. Gene therapy of X-linked severe combined immunodeficiency. Int J Hematol. 2002 Nov;76(4):295-8.

[22] Hacein-Bey-Abina S, Le Deist F, Carlier F, Bouneaud C, Hue C, De Villartay JP, et al. Sustained correction of X-linked severe combined immunodeficiency by ex vivo gene therapy. N Engl J Med. 2002 Apr 18;346(16):1185-93.

[23] Gaspar HB, Bjorkegren E, Parsley K, Gilmour KC, King D, Sinclair J, et al. Successful reconstitution of immunity in ADA-SCID by stem cell gene therapy following cessation of PEG-ADA and use of mild preconditioning. Mol Ther. 2006 Oct;14(4):505-13.

[24] Hacein-Bey-Abina S, Hauer J, Lim A, Picard C, Wang GP, Berry CC, et al. Efficacy of gene therapy for X-linked severe combined immunodeficiency. N Engl J Med. 2010 Jul 22;363(4):355-64.

[25] Gaspar HB, Cooray S, Gilmour KC, Parsley KL, Adams S, Howe SJ, et al. Long-term persistence of a polyclonal T cell repertoire after gene therapy for X-linked severe combined immunodeficiency. Sci Transl Med. 2011 Aug 24;3(97):97ra79.

[26] Hacein-Bey-Abina S, Garrigue A, Wang GP, Soulier J, Lim A, Morillon E, et al. Insertional oncogenesis in 4 patients after retrovirus-mediated gene therapy of SCID-X1. J Clin Invest. 2008 Sep;118(9):3132-42.

[27] Hacein-Bey-Abina S, von Kalle C, Schmidt M, Le Deist F, Wulffraat N, McIntyre E, et al. A serious adverse event after successful gene therapy for X-linked severe combined immunodeficiency. N Engl J Med. 2003 Jan 16;348(3):255-6.

[28] Wu X, Li Y, Crise B, Burgess SM. Transcription start regions in the human genome are favored targets for MLV integration. Science. 2003 Jun 13;300(5626):1749-51.

[29] Laufs S, Nagy KZ, Giordano FA, Hotz-Wagenblatt A, Zeller WJ, Fruehauf S. Insertion of retroviral vectors in NOD/SCID repopulating human peripheral blood progenitor cells occurs preferentially in the vicinity of transcription start regions and in introns. Mol Ther. 2004 Nov;10(5):874-81.

[30] Bushman F, Lewinski M, Ciuffi A, Barr S, Leipzig J, Hannenhalli S, et al. Genome-wide analysis of retroviral DNA integration. Nat Rev Microbiol. 2005 Nov;3(11): 848-58.

[31] Ratech H, Hirschhorn R, Greco MA. Pathologic findings in adenosine deaminase deficient-severe combined immunodeficiency. II. Thymus, spleen, lymph node, and gastrointestinal tract lymphoid tissue alterations. Am J Pathol. 1989 Dec;135(6): 1145-56.

[32] Rogers MH, Lwin R, Fairbanks L, Gerritsen B, Gaspar HB. Cognitive and behavioral abnormalities in adenosine deaminase deficient severe combined immunodeficiency. J Pediatr. 2001 Jul;139(1):44-50.

[33] Gaspar HB, Aiuti A, Porta F, Candotti F, Hershfield MS, Notarangelo LD. How I treat ADA deficiency. Blood. 2009 Oct 22;114(17):3524-32.

[34] Aiuti A, Slavin S, Aker M, Ficara F, Deola S, Mortellaro A, et al. Correction of ADA-SCID by stem cell gene therapy combined with nonmyeloablative conditioning. Science. 2002 Jun 28;296(5577):2410-3.

[35] Sakiyama Y, Ariga T, Ohtsu M. [Gene therapy for adenosine deaminase deficiency]. Nippon Rinsho. 2005 Mar;63(3):448-52.

[36] Aiuti A, Cassani B, Andolfi G, Mirolo M, Biasco L, Recchia A, et al. Multilineage hematopoietic reconstitution without clonal selection in ADA-SCID patients treated with stem cell gene therapy. J Clin Invest. 2007 Aug;117(8):2233-40.

[37] Seger RA. Modern management of chronic granulomatous disease. Br J Haematol. 2008 Feb;140(3):255-66.

[38] Malech HL, Maples PB, Whiting-Theobald N, Linton GF, Sekhsaria S, Vowells SJ, et al. Prolonged production of NADPH oxidase-corrected granulocytes after gene therapy of chronic granulomatous disease. Proc Natl Acad Sci U S A. 1997 Oct 28;94(22): 12133-8.

[39] Grez M, Reichenbach J, Schwable J, Seger R, Dinauer MC, Thrasher AJ. Gene therapy of chronic granulomatous disease: the engraftment dilemma. Mol Ther. 2011 Jan; 19(1):28-35.

[40] Stein S, Ott MG, Schultze-Strasser S, Jauch A, Burwinkel B, Kinner A, et al. Genomic instability and myelodysplasia with monosomy 7 consequent to EVI1 activation after gene therapy for chronic granulomatous disease. Nat Med. 2010 Feb;16(2):198-204.

[41] Kuhns DB, Alvord WG, Heller T, Feld JJ, Pike KM, Marciano BE, et al. Residual NADPH oxidase and survival in chronic granulomatous disease. N Engl J Med. 2010 Dec 30;363(27):2600-10.

[42] Bedard K, Krause KH. The NOX family of ROS-generating NADPH oxidases: physiology and pathophysiology. Physiol Rev. 2007 Jan;87(1):245-313.

[43] Gallego MD, Santamaria M, Pena J, Molina IJ. Defective actin reorganization and polymerization of Wiskott-Aldrich T cells in response to CD3-mediated stimulation. Blood. 1997;90(8):3089-97.

[44] Ochs HD, Thrasher AJ. The Wiskott-Aldrich syndrome. J Allergy Clin Immunol. 2006 Apr;117(4):725-38; quiz 39.

[45] Bosticardo M, Marangoni F, Aiuti A, Villa A, Roncarolo MG. Recent advances in understanding the pathophysiology of Wiskott-Aldrich syndrome. Blood. 2009 Apr 7.

[46] Moratto D, Giliani S, Bonfim C, Mazzolari E, Fischer A, Ochs HD, et al. Long-term outcome and lineage-specific chimerism in 194 patients with Wiskott-Aldrich syndrome treated by hematopoietic cell transplantation in the period 1980-2009: an international collaborative study. Blood. 2011 Aug 11;118(6):1675-84.

[47] Dupre L, Trifari S, Follenzi A, Marangoni F, Lain de Lera T, Bernad A, et al. Lentiviral vector-mediated gene transfer in T cells from Wiskott-Aldrich syndrome patients leads to functional correction. Mol Ther. 2004 Nov;10(5):903-15.

[48] Konno A, Wada T, Schurman SH, Garabedian EK, Kirby M, Anderson SM, et al. Differential contribution of Wiskott-Aldrich syndrome protein to selective advantage in T- and B-cell lineages. Blood. 2004 Jan 15;103(2):676-8.

[49] Martin F, Toscano MG, Blundell M, Frecha C, Srivastava GK, Santamaria M, et al. Lentiviral vectors transcriptionally targeted to hematopoietic cells by WASP gene proximal promoter sequences. Gene Ther. 2005 Apr;12(8):715-23.

[50] Ariga T, Kondoh T, Yamaguchi K, Yamada M, Sasaki S, Nelson DL, et al. Spontaneous in vivo reversion of an inherited mutation in the Wiskott-Aldrich syndrome. J Immunol. 2001 Apr 15;166(8):5245-9.

[51] Wada T, Konno A, Schurman SH, Garabedian EK, Anderson SM, Kirby M, et al. Second-site mutation in the Wiskott-Aldrich syndrome (WAS) protein gene causes somatic mosaicism in two WAS siblings. J Clin Invest. 2003 May;111(9):1389-97.

[52] Wada T, Schurman SH, Otsu M, Garabedian EK, Ochs HD, Nelson DL, et al. Somatic mosaicism in Wiskott--Aldrich syndrome suggests in vivo reversion by a DNA slippage mechanism. Proc Natl Acad Sci U S A. 2001 Jul 17;98(15):8697-702.

[53] Boztug K, Dewey RA, Klein C. Development of hematopoietic stem cell gene therapy for Wiskott-Aldrich syndrome. Curr Opin Mol Ther. 2006 Oct;8(5):390-5.

[54] Boztug K, Schmidt M, Schwarzer A, Banerjee PP, Diez IA, Dewey RA, et al. Stem-cell gene therapy for the Wiskott-Aldrich syndrome. N Engl J Med. 2010 Nov 11;363(20): 1918-27.

[55] Corrigan-Curay J, Cohen-Haguenauer O, O'Reilly M, Ross SR, Fan H, Rosenberg N, et al. Challenges in vector and trial design using retroviral vectors for long-term gene correction in hematopoietic stem cell gene therapy. Mol Ther. 2012 Jun;20(6):1084-94.

[56] Avedillo Diez I, Zychlinski D, Coci EG, Galla M, Modlich U, Dewey RA, et al. Development of novel efficient SIN vectors with improved safety features for Wiskott-Aldrich syndrome stem cell based gene therapy. Mol Pharm. 2011 Oct 3;8(5):1525-37.

[57] Montini E, Cesana D, Schmidt M, Sanvito F, Ponzoni M, Bartholomae C, et al. Hematopoietic stem cell gene transfer in a tumor-prone mouse model uncovers low genotoxicity of lentiviral vector integration. NatBiotechnol. 2006;24(6):687-96.

[58] Zufferey R, Dull T, Mandel RJ, Bukovsky A, Quiroz D, Naldini L, et al. Self-inactivating lentivirus vector for safe and efficient in vivo gene delivery. J Virol. 1998;72(12): 9873-80.

[59] Naldini L, Blomer U, Gallay P, Ory D, Mulligan R, Gage FH, et al. In vivo gene delivery and stable transduction of nondividing cells by a lentiviral vector. Science. 1996;272(5259):263-7.

[60] Case SS, Price MA, Jordan CT, Yu XJ, Wang L, Bauer G, et al. Stable transduction of quiescent CD34(+)CD38(-) human hematopoietic cells by HIV-1-based lentiviral vectors. Proc Natl Acad Sci U S A. 1999 Mar 16;96(6):2988-93.

[61] Montini E, Cesana D, Schmidt M, Sanvito F, Ponzoni M, Bartholomae C, et al. Hematopoietic stem cell gene transfer in a tumor-prone mouse model uncovers low genotoxicity of lentiviral vector integration. Nat Biotechnol. 2006 Jun;24(6):687-96.

[62] Gonzalez-Murillo A, Lozano ML, Montini E, Bueren JA, Guenechea G. Unaltered repopulation properties of mouse hematopoietic stem cells transduced with lentiviral vectors. Blood. 2008 Aug 6.

[63] Montini E, Cesana D, Schmidt M, Sanvito F, Bartholomae CC, Ranzani M, et al. The genotoxic potential of retroviral vectors is strongly modulated by vector design and integration site selection in a mouse model of HSC gene therapy. J Clin Invest. 2009 Apr;119(4):964-75.

[64] Zhou S, Mody D, DeRavin SS, Hauer J, Lu T, Ma Z, et al. A self-inactivating lentiviral vector for SCID-X1 gene therapy that does not activate LMO2 expression in human T cells. Blood. 2010 Aug 12;116(6):900-8.

[65] Toscano MG, Romero Z, Munoz P, Cobo M, Benabdellah K, Martin F. Physiological and tissue-specific vectors for treatment of inherited diseases. Gene Ther. 2011 Feb; 18(2):117-27.

[66] Santilli G, Almarza E, Brendel C, Choi U, Beilin C, Blundell MP, et al. Biochemical correction of X-CGD by a novel chimeric promoter regulating high levels of transgene expression in myeloid cells. Mol Ther. 2011 Jan;19(1):122-32.

[67] Barde I, Laurenti E, Verp S, Wiznerowicz M, Offner S, Viornery A, et al. Lineage- and stage-restricted lentiviral vectors for the gene therapy of chronic granulomatous disease. Gene Ther. 2011 Nov;18(11):1087-97.

[68] Frecha C, Toscano MG, Costa C, Saez-Lara MJ, Cosset FL, Verhoeyen E, et al. Improved lentiviral vectors for Wiskott-Aldrich syndrome gene therapy mimic endogenous expression profiles throughout haematopoiesis. Gene Ther. 2008 Jun;15(12): 930-41.

[69] Charrier S, Dupre L, Scaramuzza S, Jeanson-Leh L, Blundell MP, Danos O, et al. Lentiviral vectors targeting WASp expression to hematopoietic cells, efficiently transduce and correct cells from WAS patients. Gene Ther. 2007 Mar;14(5):415-28.

[70] Toscano MG, Frecha C, Benabdellah K, Cobo M, Blundell M, Thrasher AJ, et al. Hematopoietic-specific lentiviral vectors circumvent cellular toxicity due to ectopic expression of Wiskott-Aldrich syndrome protein. Hum Gene Ther. 2008 Feb;19(2): 179-97.

Chapter 3

Gene Therapy for Diabetic Retinopathy – Targeting the Renin-Angiotensin System

Qiuhong Li, Amrisha Verma, Ping Zhu, Bo Lei,
Yiguo Qiu, Takahiko Nakagawa,
Mohan K Raizada and William W Hauswirth

Additional information is available at the end of the chapter

1. Introduction

1.1. Diabetic retinopathy clinical features and current treatment options

The prevalence of diabetes has been continuously increasing for the last few decades and it is being recognized as a worldwide epidemic [1]. Diabetic retinopathy (DR) is the most common diabetic microvascular complication, and despite recent advances in therapeutics and management, DR remains the leading cause of severe vision loss in people under age of sixty [2-4]. The prevalence of DR increases with duration of diabetes, and nearly all individuals with type 1 diabetes and more than 60% of those with type 2 have some form of retinopathy after 20 years [5-7].

Diabetic retinopathy (DR) is characterized by the development of progressive pathological changes in the retinal neuro-glial cells and microvasculature. The earlier hallmarks of diabetic retinopathy include breakdown of the blood-retinal barrier (BRB), loss of pericytes, thickening of basement membrane, and the formation of microaneuryms, which are outpouchings of capillaries [8]. BRB breakdown results in increased vascular permeability and leakage of fluid into the macula causing macular edema, another significant cause of vision loss in those with diabetes. With the progression of diabetic retinopathy, hemorrhage, macular edema, cotton wool spots, all signs of retinal ischemia, and hard exudates, the result of precipitation of lipoproteins and other circulating proteins through abnormally leaky retinal vessels become increasingly apparent. More severe and later stages of diabetic retinopathy, known as proliferative diabetic retinopathy (PDR), is characterized by pathological neovascularization. Vision loss can occur from vitreous hemorrhage or from tractional retinal detachment [8, 9].

Despite recent developments in the pharmacotherapy of DR, treatment options for patients with DR are still limited. Laser photocoagulation, the primary treatment option for patients with PDR, is still considered gold standard therapy for the treatment of PDR. Although this treatment slows the loss of vision in those with PDR, it does not represent a cure, and is in itself a cell destructive therapy. Corticosteroids and anti-VEGF agents have shown promising results with regard to prevention of neovascularization, but remain limited in use due to their short-duration effects. More importantly, none of these agents have been able to substitute for the durability and effectiveness of laser mediated panretinal photocoagulation in preventing vision loss in the late stages of DR.

1.2. RAS and diabetic complications

The renin-angiotensin system (RAS) plays a vital role in the cardiovascular homeostasis by regulating vascular tone, fluid and electrolyte balance, and in the sympathetic nerve system. Angiotensin II (Ang II), a peptide hormone of RAS, has been known to regulate a variety of hemodynamic physiological responses, including fluid homeostasis, renal function, and contraction of vascular smooth muscle [10]. In addition, Ang II is capable of inducing a multitude of non-hemodynamic effects, such as the induction of reactive oxygen species (ROS), cytokines, and the stimulation of collagen synthesis [11-14]. Most of the pathophysiological actions of Ang II are mediated via activation of Ang II type 1 receptors (AT1R), G protein–coupled receptors (GPCRs) that couple to many signaling molecules, including small G proteins, phospholipases, mitogen-activated protein (MAP) kinases, phosphatases, tyrosine kinases, NADPH oxidase, and transcription factors to stimulate vascular smooth muscle cell growth, inflammation, and fibrosis [11, 15, 16]. Dysregulation of RAS has been implicated in a number of major cardiovascular and metabolic diseases, including endothelial dysfunction, atherosclerosis, hypertension, renal disease, diabetic complications, stroke, myocardial infarction and congestive heart failure [17, 18]. RAS blockade produces beneficial cardiovascular and renal effects in numerous clinical trials [19-21].

1.3. Recent advances in RAS research

Recent discoveries have revealed that the RAS hormonal signaling cascade is more complex than initially conceived with multiple enzymes, effector molecules, and receptors that coordinately regulate the effects of the RAS. Recent studies have identified additional peptides with important physiological and pathological roles, new enzymatic cascades that generate these peptides and more receptors and signaling pathways that mediate their function [22, 23].

Discovery of angiotensin-converting enzyme 2 (ACE2) has resulted in the establishment of a novel axis of the RAS involving ACE2/Ang-(1-7)/Mas [24-27]. ACE2, like ACE, is a zinc-metallopeptidase, exhibiting approximately 42% amino acid identity with ACE in its catalytic domain. However, unlike somatic ACE, ACE2 only contains a single catalytic site and functions as a carboxymonopeptidase, cleaving a single C-terminal residue from peptide substrates, thus ACE2 is able to cleave Ang II to form Ang (1-7). Ang (1-7), a biologically active component of the RAS [28-30] binds to a G-protein coupled receptor, Mas receptor [31], and plays a counter-regulatory role in the RAS by opposing the vascular and proliferative effects of Ang II [32]. A current view of RAS consists of at least two axis with counteracting biologic effects (Figure 1).

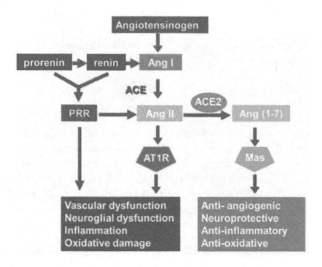

Figure 1. Schematic diagram depicting the key components of the Renin Angiotensin System. Angiotensinogen is cleaved by renin to form angiotensin I (Ang I). Angiotensin converting enzyme (ACE) converts Ang I into Angiotensin II (Ang II) the main effector peptide of the RAS. Ang II elicits is cellular effects by activating the main receptor, Angiotensin II receptor 1 (AT1R), as well as other receptors (not shown). Angiotensin II-converting enzyme 2 (ACE2), a recently discovered component of RAS, cleaves Ang II to form Angiotensin (1-7) (Ang 1-7), which activate Mas receptor to produce counteracting effects mediated by Ang II. All these components are expressed locally in various cell types in the eye, regulating metabolism, cell survival, and other local neuronal-vascular and immune-modulating functions in the retina.

This vasoprotective axis of RAS counteracts the traditional proliferative, fibrotic, proinflammatory and hypertrophic effects of the ACE/Ang II/AT1R axis of the RAS [24]. The importance of the vasodeleterious axis of the RAS [ACE/angiotensin II (Ang II)/ AT1R] in cardiovascular disease, as well as in diabetes and diabetic complications, is well established since ACE inhibitors (ACEi) and angiotensin receptor blockers (ARBs) are leading therapeutic strategies [20, 33-35]. However, the impact of the vasoprotective axis of the RAS remains poorly understood [24, 36-38]. The concept that shifting the balance of the RAS towards the vasodilatory axis by activation of ACE2 or its product, Ang-(1-7) is beneficial has been supported by many studies in cardiac, pulmonary, and vascular fibrosis [24, 39-43]. Indeed, ACE2/Ang-(1-7) activation is now considered to be a critical part of the beneficial actions of ACEi and ARB drugs [24, 36].

1.4. Tissue RAS in end-organ damage

The classical (endocrine) RAS has been traditionally regarded as systemic hormonal system. Ang II is formed from liver-synthesized angiotensinogen via a series of proteolytic cleavage events. Circulating Ang II activates AT1 and AT2 receptors in various tissues, such as the brain, adrenal and vascular tissues to modulate cardiovascular and hydromineral homeostasis.

However, most components of RAS have also been identified in essentially every organ including kidney, heart, liver, brain, adipose tissue, reproductive tissue, hematopoietic tissue, immune cells and eye, and increasing evidence supports the existence of tissue- specific RAS that exerts diverse physiological effects locally and independently of circulating Ang II [44-46]. These tissue- specific paracrine, intracrine andautocrine actions of RAS may contribute to end-organ damage in many pathological conditions including diabetic complications and maybe the basis for the reported limited beneficial effects of RAS blockade.

2. Ocular RAS in pathogenesis of diabetic retinopathy

Increasing evidence continues to implicate the involvement of the local renin-angiotensin-system (RAS) in retinal vascular dysfunctions. Various components of RAS have been detected in the different cell types of the eye (Table 1).

RAS components	Retinal Localization	Reference
Angiotensinogen	Retinal microvasculature, RGCs, RPE	[47, 48]
Angiotensin I	Aqueous, vitreous, and subretinal fluid	[49]
Angiotensin II	Aqueous, vitreous, and subretinal fluid, RGCs, retinal endothelial cells and photoreceptors	[49-51]
Angiotensin 1-7	Muller cells	[50]
Renin	Muller cells and vitreous fluid	[52, 53]
Renin receptor	Retinal microvasculature, microglia, astrocytes, RGCs, RPE	[54-58]
ACE	Muller cells, RGCs, retinal endothelial cells, photoreceptors, and vitreous	[51, 59-61]
ACE2	Retina	[50]
AT1R	Muller cells, retinal blood vessels, photoreceptors and RGCs	[50, 51]
AT2R	Muller cells, nuclei of some inner, nuclear layer neurons, and ganglion cells	[50]
Mas receptor	RGCs, retinal microvasculature, microglia, subset of astrocytes	unpublished results

GC: retinal ganglion cells; RPE: retinal pigment epithelium.

Table 1. All components of RAS are expressed locally in the eye.

Hyperglycemia has been shown to directly stimulate angiotensin gene expression via the hexominase pathway, thus contributing to increased Ang II synthesis [62]. Elevated levels of renin, prorenin, and Ang II have been found in patients with DR. In fact, ACE inhibitors and angiotensin receptor blockers (ARBs) have been shown to improve diabetes-induced vascular, neuronal, and glial dysfunction [61, 63-66]. Recent clinical studies have also clearly demonstrated the beneficial effects of RAS inhibition in both type 1 and type 2 diabetic patients with retinopathy [67-71]. Despite these positive outcomes, RAS blockers are not completely retinoprotective and retinopathy still progresses to more advanced stages. This could be attributed to the existence of local Ang II formation and that current therapeutic agents are unable to cross the blood-retina barrier (BRB) in a concentration sufficient to influence the local RAS in the eye. In addition, increasing evidence suggests that Ang II can be generated via multiple pathways, many of which may not be blocked by classic inhibitors of ACE [72-75]. Furthermore, additional components of RAS that contribute to end-organ damage, such as receptors for renin and prorenin (PRR), have been recently identified [76]. Activation of prorenin/PRR signaling pathway can initiate the RAS cascade independent of Ang II [76].

Ang II may contribute to development and progression of DR by several mechanisms. First, Ang II has been shown to increase VEGF expression directly via activation of AT1R signaling and indirectly by PCK activation [77] to enhance the role of VEGF induced vascular permeability and angiogenesis. Treatment with ACE inhibitors reduces vitreous levels of VEGF and attenuates VEGF-mediated BRB breakdown [78, 79]. Second, Ang II, mediated via AT1R, also contributes to diabetes-induced retinal inflammation by activation of nuclear factor-κβ signaling pathway within retinal endothelial cells [80, 81] leading to the release of inflammatory cytokines which perpetuates the inflammatory cycle. Pro-inflammatory cytokines, chemokines and other inflammatory mediators play an important role in the pathogenesis of DR [82, 83]. These lead to persistent low-grade inflammation, the adhesion of leukocytes to the retinal vasculature (leukostasis), breakdown of BRB and neovascularization with subsequent sub-retinal fibrosis or disciform scarring [84-88]. Third, Ang II may contribute to increased oxidative stress in diabetic retina. Ang II induces reactive oxygen species (ROS) production by activation of NADPH oxidases [89], which has been implicated in diabetic complications [90, 91]. Ang II also induces mitochondrial ROS production, which further stimulate of NADPH oxidases leading to vicious cycle and contributing tissue damage [92, 93].

Fourth, Ang II may also contribute to neuronal dysfunction induced by diabetes [94]. Receptors for Ang II are also expressed in the inner retinal neurons (Table 1). Ang II induced AT1R signaling may cause neuronal dysfunction by reducing the synaptophysin protein in the synaptic vesicles [94].

3. Protective role of the ACE2/Ang1-7-Mas axis of RAS in diabetic complications

The discovery of ACE2- mediated degradation of Ang II into the protective peptide Ang 1-7 thereby negatively regulating the classic RAS, has instigated stimulated interest regarding the potential of ACE2 as a therapeutic target [88, 89], and strategies aimed at enhancing

ACE2 action may have important therapeutic potential for cardiovascular disorders as well as for diabetic complications [40, 95-99]. Ang (1-7) has been shown to prevent diabetes-induced cardiovascular dysfunction [100] and nephropathy [101]. The protective effect of Ang 1-7 signaling is at least in part mediated by direct inhibition of diabetes-induced ROS production due to elevated NADPH oxidase activity [101, 102] and reduction in PPAR-gamma and catalase activities [102]. Adenovirus mediated gene delivery of human ACE2 in pancreas improved fasting blood glucose, beta-cell dysfunction and apoptosis occurring in type 2 diabetes mouse model [103]. The importance of ACE2 as a negative regulator of RAS in diabetic complications is supported by the facts that ACE2 deficiency exacerbates diabetic complications [104, 105] and enhancing ACE2 action counteracts the deleterious effects of Ang II and produces protective effects [96-99, 106].

3.1. Diabetes induced changes in the expression of the retinal RAS genes in the mouse retina during the progression of diabetes

We have previously shown that diabetes induced by STZ treatment in eNOS$^{-/-}$ mice results in more severe, accelerated retinopathy than diabetes in untreated eNOS$^{+/+}$ animals [107]. Thus it became critical to compare retinal mRNA levels of the RAS genes in control and diabetic animals during the progression of diabetes. We observed significant (3-10 fold) increases in the mRNA levels of the vasodeleterious axis of the RAS (angiotensinogen, renin, pro/renin receptor, ACE and AT1 receptor subtypes) following STZ treatment (Figure 2) [108]. In contrast, there was ~ 30% reduction in ACE2 mRNA following an initial stimulatory response. As a result the ACE/ACE2 mRNA ratio was increased by 10-fold, while AT1R/Mas ratio was increased by 3-fold following one month of diabetes (Figure 2). These observations were our initial indication that DR is associated with a shifting balance of the retinal RAS towards vasodeleterious axis.

3.2. Enhancing ACE2/Ang1-7-Mas axis by AAV-mediated gene delivery

3.2.1. Characterization of AAV vectors expressing ACE2 and Ang-(1-7)

AAV vector expressing the secreted form of human ACE2 was constructed under the control of the chicken-beta-actin (CBA) promoter (Figure 3A). This secreted form of ACE2 has been previously characterized and shown to be active enzymatically [109]. Since Ang-(1-7) peptide contains only 7 amino acids and small peptides are usually difficult to express in mammalian cells, we designed an expression construct in which the Ang-(1-7) peptide is expressed as part of the secreted fusion GFP protein, and is subsequently cleaved upon secretion into the active peptide. Expression of the fusion sGFP-FC-Ang-(1-7) is under the control of the CBA promoter in the AAV vector (Figure 3A) and was confirmed by tranfecting HEK293 cells using this plasmid DNA (Figure 3B). To ensure that the fusion protein was indeed secreted, proteins isolated from the culture supernatants as well as cell lysates from transfected, sham-transfected or untransfected cells were analysized by western blotting (Figure 3B). Mass spectrometry analysis of Ang (1-7) peptide in supernatant samples of HEK293 cells transfected with the sGFP-FC-Ang-(1-7) plasmid DNA was also performed. The Ang-(1-7) peptide is detectable in supernatant isolated from cells transfected with sGFP-FC-Ang-(1-7) plasmid DNA, but not detectable in samples isolated from un-transfected cells, or cells transfected with the control plasmid expressing only the cytoplasmic GFP protein (data not shown). Intravitreal administration of AAV-Ang-(1-7) resulted in a robust transduction of retinal cells primarily within the inner retinal layer (Figure 3C-F). This was associated with an increase in both cellular and secreted Ang-(1-7) (Figure 3G-H). Similarly, ACE2 protein level was increased in the retina following transduction with AAV-ACE2 (Figure 3G).

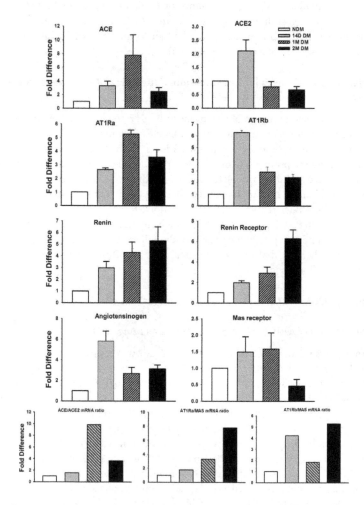

Figure 2. Real-time RT-PCR analysis of retinal mRNA for renin-angiotensin system genes. Values represent fold difference compared to age matched non-diabetic retinal samples for each gene at each time point (14 day and 1 month after induced diabetes). DM: diabetic. NDM: non-diabetic. At least 4 eyes were analyzed at each time point. *p<0.01 (versus NDM group). (From [108] with permission of Mol. Therapy).

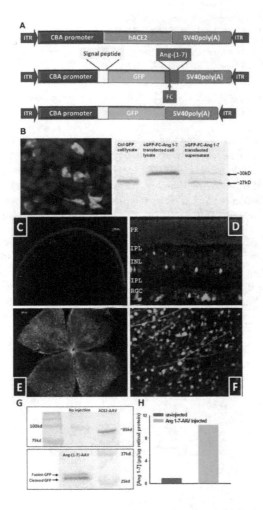

Figure 3. Construction and characterization of AAV vectors expressing ACE2 and Ang-(1-7).A: Maps of the AAV vector expressing the human ACE2 gene (hACE2) and the AAV vector expressing Ang-(1-7) gene. The Ang-(1-7) peptide is expressed as part of fusion protein, and cleaved in vivo upon secretion at the furin cleavage (FC) site. ITR: inverted terminal repeat; CBA: CMV- chicken-β-actin promoter. A control vector contains the coding region for the secreted GFP without the Ang-(1-7) peptide coding sequence. B: Expression and cleavage of the fusion protein. In cultured HEK293 cells transfected with the plasmid sGFP-FC-Ang-(1-7), or infected with AAV-sGFP-FC-Ang-(1-7), there was robust expression of GFP as expected. Proteins isolated from cell lysates contained a single protein band with molecular weight ~30 kd, as predicted for the precursor (fusion protein), but culture supernatants contained two protein bands (30kd and a 27kd), indicating that the secreted protein is cleaved at the furin cleavage site as predicted. C-F: Transduction of mouse retina with AAV vector expressing sGFP-FC-Ang-(1-7) and hACE2. A single intravitreal injection of 1µl AAV vector (10⁹ vg/eye) resulted in efficient transduction of inner retinal cells, primarily retinal ganglion cells. C. Low magnification of cross section of a mouse eye that received AAV2-sGFP-FC-Ang-(1-7) injection. D. Higher magnification of the same eye. E. A retinal whole mount showing GFP expression. F. Higher magnification of the same retinal whole mount. G: Western blot of proteins isolated from an uninjected eye and an eye injected with AAV2-ACE2 (top)

and AAV2-sGFP-FC-Ang-(1-7) (bottom) compared to a molecular weight standard (right lane). H: Ang-(1-7) peptide levels in the retina with and without AAV-sGFP-FC-Ang-(1-7) injection. There was more than a 10-fold increase in Ang-(1-7) peptide level detected by using an Ang-(1-7) specific EIA kit (Bachem, San Carlos, CA) in retinas receiving injection of AAV-sGFP-FC Ang-(1-7). PR: photoreceptor; OPL: outer plexiform layer; INL: inner nuclear layer; IPL: inner plexiform layer; RGC: retinal ganglion cells. (From [108] with permission of Mol. Therapy).

3.2.2. Ocular gene delivery of ACE2/Ang-(1-7) via the AAV vector in the retina results increased ACE2 activities and Ang-(1-7) peptide levels

Diabetes induced more than a 5-fold increase in ACE activity in the retinas of eNOS$^{-/-}$ mice, whereas ACE2 activity was relatively unchanged (Figure 4A). AAV2-ACE2 injected retinas show more than a two-fold increase in ACE2 enzymatic activity (Figure 4A) and this is associated with a reduced level of Ang II and increased Ang-(1-7) peptide level (Figure 4B), but has only a marginal effect on ACE activity (Figure 4A). Injection of AAV2-Ang-(1-7) has no effect on ACE2 activity, but significantly decreased ACE activity (Figure 4A).

We also determined Ang II and Ang-(1-7) peptide levels using a commercial EIA kit (Bachem, San Carlos, CA). STZ induced diabetes resulted in more than a 2-fold increase in Ang II levels whereas the Ang-(1-7) level was unchanged in the retinas of eNOS-/- mice (Figure 4B). This increase of Ang II was completely normalized in retinas injected with AAV-ACE2 but was unchanged in retinas injected with AAV-Ang-(1-7) vector (Figure 4B).

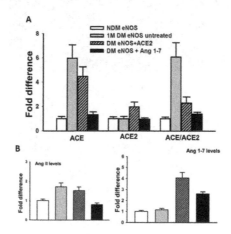

Figure 4. ACE, ACE2 activities and angiotensin peptide levels in the mouse retina.A: ACE and ACE2 enzymatic activities and ACE/ACE2 ratios in non-diabetic (NDM), 1 month diabetic (1M DM), and 1 month diabeticeNOS-/- mouse retinas treated with AAV-ACE2/Ang-(1-7). Values are expressed as fold differences compared with age-matched non-diabetic group. *p<0.01 (versus untreated DM group, N=6/group). B: Ang II and Ang-(1-7) peptide levels in non-diabetic (NDM), 1 month diabetic (1M DM), and 1 month diabetic eNOS-/- retinas treated with AAV-ACE2/Ang-(1-7), measured by ELISA using a commercial kit. *p<0.01 (versus untreated DM group). Values represent fold difference compared with age-matched non-diabetic group. Three retinas were pooled for each measurement, each measurement was done in duplicates, and three separate pools were averaged for each group. (From [108] with permission of Mol. Therapy).

3.3. Protective role of ACE2/Ang (1-7) AAV gene delivery in mouse model of DR

3.3.1. Enhanced ACE2/Ang1-7 expression in the retina reduced diabetes-induced retinal vascular leakage

We investigated if elevated expression of retinal ACE2 or Ang-(1-7) would overcome the vasodeleterious effect of the ACE/AT1R axis and prevent the development of diabetes-induced retinopathy. Effects of increased ACE2 and Ang-(1-7) expression on retinal vascular permeability were evaluated by FITC-labeled albumin extravasations and quantified by measuring its fluorescence intensity in serial sections from non-diabetic, untreated, ACE2 treated diabetic eNOS$^{-/-}$ mice and Ang 1-7 treated diabetic eNOS$^{-/-}$ mice. Induction of diabetes for 2 month in eNOS$^{-/-}$ mice resulted in a 2-fold increase in vascular permeability. This pathophysiology was significantly reduced in diabetic retinas which received ACE2/Ang-(1-7) vector treatments (Figure 5), but not in the retinas receiving control vector containing the coding sequence for secreted GFP without Ang-(1-7) or ACE2 (data not shown).

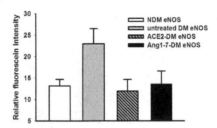

Figure 5. Effects of ocular treatments with ACE2 and Ang-(1-7)-AAV2 on retinal vascular permeability in diabetic eNOS$^{-/-}$ mice. Retinal vascular permeability was evaluated by FITC-labeled albumin extravasations and quantified by measuring the fluorescence intensity in serial sections from eNOS$^{-/-}$ mice at 1 month after induced diabetes. Data are presented as mean ± SD from 6 eyes in each group. *p<0.01 (versus untreated DM group). NDM: non-diabetes; DM: diabetes. (From [108] with permission of Mol. Therapy).

3.3.2. Increased expression of ACE2 and Ang1-7 resulted in reduced ocular inflammation in diabetic retina

Diabetes-induced ocular inflammation, as demonstrated by increased infiltrating CD45 positive macrophages and activation of CD11b positive microglial cells, was significantly reduced in eyes treated with ACE2 and Ang-(1-7) expression vectors (Figure 6).

3.3.3. Increased ACE2/Ang1-7 expression reduced the number of acellular capillaries in the diabetic retina

Induction of diabetes for 2 month in eNOS-/- mice resulted in a >10-fold increase in the formation of acellular capillaries that was significantly reduced in diabetic retinas which received ACE2/Ang-(1-7) vector treatments (Figure 7). Furthermore, increasing the level of ACE2 also prevented basement membrane thickening in diabetic eNOS$^{-/-}$ retina (Figure 8).

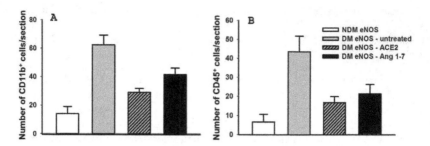

Figure 6. Intravitreal administration of ACE2 or Ang-(1-7)-AAV reduces diabetes-induced ocular inflammation. A. Quantification of CD45positive inflammatory cells in the retinas from untreated non-diabetic, ACE2 treated and Ang-(1-7) treated diabetic eNOS[-/-] mouse retinas at 1 month after induced diabetes or the equivalent age in untreated controls. B. Quantification of CD11b positive inflammatory cells in the retinas from untreated non-diabetic, ACE2 treated and Ang-(1-7) treated diabetic eNOS[-/-] mouse retinas at 1 month after induced diabetes or the equivalent age in untreated controls. N=4 for each group. *p<0.01 (versus untreated DM group). (From [108] with permission of Mol. Therapy).

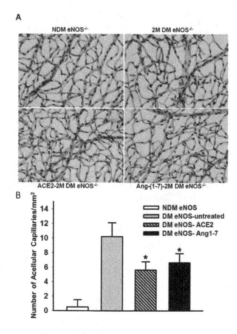

Figure 7. Evaluation of acellular capillary formation in untreated and AAV-ACE2/Ang-(1-7) treated retinas of diabetic mice. Treatments with ACE2 and Ang 1-7 vectors in the diabetic eNOS-/- mouse retinas reduced acellular capillaries. A: Representative images of trypsin-digested retinal vascular preparations from untreated non-diabetic eNOS-/-, ACE2 and Ang-(1-7) treated diabetic eNOS[-/-] mouse retinas (2 months after induced diabetes or the equivalent age in untreated controls. Arrows indicate the acellular capillaries. B. Quantitative measurements of acellular capillaries. The values on Y-axis represent the number of acellular capillaries per mm[2] retina. NDM: non-diabetes; DM: diabetes. N=6. *p<0.01 (versus untreated DM group). (From [108] with permission of Mol. Therapy).

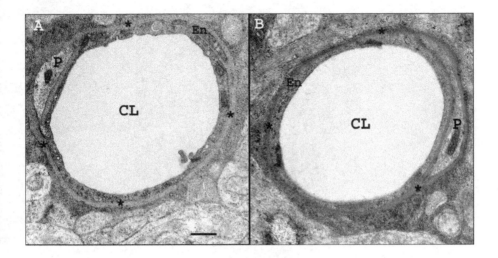

Figure 8. Transmission electron micrographs of retinal capillaries from a untreated 2 month diabetic eNOS$^{-/-}$ mouse eye (A), and an eye that received AAV-ACE2 treatment 2 weeks before STZ-induction of diabetes (B). CL: capillary lumen; En: endothelial cell; P: pericyte; * indicates the capillary basement membrane. Scale bar = 500nm. We have previously shown that the basement membranes of retinal capillaries from the diabetic eNOS$^{-/-}$ animals at two months after STZ induction of diabetes was significantly thicker than those from age-matched, non-diabetic animals [107]. The thickening of the basement membrane was prevented in the AAV-ACE2 treated eyes (73.81+17nm, versus 95.72+20 nm in untreated DM eye).

3.4. Protective role of ACE2/Ang (1-7) AAV gene delivery in a rat model of DR

3.4.1. Increased ACE2/Ang1-7 expression reduced the number of acellular capillaries in the diabetic rat retina

We also used STZ-induced diabetic SD rats as an additional animal model of diabetes to provide conceptual validation. We observed more than a 5-fold increase in the number of acellular capillaries in STZ-induced diabetic rat retinas at 14 month of diabetes. This increase was almost completely prevented by gene delivery of either ACE2 or Ang-(1-7) (Figure 9).

3.4.2. Increased expression of ACE2/Ang-(1-7) reduces oxidative damage in diabetic retina

Diabetes and its complications are associated with increased oxidative stress. We assessed oxidative damage measuring the levels of thiobarbituric acid-reactive substances (TBARs, is a marker for oxidative damage [110]) in the retina). Diabetes induced a significant increase in TBARs (Figure 10A) in eNOS$^{-/-}$ mouse retinas (Figure 10A). This increase is completely prevented by AAV-ACE2 or Ang-(1-7) treatment. Similar results were also obtained in SD rat retinas (Figure 10B).

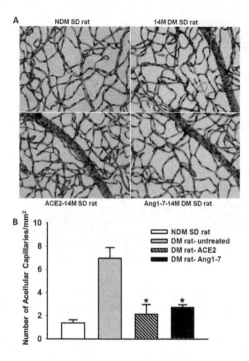

Figure 9. Evaluation of acellular capillary formation in untreated and ACE2/Ang-(1-7) AAV2 vector treated retinas of diabetic SD rats. (A) Representative images of trypsin-digested retinal vascular preparations from non-diabetic SD rat, untreated, ACE2 and Ang-(1-7) treated diabetic SD rat retinas (14 months after induced diabetes). (B) Quantitative measurements of acellular capillaries. Values on Y-axis represent the number of acellular capillaries per mm^2 of retina. NDM: non-diabetes; DM: diabetes. N=6. *p<0.01(versus untreated DM group). (From [108] with permission of Mol. Therapy).

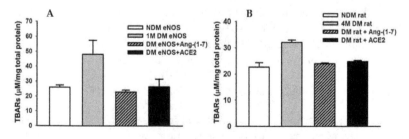

Figure 10. TBARs levels in eNOS-/- mouse retinas (A) and SD rat retinas (B). Diabetes resulted in increased TBARs levels in both eNOS$^{-/-}$ mouse retinas at 1 month of diabetes and SD rat retinas at 4 months of diabetes. These increases were prevented by AAV-ACE2/Ang-(1-7) treatments. NDM: non-diabetes; DM: diabetes. N=6/group. *p<0.01(vs untreated DM). (From [108] with permission of Mol. Therapy).

3.5. Possible mechanisms of protective action of ACE2/Ang (1-7) in diabetic retina

We demonstrate that all the genes within the RAS are expressed in the retina, consistent with various previous reports (reviewed in [111] and references therein), and the expression levels of genes in the vasoconstrictive arm of RAS (renin, ACE, AT1R) are highly elevated in diabetic retinas, whereas there is initial increase in the expression of genes in the vasodilative axis (ACE2 and MAS) earlier in diabetes that attenuate over time with the progression of diabetes, thus tipping the balance towards more vasoconstrictive, proinflammatory, hypertrophic effects of RAS mediated by ACE/Ang II/AT1R axis. This is associated with increased ACE activity and Ang II levels in diabetic retinas, whereas ACE2 activity and Ang-(1-7) levels are not significantly changed, while the mRNA levels for ACE2 and Mas receptor are reduced under these conditions.

Furthermore, we show that enhanced expression of either ACE2 or Ang-(1-7) via AAV vector mediated gene delivery in the retina prevents diabetes-induced retinal vascular permeability, thickening of basement membrane, retinal inflammation, formation of acellular capillaries, and oxidative damage in both mouse and rat models of diabetic retinopathy. More importantly, these beneficial effects occur in the absence of systemic control of glucose, blood pressure, which is elevated in eNOS-/- mice [107], and other diabetic complications [112], suggesting that local RAS activation plays a significant role of pathogenesis of diabetic retinopathy, and can be modulated locally to restore the balance between the two counter-acting arms by enhancing the ACE2/Ang-(1-7)/MAS axis. These observations provide conceptual support that enhancing ACE2/ Ang-(1-7) axis maybe an effective strategy for the treatment of DR.

Although various components of RAS have been detected in retina, our study is the first to examine the expression levels of all known RAS genes during the progression of diabetes in the eNOS-/- mice, which exhibit accelerated retinopathy [107]. We show that increased expression of genes in the vasoconstrictive, proinflammatory axis of RAS (ACE, AT1R, renin, renin receptor) occur early, 14 days after STZ-induced diabetes. We have previously shown that increased retinal vascular permeability and gliosis are already detectable at this time point in diabetic eNOS-/- mouse retina, suggesting that local hyperactivity of the deleterious axis (ACE/Ang II/AT1R) may contribute to these pathological changes. We also measured ACE and ACE2 activities in diabetic eNOS-/- mouse retina. In contrast to a previous report which showed that ACE enzyme activity was decreased, whereas ACE2 enzyme activity was increased in diabetic rat retinas [113], we found that ACE activity is highly increased in diabetic retinas, whereas ACE2 activity remains unchanged. This discrepancy may be due to the difference in animal models or the time points at which these assays were performed.

The importance of the vasodeleterious axis of the RAS (ACE/ Ang II/ AT1R) in cardiovascular disease, as well as in diabetes and diabetic complications, is well established since ACE inhibitors (ACEi) and angiotensin receptor blockers (ARBs) are leading therapeutic strategies [20, 33-35]. However, the impact of the vasoprotective axis of the RAS remains poorly understood, particularly in the eye. The concept that shifting the balance of the RAS towards the vasodilatory axis by activation of ACE2 or its product, Ang-(1-7) is beneficial has been supported by many studies in cardiac, pulmonary, and vascular fibrosis [24, 36-38]. We show that increased expression of either ACE2 or Ang-(1-7) is protective in both eNOS[-/-] mouse and rat models of diabetic retinopathy. However the action of ACE2 and Ang-(1-7) may be different. The protective effect of ACE2 may result from reduced Ang II, by catalyzing its conversion to Ang-(1-7), thus increasing the level of Ang-(1-7), or combination of both. Indeed, in the AAV-ACE2 treated retina diabetes-induced elevation of Ang II is reduced and this is associated with an increased level of Ang-(1-7). On other hand, the fact that increased Ang-(1-7) expressed from AAV vector in the retina is also protective and that the Ang II level remained high in AAV-Ang-(1-7) treated retinas suggest that Ang-(1-7) can produce physiological responses that direct counteract these of Ang II, consistent with well-established effects of Ang-(1-7) [114].

It is interesting to note that ACE2 over-expression resulted in reduced Ang II and increased Ang-(1-7) levels as expected, but has no effect on ACE activity. However, over-expression of Ang-(1-7) had no effect on endogenous ACE2 activity, but significantly reduced ACE activity. Paradoxically, despite reduced ACE activity in AAV-Ang-(1-7) treated retinas, Ang II levels remained high. It is possible that other enzymes/pathways may be involved in Ang II formation in addition to ACE. One such candidate is chymase, which has been detected in vascular systems and other tissues including eye [115]. Another candidate is the receptor for prorenin and renin (pro/renin). It has been recently demonstrated that binding of pro/renin to its receptor, pro/renin receptor (PRR), causes its prosegment to unfold, thereby activating prorenin so that it is able to generate angiotensin peptides that stimulate the Ang II-dependent pathway [76]. Considering the fact that retina contains high level of prorenin, and its level is further increased in patients with diabetic retinopathy [52], this pathway likely contributes to increased Ang II level under diabetic conditions. The existence of multiple pathways for Ang II formation at the tissue level may explain the limited beneficial effects of classic RAS blockers, and may also lend support for thtoe notion that enhancing the protective axis of RAS (ACE2/Ang-(1-7)/Mas) may represent a more effective strategy for treatment of diabetic retinopathy and other diabetic complications.

AAV vector mediated gene therapy for ocular diseases has been studied in animal models for more than a decade. Reports focusing on retinal therapy include a wide variety of retinal degenerative animal models of corresponding human retinopathies, as well as the therapeutic effects of AAV-vector mediated expression of neuroprotective, anti-apoptotic, and anti-angiogenic agents in the retina [116]. In view of recent clinical trials in which AAV delivered RPE65 gene led to restoration of vision in human patients and other reports on successful trials on treatment of ocular diseases and inherited immune deficiencies (reviewed in [117] and references therein), gene therapy has emerged as promising approach and may become a standard treatment option for a wide range of diseases in the future. In particular, when considering that the diabetic individual experience this serious ocular complication for decades, a therapeutic strategy that is long-lasting and does not require patient compliance is particularly desirable. Thus, the delivery of ACE2 and/or Ang-(1-7) could serve as a novel gene therapeutic target for DR in combination with existing strategies to control hyperglycemic and insulin resistance states.

4. Summary

All genes of the RAS are locally expressed in the retina, establishing the existence of an intrinsic retinal RAS. It is clear that the expression of genes of the vasoconstrictive/pro-inflammatory/ proliferative/fibrotic (i.e., vasodeleterious) axis (ACE/Ang II/AT1R) is highly elevated, while the vasoprotective axis [ACE2/Ang-(1-7)/Mas] is decreased in the diabetic retina. We have demonstrated that increased expression of ACE2 or Ang-(1-7), two key members of the vasoprotective axis, via AAV-mediated gene delivery to the retina attenuates diabetes-induced retinal vascular pathology. Moreover, these beneficial effects of gene transfer occur without influencing the systemic hyperglycemic status. Thus, strategies enhancing the protective ACE2/Ang-(1-7) axis of RAS could serve as a novel therapeutic target for DR.

5. Implications and future challenges

Hyperactivity of RAS, resulting in elevated concentrations of the principal effector peptide Ang II, is central to pathways leading to increased vascular inflammation, oxidative stress, endothelial dysfunction and tissue remodeling in variety of conditions including heart failure, stroke, renal failure, diabetes and its associated complications including DR. As a result, RAS inhibitors are one of the first-line therapeutic agents for treating patients with cardiovascular diseases, metabolic syndrome, diabetes and diabetic complications. Ang II blockade has shown to be antiangiogenic [66, 118, 119], anti-inflammatory [120] and improves retinal function [65], and indeed Ang II blockade therapy for retinopathy is in several clinical trials [67, 68, 121]. Despite the clear beneficial effects of RAS blockers (ACE inhibitors [ACEi] and angiotensin receptor blockers [ARBs]) [70, 71, 122], end-organ damage still ensue in patients with diabetes. Overwhelming evidence now supports the notion thatactivation of RAS at tissue levels contributes to the development and progression of diabetic complications including DR, independent of circulating RAS regulation. However the precise molecular and cellular mechanisms as to how retinal RAS contributes to the development and progression of DR remain to be elucidated. Recent studies have also revealed the evolving complexity of RAS with a myriad cellular and intracellular pathways leading to formation of Ang II, as well as Ang II- independent signaling pathways resulting in hyperactivity of tissue RAS. The physiological implications of many of these components are still not well understood and new antagonists/agonists specific to these new components remain to be discovered. Nevertheless, our results clearly demonstrate that enhancing the protective axis of RAS (ACE2/Ang1-7/Mas) locally may be a better strategy for counteracting the effects of the pathological RAS activation than present systemic approaches. Furthermore, since AAV vector mediated gene delivery has been shown to be safe, and improve vision for extended periods of time after a single administration in several clinical trials, enhancing the endogenous protective axis of RAS (ACE2/Ang1-7/Mas) by local gene delivery, in combination with combination with existing strategies to control hyperglycemic and insulin resistance states may represent a better strategy for preventing and treating diabetic complications such as diabetic retinopathy.

Acknowledgments

Supported in part by grants from American Diabetes Association, American Heart Association, Research to Prevent Blindness, NIH grants EY021752 and EY021721.

Author details

Qiuhong Li[1], Amrisha Verma[1], Ping Zhu[1], Bo Lei[1], Yiguo Qiu[1,2], Takahiko Nakagawa[3], Mohan K Raizada[4] and William W Hauswirth[1]

*Address all correspondence to: qli@ufl.edu

1 Departments of Ophthalmology, University of Florida, Gainesville, FL, USA

2 The First Affiliated Hospital of Chongqing Medical University, Chongqing Key Laboratory of Ophthalmology, Chongqing Eye Institute, China

3 Division of Renal Disease and Hypertension, University of Colorado Denver, Aurora, CO, USA

4 Department of Physiology & Functional Genomics, University of Florida, Gainesville, FL, USA

References

[1] Shaw, J.E., R.A. Sicree, and P.Z. Zimmet, Global estimates of the prevalence of diabetes for 2010 and 2030. Diabetes Res ClinPract, 2010. 87(1): p. 4-14.

[2] Cheung, N., P. Mitchell, and T.Y. Wong, Diabetic retinopathy. Lancet, 2010. 376(9735): p. 124-36.

[3] Klein, B.E., Overview of epidemiologic studies of diabetic retinopathy. Ophthalmic Epidemiol, 2007. 14(4): p. 179-83.

[4] Yau, J.W., et al., Global prevalence and major risk factors of diabetic retinopathy. Diabetes Care, 2012. 35(3): p. 556-64.

[5] Fong, D.S., et al., Retinopathy in diabetes. Diabetes Care, 2004. 27 Suppl 1: p. S84-7.

[6] Fong, D.S., et al., Diabetic retinopathy. Diabetes Care, 2004. 27(10): p. 2540-53.

[7] Williams, R., et al., Epidemiology of diabetic retinopathy and macular oedema: a systematic review. Eye, 2004. 18(10): p. 963-83.

[8] Frank, R.N., Diabetic retinopathy. N Engl J Med, 2004. 350(1): p. 48-58.

[9] Watkins, P.J., Retinopathy. BMJ, 2003. 326(7395): p. 924-6.

[10] Hunyady, L. and K.J. Catt, Pleiotropic AT1 receptor signaling pathways mediating physiological and pathogenic actions of angiotensin II.MolEndocrinol, 2006. 20(5): p. 953-70.

[11] Mehta, P.K. and K.K. Griendling, Angiotensin II cell signaling: physiological and pathological effects in the cardiovascular system. Am J Physiol Cell Physiol, 2007.292(1): p. C82-97.

[12] Marchesi, C., P. Paradis, and E.L. Schiffrin, Role of the renin-angiotensin system in vascular inflammation. Trends PharmacolSci, 2008. 29(7): p. 367-74.

[13] de Cavanagh, E.M., et al., From mitochondria to disease: role of the renin-angiotensin system. Am J Nephrol, 2007.27(6): p. 545-53.

[14] de Cavanagh, E.M., et al., Angiotensin II, mitochondria, cytoskeletal, and extracellular matrix connections: an integrating viewpoint. Am J Physiol Heart CircPhysiol, 2009.296(3): p. H550-8.

[15] Touyz, R.M. and E.L. Schiffrin, Signal transduction mechanisms mediating the physiological and pathophysiological actions of angiotensin II in vascular smooth muscle cells.Pharmacol Rev, 2000. 52(4): p. 639-72.

[16] Nguyen Dinh Cat, A. and R.M. Touyz, Cell signaling of angiotensin II on vascular tone: novel mechanisms.CurrHypertens Rep, 2011. 13(2): p. 122-8.

[17] Carey, R.M. and H.M. Siragy, Newly recognized components of the renin-angiotensin system: potential roles in cardiovascular and renal regulation.Endocr Rev, 2003. 24(3): p. 261-71.

[18] Putnam, K., et al., The renin-angiotensin system: a target of and contributor to dyslipidemias, altered glucose homeostasis, and hypertension of the metabolic syndrome. Am J Physiol Heart CircPhysiol, 2012.302(6): p. H1219-30.

[19] Nakao, Y.M., et al., Effects of renin-angiotensin system blockades on cardiovascular outcomes in patients with diabetes mellitus: A systematic review and meta-analysis. Diabetes Res ClinPract, 2012. 96(1): p. 68-75.

[20] Perret-Guillaume, C., et al., Benefits of the RAS blockade: clinical evidence before the ONTARGET study. J Hypertens, 2009. 27 Suppl 2: p. S3-7.

[21] Ostergren, J., Renin-angiotensin-system blockade in the prevention of diabetes. Diabetes Res ClinPract, 2007. 76 Suppl 1: p. S13-21.

[22] Crowley, S.D. and T.M. Coffman, Recent advances involving the renin-angiotensin system.Exp Cell Res, 2012. 318(9): p. 1049-56.

[23] Nguyen Dinh Cat, A. and R.M. Touyz, A new look at the renin-angiotensin system--focusing on the vascular system. Peptides, 2011. 32(10): p. 2141-50.

[24] Ferreira, A.J., et al., Therapeutic implications of the vasoprotective axis of the renin-angiotensin system in cardiovascular diseases. Hypertension, 2010. 55(2): p. 207-13.

[25] Ferrario, C.M., A.J. Trask, and J.A. Jessup, Advances in biochemical and functional roles of angiotensin-converting enzyme 2 and angiotensin-(1-7) in regulation of cardiovascular function. Am J Physiol Heart CircPhysiol, 2005.289(6): p. H2281-90.

[26] Donoghue, M., et al., A novel angiotensin-converting enzyme-related carboxypeptidase (ACE2) converts angiotensin I to angiotensin 1-9.Circ Res, 2000. 87(5): p. E1-9.

[27] Tipnis, S.R., et al., A human homolog of angiotensin-converting enzyme. Cloning and functional expression as a captopril-insensitive carboxypeptidase. J BiolChem, 2000. 275(43): p. 33238-43.

[28] Ferreira, A.J. and R.A. Santos, Cardiovascular actions of angiotensin-(1-7).Braz J Med Biol Res, 2005. 38(4): p. 499-507.

[29] Varagic, J., et al., New angiotensins. J Mol Med, 2008. 86(6): p. 663-71.

[30] Mercure, C., et al., Angiotensin(1-7) blunts hypertensive cardiac remodeling by a direct effect on the heart.Circ Res, 2008. 103(11): p. 1319-26.

[31] Santos, R.A., et al., Angiotensin-(1-7) is an endogenous ligand for the G protein-coupled receptor Mas.ProcNatlAcadSci U S A, 2003. 100(14): p. 8258-63.

[32] Santos, R.A., A.J. Ferreira, and E.S.A.C. Simoes, Recent advances in the angiotensin-converting enzyme 2-angiotensin(1-7)-Mas axis.ExpPhysiol, 2008. 93(5): p. 519-27.

[33] Sica, D.A., The practical aspects of combination therapy with angiotensin receptor blockers and angiotensin-converting enzyme inhibitors. J Renin Angiotensin Aldosterone Syst, 2002. 3(2): p. 66-71.

[34] Ribeiro-Oliveira, A., Jr., et al., The renin-angiotensin system and diabetes: an update.Vasc Health Risk Manag, 2008. 4(4): p. 787-803.

[35] Perkins, J.M. and S.N. Davis, The renin-angiotensin-aldosterone system: a pivotal role in insulin sensitivity and glycemic control.CurrOpinEndocrinol Diabetes Obes, 2008. 15(2): p. 147-52.

[36] Keidar, S., M. Kaplan, and A. Gamliel-Lazarovich, ACE2 of the heart: From angiotensin I to angiotensin (1-7).Cardiovasc Res, 2007. 73(3): p. 463-9.

[37] Iwai, M. and M. Horiuchi, Devil and angel in the renin-angiotensin system: ACE-angiotensin II-AT1 receptor axis vs. ACE2-angiotensin-(1-7)-Mas receptor axis.Hypertens Res, 2009. 32(7): p. 533-6.

[38] Der Sarkissian, S., et al., ACE2: A novel therapeutic target for cardiovascular diseases.ProgBiophysMolBiol, 2006. 91(1-2): p. 163-98.

[39] Huentelman, M.J., et al., Protection from angiotensin II-induced cardiac hypertrophy and fibrosis by systemic lentiviral delivery of ACE2 in rats.ExpPhysiol, 2005. 90(5): p. 783-90.

[40] Hernandez Prada, J.A., et al., Structure-based identification of small-molecule angiotensin-converting enzyme 2 activators as novel antihypertensive agents. Hypertension, 2008. 51(5): p. 1312-7.

[41] Ferreira, A.J., et al., Evidence for angiotensin-converting enzyme 2 as a therapeutic target for the prevention of pulmonary hypertension.Am J RespirCrit Care Med, 2009. 179(11): p. 1048-54.

[42] Fraga-Silva, R.A., et al., ACE2 activation promotes antithrombotic activity.Mol Med, 2010. 16(5-6): p. 210-5.

[43] Der Sarkissian, S., et al., Cardiac overexpression of angiotensin converting enzyme 2 protects the heart from ischemia-induced pathophysiology. Hypertension, 2008. 51(3): p. 712-8.

[44] Paul, M., A. PoyanMehr, and R. Kreutz, Physiology of local renin-angiotensin systems.Physiol Rev, 2006. 86(3): p. 747-803.

[45] Bader, M., et al., Tissue renin-angiotensin systems: new insights from experimental animal models in hypertension research. J Mol Med, 2001. 79(2-3): p. 76-102.

[46] Baltatu, O.C., L.A. Campos, and M. Bader, Local renin-angiotensin system and the brain--a continuous quest for knowledge. Peptides, 2011. 32(5): p. 1083-6.

[47] Wagner, J., et al., Demonstration of renin mRNA, angiotensinogen mRNA, and angiotensin converting enzyme mRNA expression in the human eye: evidence for an intraocular renin-angiotensin system. Br J Ophthalmol, 1996. 80(2): p. 159-63.

[48] Sarlos, S. and J.L. Wilkinson-Berka, The renin-angiotensin system and the developing retinal vasculature. Invest Ophthalmol Vis Sci, 2005. 46(3): p. 1069-77.

[49] Danser, A.H., et al., Angiotensin levels in the eye. Invest Ophthalmol Vis Sci, 1994. 35(3): p. 1008-18.

[50] Senanayake, P., et al., Angiotensin II and Its Receptor Subtypes in the Human Retina. Invest Ophthalmol Vis Sci, 2007. 48(7): p. 3301-11.

[51] Savaskan, E., et al., Immunohistochemical localization of angiotensin-converting enzyme, angiotensin II and AT1 receptor in human ocular tissues. Ophthalmic Res, 2004. 36(6): p. 312-20.

[52] Danser, A.H., et al., Renin, prorenin, and immunoreactive renin in vitreous fluid from eyes with and without diabetic retinopathy. J ClinEndocrinolMetab, 1989. 68(1): p. 160-7.

[53] Berka, J.L., et al., Renin-containing Muller cells of the retina display endocrine features. Invest Ophthalmol Vis Sci, 1995. 36(7): p. 1450-8.

[54] Alcazar, O., et al., (Pro)renin receptor is expressed in human retinal pigment epithelium and participates in extracellular matrix remodeling.Exp Eye Res, 2009. 89(5): p. 638-47.

[55] Satofuka, S., et al., Role of nonproteolytically activated prorenin in pathologic, but not physiologic, retinal neovascularization. Invest Ophthalmol Vis Sci, 2007. 48(1): p. 422-9.

[56] Satofuka, S., et al., (Pro)renin receptor promotes choroidal neovascularization by activating its signal transduction and tissue renin-angiotensin system. Am J Pathol, 2008.173(6): p. 1911-8.

[57] Satofuka, S., et al., (Pro)renin receptor-mediated signal transduction and tissue renin-angiotensin system contribute to diabetes-induced retinal inflammation. Diabetes, 2009. 58(7): p. 1625-33.

[58] Wilkinson-Berka, J.L., et al., RILLKKMPSV influences the vasculature, neurons and glia, and (pro)renin receptor expression in the retina. Hypertension, 2010. 55(6): p. 1454-60.

[59] Maruichi, M., et al., Measurement of activities in two different angiotensin II generating systems, chymase and angiotensin-converting enzyme, in the vitreous fluid of vitreoretinal diseases: a possible involvement of chymase in the pathogenesis of macular hole patients.Curr Eye Res, 2004. 29(4-5): p. 321-5.

[60] Kida, T., et al., Renin-angiotensin system in proliferative diabetic retinopathy and its gene expression in cultured human muller cells.Jpn J Ophthalmol, 2003. 47(1): p. 36-41.

[61] Zhang, J.Z., et al., Captopril inhibits glucose accumulation in retinal cells in diabetes. Invest Ophthalmol Vis Sci, 2003. 44(9): p. 4001-5.

[62] Hsieh, T.J., et al., High glucose stimulates angiotensinogen gene expression and cell hypertrophy via activation of the hexosamine biosynthesis pathway in rat kidney proximal tubular cells. Endocrinology, 2003. 144(10): p. 4338-49.

[63] Zhang, J.Z., et al., Captopril inhibits capillary degeneration in the early stages of diabetic retinopathy.Curr Eye Res, 2007. 32(10): p. 883-9.

[64] Moravski, C.J., et al., The renin-angiotensin system influences ocular endothelial cell proliferation in diabetes: transgenic and interventional studies. Am J Pathol, 2003.162(1): p. 151-60.

[65] Phipps, J.A., J.L. Wilkinson-Berka, and E.L. Fletcher, Retinal dysfunction in diabetic ren-2 rats is ameliorated by treatment with valsartan but not atenolol. Invest Ophthalmol Vis Sci, 2007. 48(2): p. 927-34.

[66] Wilkinson-Berka, J.L., et al., Valsartan but not atenolol improves vascular pathology in diabetic Ren-2 rat retina. Am J Hypertens, 2007.20(4): p. 423-30.

[67] Chaturvedi, N., et al., Effect of candesartan on prevention (DIRECT-Prevent 1) and progression (DIRECT-Protect 1) of retinopathy in type 1 diabetes: randomised, placebo-controlled trials. Lancet, 2008. 372(9647): p. 1394-402.

[68] Sjolie, A.K., et al., Effect of candesartan on progression and regression of retinopathy in type 2 diabetes (DIRECT-Protect 2): a randomised placebo-controlled trial. Lancet, 2008. 372(9647): p. 1385-93.

[69] Mauer, M., et al., Renal and retinal effects of enalapril and losartan in type 1 diabetes. N Engl J Med, 2009. 361(1): p. 40-51.

[70] Ghattas, A., P.L. Lip, and G.Y. Lip, Renin-angiotensin blockade in diabetic retinopathy.Int J ClinPract, 2011. 65(2): p. 113-6.

[71] Wright, A.D. and P.M. Dodson, Diabetic retinopathy and blockade of the renin-angiotensin system: new data from the DIRECT study programme. Eye (Lond), 2010. 24(1): p. 1-6.

[72] Miyazaki, M. and S. Takai, Tissue angiotensin II generating system by angiotensin-converting enzyme and chymase. J PharmacolSci, 2006. 100(5): p. 391-7.

[73] Cristovam, P.C., et al., ACE-dependent and chymase-dependent angiotensin II generation in normal and glucose-stimulated human mesangial cells.ExpBiol Med (Maywood), 2008. 233(8): p. 1035-43.

[74] Kumar, R. and M.A. Boim, Diversity of pathways for intracellular angiotensin II synthesis.CurrOpinNephrolHypertens, 2009. 18(1): p. 33-9.

[75] Shiota, N., et al., Angiotensin II-generating system in dog and monkey ocular tissues.ClinExpPharmacolPhysiol, 1997. 24(3-4): p. 243-8.

[76] Nguyen, G., et al., Pivotal role of the renin/prorenin receptor in angiotensin II production and cellular responses to renin. J Clin Invest, 2002. 109(11): p. 1417-27.

[77] Malhotra, A., et al., Angiotensin II promotes glucose-induced activation of cardiac protein kinase C isozymes and phosphorylation of troponin I. Diabetes, 2001. 50(8): p. 1918-26.

[78] Kim, H.W., et al., Enalapril alters expression of key growth factors in experimental diabetic retinopathy.Curr Eye Res, 2009. 34(11): p. 976-87.

[79] Kim, J.H., et al., Blockade of angiotensin II attenuates VEGF-mediated blood-retinal barrier breakdown in diabetic retinopathy. J Cereb Blood Flow Metab, 2008.

[80] Li, X.C. and J.L. Zhuo, Nuclear factor-kappaB as a hormonal intracellular signaling molecule: focus on angiotensin II-induced cardiovascular and renal injury.CurrOpinNephrolHypertens, 2008. 17(1): p. 37-43.

[81] Brasier, A.R., et al., Angiotensin II induces gene transcription through cell-type-dependent effects on the nuclear factor-kappaB (NF-kappaB) transcription factor.Mol Cell Biochem, 2000. 212(1-2): p. 155-69.

[82] Adamis, A.P., Is diabetic retinopathy an inflammatory disease? Br J Ophthalmol, 2002. 86(4): p. 363-5.

[83] Joussen, A.M., et al., Nonsteroidal anti-inflammatory drugs prevent early diabetic retinopathy via TNF-alpha suppression. FASEB J, 2002. 16(3): p. 438-40.

[84] Tang, J. and T.S. Kern, Inflammation in diabetic retinopathy.ProgRetin Eye Res, 2012. 30(5): p. 343-58.

[85] Joussen, A.M., et al., A central role for inflammation in the pathogenesis of diabetic retinopathy. FASEB J, 2004. 18(12): p. 1450-2.

[86] Adamis, A.P. and A.J. Berman, Immunological mechanisms in the pathogenesis of diabetic retinopathy.SeminImmunopathol, 2008. 30(2): p. 65-84.

[87] Kern, T.S., Contributions of inflammatory processes to the development of the early stages of diabetic retinopathy.Exp Diabetes Res, 2007. 2007: p. 95103.

[88] Kurihara, T., et al., Renin-Angiotensin system hyperactivation can induce inflammation and retinal neural dysfunction.Int J Inflam, 2012. 2012: p. 581695.

[89] Lavoie, J.L. and C.D. Sigmund, Minireview: overview of the renin-angiotensin system--an endocrine and paracrine system. Endocrinology, 2003. 144(6): p. 2179-83.

[90] Sedeek, M., et al., Oxidative stress, nox isoforms and complications of diabetes-potential targets for novel therapies. J CardiovascTransl Res, 2012. 5(4): p. 509-18.

[91] Gao, L. and G.E. Mann, Vascular NAD(P)H oxidase activation in diabetes: a double-edged sword in redox signalling.Cardiovasc Res, 2009. 82(1): p. 9-20.

[92] Dikalov, S., Cross talk between mitochondria and NADPH oxidases. Free RadicBiol Med, 2011. 51(7): p. 1289-301.

[93] Dikalov, S.I. and R.R. Nazarewicz, Angiotensin II-Induced Production of Mitochondrial Reactive Oxygen Species: Potential Mechanisms and Relevance for Cardiovascular Disease.Antioxid Redox Signal, 2012.

[94] Kurihara, T., et al., Angiotensin II type 1 receptor signaling contributes to synaptophysin degradation and neuronal dysfunction in the diabetic retina. Diabetes, 2008. 57(8): p. 2191-8.

[95] Katovich, M.J., et al., Angiotensin-converting enzyme 2 as a novel target for gene therapy for hypertension.ExpPhysiol, 2005. 90(3): p. 299-305.

[96] Oudit, G.Y., et al., Human recombinant ACE2 reduces the progression of diabetic nephropathy. Diabetes, 2010. 59(2): p. 529-38.

[97] Oudit, G.Y. and J.M. Penninger, Recombinant human angiotensin-converting enzyme 2 as a new renin-angiotensin system peptidase for heart failure therapy.Curr Heart Fail Rep, 2011. 8(3): p. 176-83.

[98]   Zhong, J., et al., Angiotensin-converting enzyme 2 suppresses pathological hypertrophy, myocardial fibrosis, and cardiac dysfunction. Circulation, 2010. 122(7): p. 717-28, 18 p following 728.

[99]   Zhong, J., et al., Prevention of angiotensin II-mediated renal oxidative stress, inflammation, and fibrosis by angiotensin-converting enzyme 2. Hypertension, 2011. 57(2): p. 314-22.

[100] Benter, I.F., et al., Angiotensin-(1-7) prevents diabetes-induced cardiovascular dysfunction. Am J Physiol Heart CircPhysiol, 2007.292(1): p. H666-72.

[101] Moon, J.Y., et al., Attenuating effect of angiotensin-(1-7) on angiotensin II-mediated NAD(P)H oxidase activation in type 2 diabetic nephropathy of KK-Ay/Ta mice. Am J Physiol Renal Physiol, 2011.

[102] Dhaunsi, G.S., et al., Angiotensin-(1-7) prevents diabetes-induced attenuation in PPAR-gamma and catalase activities.Eur J Pharmacol, 2010. 638(1-3): p. 108-14.

[103] Bindom, S.M., et al., Angiotensin I-converting enzyme type 2 (ACE2) gene therapy improves glycemic control in diabetic mice. Diabetes, 2010. 59(10): p. 2540-8.

[104] Patel, V.B., et al., Loss of angiotensin-converting enzyme-2 exacerbates diabetic cardiovascular complications and leads to systolic and vascular dysfunction: a critical role of the angiotensin II/AT1 receptor axis.Circ Res, 2012. 110(10): p. 1322-35.

[105] Wong, D.W., et al., Loss of angiotensin-converting enzyme-2 (Ace2) accelerates diabetic kidney injury. Am J Pathol, 2007.171(2): p. 438-51.

[106] Lo, J., et al., Angiotensin Converting Enzyme 2 antagonizes Ang II-induced pressor response and NADPH oxidase activation in WKY rats and in SHR model.ExpPhysiol, 2012.

[107] Li, Q., et al., Diabetic eNOS-knockout mice develop accelerated retinopathy. Invest Ophthalmol Vis Sci, 2010. 51(10): p. 5240-6.

[108] Verma, A., et al., ACE2 and Ang-(1-7) confer protection against development of diabetic retinopathy.MolTher, 2012. 20(1): p. 28-36.

[109] Huentelman, M.J., et al., Cloning and characterization of a secreted form of angiotensin-converting enzyme 2.RegulPept, 2004. 122(2): p. 61-7.

[110] Dawn-Linsley, M., et al., Monitoring thiobarbituric acid-reactive substances (TBARs) as an assay for oxidative damage in neuronal cultures and central nervous system. J Neurosci Methods, 2005. 141(2): p. 219-22.

[111] Fletcher, E.L., et al., The renin-angiotensin system in retinal health and disease: Its influence on neurons, glia and the vasculature.ProgRetin Eye Res, 2010: p. 1-28.

[112] Nakagawa, T., et al., Diabetic endothelial nitric oxide synthase knockout mice develop advanced diabetic nephropathy. J Am SocNephrol, 2007. 18(2): p. 539-50.

[113] Tikellis, C., et al., Identification of angiotensin converting enzyme 2 in the rodent retina.Curr Eye Res, 2004. 29(6): p. 419-27.

[114] Ferrario, C.M., et al., Counterregulatory actions of angiotensin-(1-7). Hypertension, 1997. 30(3 Pt 2): p. 535-41.

[115] Lorenz, J.N., Chymase: the other ACE? Am J Physiol Renal Physiol, 2010.298(1): p. F35-6.

[116] Hauswirth, W.W., et al., Range of retinal diseases potentially treatable by AAV-vectored gene therapy. Novartis Found Symp, 2004. 255: p. 179-88; discussion 188-94.

[117] Herzog, R.W., O. Cao, and A. Srivastava, Two decades of clinical gene therapy--success is finally mounting.Discov Med, 2010. 9(45): p. 105-11.

[118] Sarlos, S., et al., Retinal angiogenesis is mediated by an interaction between the angiotensin type 2 receptor, VEGF, and angiopoietin. Am J Pathol, 2003.163(3): p. 879-87.

[119] Moravski, C.J., et al., Retinal neovascularization is prevented by blockade of the renin-angiotensin system. Hypertension, 2000. 36(6): p. 1099-104.

[120] Nagai, N., et al., Suppression of diabetes-induced retinal inflammation by blocking the angiotensin II type 1 receptor or its downstream nuclear factor-kappaB pathway. Invest Ophthalmol Vis Sci, 2007. 48(9): p. 4342-50.

[121] Chaturvedi, N., et al., Effect of lisinopril on progression of retinopathy in normotensive people with type 1 diabetes. The EUCLID Study Group. EURODIAB Controlled Trial of Lisinopril in Insulin-Dependent Diabetes Mellitus. Lancet, 1998. 351(9095): p. 28-31.

[122] Sjolie, A.K., P. Dodson, and F.R. Hobbs, Does renin-angiotensin system blockade have a role in preventing diabetic retinopathy? A clinical review.Int J ClinPract, 2011. 65(2): p. 148-53.

Chapter 4

Gene Therapy for the *COL7A1* Gene

E. Mayr, U. Koller and J.W. Bauer

Additional information is available at the end of the chapter

1. Introduction

1.1. Epidermolysis bullosa

Epidermolysis bullosa (EB) is a genetically and clinically variable disease characterized by blister formation and erosions of the skin and mucous membranes after minor trauma [1]. The inheritance of the affected genes can occur in a dominant or recessive way depending on the subform of the disease. In general, epidermolysis bullosa is caused by mutations in genes encoding structural proteins within the basal membrane zone of the skin. Absence or functional loss of one of these proteins results in a lack of stability of the microarchitecture of the connection between dermis and epidermis leading to a loss of coherence [1]. The basement membrane between the dermis and the epidermis is a complex membrane produced by basal keratinocytes and dermal fibroblasts that acts as mechanical support for the connection of both skin layers. The basal membrane also regulates the metabolic exchange between the two skin compartments [2]. Up to date, there are at least 15 genes associated with EB causing different forms of the disease. Numerous mutations in these genes that encode for structural proteins within keratinocytes or within mucocutaneous basement membranes have been identified up to now [1].

Mutations in the genes, encoding for the keratins 5 and 14 and plectin, lead to epidermolysis bullosa simplex (EBS) characterized by the cytolysis within basal keratinocytes. Junctional epidermolysis bullosa (JEB) is caused by the absence or loss of function of laminin-332, type XVII collagen or integrin-β4. JEB is a severe EB form and is characterized by the separation of the skin within the lamina lucida. Mutations in type VII collagen (encoded by *COL7A1*) lead to the dystrophic form of epidermolysis bullosa, characterized by skin separation below the lamina densa. The severity and clinical manifestation of the disease depend on the mutation type (missense mutation, nonsense mutation, splice site mutations, deletion or insertion), the mode of inheritance and the localization of the mutation within the gene. Due to this fact, diagnosis, course of disease and therapy vary significantly depending on the present EB subform [3]. Blister formation can be restricted to the soles of the feet or occur generalized. Severe systemic complications and extracutaneous manifestations including blistering and erosions of the cornea and mucosal tissues, stenoses or strictures of respiratory, gastrointestinal and urogenital tracts, pylorus atresia, muscular dystrophy and skin cancer are certain complications associated with different EB subtypes [1]. So far over 30 distinctive subtypes have been described and classified in a system, which was recently revised [4]. See Table 1.

A: Classification scheme for the major EB subtypes

Major EB type	Major EB subtypes	Affected proteins
EB simplex (EBS)	Suprabasal EBS	plakophilin-1, desmoplakin;
		others?
	Basal EBS	keratins 5 & 14; plectin,
		α6β4 integrin, BPAG1
Junctional EB (JEB)	JEB, Herlitz (JEB-H)	laminin-332, (laminin-5)
	JEB, other	laminin-332, type XVII collagen
		α6β4 integrin, α3 integrin
Dystrophic EB (DEB)	Dominant DEB (DDEB)	type VII collagen
	Recessive DEB (RDEB)	type VII collagen
Kindler syndrome		kindlin-1

B: Classification scheme for all known EB simplex subtypes

Major types	EBS subtypes	Affected proteins
EBS suprabasal	*lethal acantholytic EB*	desmoplakin
	plakophilin deficiency	plakophilin-1
	EBS superficialis	?
EBS basal	EBS, localized (EBS-loc)[a]	K5, K14
	EBS, Dowling Meara (EBS-DM)	K5, K14
	EBS, other generalized (EBS,gen-nonDM)[b]	K5, K14, BPAG1
	EBS with mottled pigmentation(EBS-MP)	K5
	EBS with muscular dystrophy (EBS-MD)	plectin
	EBS with pylorus atresia (EBS-PA)	plectin, α6β4 integrin
	EBS, autosomal recessive (EBS-AR)	K14
	EBS, ogna (EBS-Og)	plectin
	EBS, migratory circinate (EBS-migr)	K5

(rare variants in italics)

[a] Previously called EBS, Weber-Cockayne

[b] Includes patients previously classified as EBS-Koebner

C: Classification scheme for all known junctional subtypes

Major JEB subtype	Subtypes	Affected proteins
JEB, Herlitz (JEB-H)		laminin-332
JEB, other (JEB-O)	JEB, non-Herlitz, generalized (JEB-nH gen)[a]	laminin-332, type XVII collagen

	JEB, non-Herlitz localized (JEB-nH loc)	typeXVII collagen
	JEB with pyloric atresia (JEB-PA)	α6β4 integrin
	JEB, inversa (JEB-I)	laminin-332
	JEB, late onset (JEB-lo)[b]	
	LOC syndrome (laryngo-onycho-cutaneous syndrome)	laminin-332 α3 chain
	?	α3 integrin
(rare variants in italics)		
[a] Formerly known as generalized atrophic benign EB (GABEB)		
[b] Formerly known as EB progressive		
D: Classification scheme for all known dystrophic EB subtypes		
Major DEB subtype	Subtypes	Affected protein
DDEB	DDEB, generalized (DDEB-gen)	type VII collagen
	DDEB, acral (DDEB-ac)	
	DDEB, pretibial (DDEB-Pt)	
	DDEB, pruriginosa (DDEB-Pr)	
	DDEB, nails only (DDEB-no)	
	DDEB, bullous dermolysis of the newborn (DDEB-BDN)	
RDEB	RDEB, severe generalized (RDEB-sev gen)[a]	type VII collagen
	RDEB, generalized other (RDEB-O)	
	RDEB, inversa (RDEB-I)	
	RDEB, pretibial (RDEB-Pt)	
	RDEB pruriginosa (RDEB-Pr)	
	RDEB, centripetalis (RDEB-Ce)	
	RDEB, bullous dermolysis of the Newborn (RDEB-BDN)	
(rare variants in italics)		
[a] Previously called RDEB, Hallopeau-Siemens		

Table 1. Classification system for inherited epidermolysis bullosa. Based on Fine et al. [4].

2. Dystrophic epidermolysis bullosa (DEB)

Mutations in the gene *COL7A1*, encoding for type VII collagen, cause the dystrophic form of epidermolysis bullosa (DEB). Type VII collagen is the major constituent of the basement membrane's anchoring fibrils and belongs to the superfamily of collagens [5]. *COL7A1* comprises 118 exons and mostly short intervening introns resulting in a size of the entire *COL7A1* gene of 32kb encoding an mRNA of over 9kb [6,7]. The remarkable number of *COL7A1* mutations and the variable genotype-phenotype correlation hamper the finding of an optimal therapy for DEB patients. Nevertheless severity of clinical manifestations can often be defined by the type of the mutation and its localization within the *COL7A1* gene [3]. DEB is divided into two main subtypes according to the mode of inheritance. Dominant dystrophic EB (DDEB) is inherited in an autosomal dominant way, whereas recessive dystrophic EB (RDEB) is transmitted in an autosomal recessive mode [8]. RDEB is classified in severe generalized RDEB (RDEB-sev gen) – formerly called RDEB, Hallopeau Siemens - and RDEB-generalized other (RDEB-O) – formerly called RDEB-non Hallopeau Siemens [3].

The DDEB phenotype is mostly generalized but mild and clinically characterized by recurrent blistering, milia, atrophic scarring, nail dystrophy and eventual loss of nails [3]. See Figure 1A,B. The fact that the defective and wildtype alleles are expressed equally explains the relative mild phenotype in comparison to RDEB [3]. Missense mutations or in frame deletions in *COL7A1* causing RDEB disturb the assembly and aggregation of type VII collagen into anchoring fibrils. As a result, the number of anchoring fibrils and their morphology is altered significantly. The resulting subforms of RDEB are classified as RDEB, generalized other [3]. RDEB-sev gen is caused by nonsense mutations in both alleles, resulting in a complete loss of type VII collagen within the basal membrane zone of the skin. Clinical manifestations of RDEB are generalized blistering, erosions, crusts, atrophic scarring, onychodystrophy, loss of nails, mutilating pseudosyndactyly of hands and feet and functionally disabling contractures in hands, feet, elbows and knees. See Figure 1C-H. Additionally, severe extracutaneous complications as gastrointestinal and urogenital tracts involvement, external eye, chronic anaemia, growth retardation and a high risk for the development of aggressive squamous cell carcinoma decrease (Figure 1 I) the life quality of the patient [3,9-14].

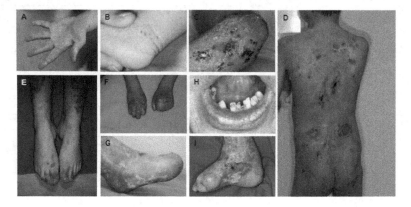

Figure 1. Clinical phenotype of DEB. **A,B:** DDEB with milia formation and atrophy. **C:** Atrophic scar with crusts and erosions in RDEB. **D:** Boy with severe-generalized RDEB leading to ulcerations and large non healing wounds with atrophic scarring at the back; **E:** Nail dystrophy on both feet. **F,G:** Mitten formation in hands and feet. **H:** Severe caries **I:** Squamous cell carcinoma on the foot (Photos: R. Hametner)

3. The dermal epidermal junction

The blisters characteristic for EB arise within the dermal-epidermal junction. Having a look at this compartment of the skin helps to understand the cause of blistering in EB. The dermal-epidermal junction is a complex basement membrane synthesized by dermal fibroblasts and basal keratinocytes. Adhesion of the epidermis to the underlying dermis is mechanically supported by the so called basement membrane zone (BMZ). Moreover it regulates the metabolic exchange between these two compartments. Up to now more than 20 macromolecules situated in the dermal-epidermal-junction have been detected and characterized at biochemical and genomic level [2].

Three protein-junction complexes stabilize the adherence of the basal keratinocytes to the dermis. See Figure 2. The hemidesmosomes built up by plectin, the bullous pemphigoid antigen 1 (BPAG1), α6β4 integrin and type XVII collagen (bullous pemphigoid antigen 2 - BPAG2) link the basal keratinocytes with the basement membrane, spanning the lamina lucida and anchored in the lamina densa [2]. Different laminin isoforms are located in the lamina lucida (laminin-332, laminin 6, laminin 10) and contribute along with BPAG2 to the formation of the anchoring filaments. The lamina densa is mainly built up by type VII collagen anchoring the lamina densa to the underlying dermis by the formation of anchoring fibrils [2]. Some other antigens as uncein (19-DEJ-1 antigen), NU-T2 antigen, KF1 antigen, LDA1 antigen, nidogen, heparin-sulfate, proteoglycan, antigens AF1 and AF2, thrombospondin, type V collagen and osteonectin/BM-40 have been detected in the lamina densa but have not yet been adequately characterized [2].

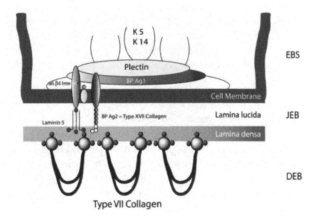

Figure 2. Schematic setup of the cutaneous dermal-epidermal junction zone and localization of structural proteins affected in inherited EB (Diagram by R. Hametner). laminin 5 = laminin 332; EBS = epidermolysis bullosa simplex; JEB = junctional epidermolysis bullosa; DEB = dystrophic epidermolysis bullosa

4. Type VII collagen

Type VII collagen is classified in the superfamily of collagens [7]. A protein domain in triple-helical conformation, which provides stability and integrity between connective tissues, is a common structural feature of all collagens [7]. Type VII collagen is a minor collagen in human skin and demonstrates spatially restricted location but it plays a critical role in providing integral stability to the skin because it is the major component of the anchoring fibrils [6,7].

5. Biology of type VII collagen

Type VII collagen molecules are characterized by the two non-collagenous NC-1 and NC-2 domains flanking a central collagenous, triple-helical segment [7]. In contrast to other interstitial collagens the repeating Gly-X-Y collagenous sequence is interrupted by 19 imperfections due to insertions or deletions of amino acids. There is a 39 amino acid non-collagenous hinge region susceptible to proteolytic digestion with pepsin in the middle of the triple-helical domain [15]. The amino terminal NC-1 domain (approximately 145kD in size), is built up of sub-modules with homology to known adhesive proteins, including segments with homology to cartilage matrix protein (CMP), nine consecutive fibronectin type III-like (FN-III) domains, a segment with homology to the A domain of von Willebrand factor, and a short cysteine and proline-rich region [15]. The C-terminal non-collagenous NC-2 domain is with 30kD in size relatively small, and contains a segment with homology to Kuniz protease inhibitor molecule [16,17].

The 32kb gene encoding a 9,2kb mRNA has been mapped to the short-arm of chromosome 3p21.1 [18]. The encoding primary sequence and the gene structure of type VII collagen are well conserved. The mouse gene shows 90.4% identity at the protein level and 84.7% homology at the nucleotide level, indicating the importance of type VII collagen as a structural protein [19].

The expression pattern of COL7A1 is tissue specific and restricted. Type VII collagen has been detected by immunomapping to a selected number of epithelia, including the dermal-epidermal BMZ of skin, the amniotic epithelial BMZ of the chorioamnion, the corneal epithelial basement membrane (Bowman's membrane) and the epithelial basement membrane of oral mucosa and cervix. Moreover the presence of type VII collagen correlates with the presence of ultrastructurally detected anchoring fibrils [6]. A number of cytokines modulate type VII collagen expression. Especially transforming growth factor-β is a powerful upregulator of COL7A1 at transcription level in fibroblasts and keratinocytes [20,21].

6. Type VII collagen – A major component of the anchoring fibrils

Type VII collagen is synthesized by two cell types in the skin: keratinocytes and fibroblasts [22]. After synthesis of complete pro-α1 (VII) polypeptides, three polypeptides are associated through their carboxy-terminal ends to a trimer molecule, which is then folded in its collagenous segment into the triple-helical formation. Past to secretion into the extracellular milieu two type VII collagen molecules are aligned into an anti-parallel dimer with the amino-terminal domains present at both ends of the molecule [6]. During dimer-assembly stabilization by inter-molecular disulfide bond formation and a proteolytic removal of a part of the carboxy-terminal ends (NC-2 domain) of both type VII collagen molecules take place [23]. Large numbers of these anti-parallel dimers aggregate laterally to form anchoring fibrils, which then can be identified by their characteristic, centro-symmetric banding patterns in transmission electron microscopy [7].

The affinity of the NC-1 domain to bind the principal components of the cutaneous basement membrane, laminin-332, laminin-311 and type IV collagen provides stability to the dermo-epidermal adhesion on the dermal site at the lamina lucida/papillary dermis interface [6,24,25]. Arg-Gly-Asp sequences in the NC-1 domain serve as integrin mediated attachment sites for cells to adhere to extracellular matrix components such as fibronectin [26].

7. Mutations in *COL7A1*

Mutations in *COL7A1* have clinical consequences in terms of disrupted integrity of the skin, due to the complexity of the *COL7A1* gene, type VII collagen protein structures and the critical importance of its distinct domains in macromolecular interactions [7]. At least 324 pathogenic mutations have been detected within *COL7A1* in different variants of DEB up to now including 43 nonsense, 127 missense, 65 deletion, 28 insertion, 9 insertion-deletion, 51 splicesite and 1 regulatory mutations [27]. See Figure 3-5. Exon 73 constitutes a region with a high frequency of mutations, what suggests being a region in which mutations commonly affect the function of anchoring fibrils [28]. RDEB is caused by nonsense, splice-site, deletions or insertions, silent glycine substitutions within the triple helix and non-glycine missense mutations within the triple-helix or non-collagenous NC-2 domain [29]. RDEB-severe generalized originates from nonsense, frameshift or splice-site mutations on both alleles leading to premature termination codons (PTCs) [30], which result in nonsense mediated mRNA decay or truncated proteins, leading to a reduced number of collagen VII monomers, which are unable to assemble into functional anchoring fibrils [29,30]. PTC mutations do not cause a clinical phenotype if they appear in the heterozygous state, but if they are homozygous or combined with another PTC mutation they are causing severe generalized RDEB [27]. Two missense mutations or compound heterozygosity of a missense and a PTC mutation lead to severe generalized RDEB in very rare cases [31].

RDEB, generalized other, the milder phenotype, is mostly caused by PTCs, small deletions, substitutions of glycine residues in the collagenous domain, splice-site mutations within NC-2 [32-35], delayed termination codons [36], in frame exon skipping [29,36], or missense substitution mutations involving amino acids other than glycine [29,37,38], the majority involving arginine residues resulting either in the loss of an ionic charge or in the introduction of a bulky chain at an external position of the triple helix [27]. Thereby these mutations usually concern a critical amino acid and change the conformation of the protein, which then might still be able to assemble into a small number of anchoring fibrils but is likely to be unstable when they laterally aggregate. Anyhow some full length type VII collagen polypeptides can still be built up [39].

DDEB is caused by glycine substitutions within the triple helical domain of *COL7A1* or other missense mutations, deletions or splice site mutations in some cases [5,26,40-44]. Critical ami-

Diverse Applications of Gene Therapy

no acids in the structure of the triple helix are affected by these mutations and therefore the overall stability of the anchoring fibrils is disturbed. More than 100 missense mutations resulting in a Gly-Xaa substitution have been detected in the collagenous domain of *COL7A1*; half of these are situated in amino acids 1522-2791 and have a dominant negative effect [27].

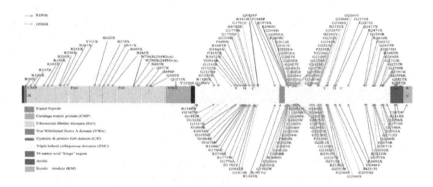

Figure 3. Missense and nonsense mutations in DEB patients. The red lettering signifies dominant and the black signifies recessive inheritance. (Dang et al. [27] © 2008 Blackwell Munksgaard, Experimental Dermatology)

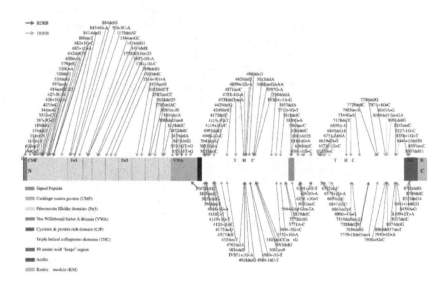

Figure 4. *COL7A1* deletions, insertions and splice site mutations in DEB patients. The red lettering signifies dominant and the black signifies recessive inheritance. (Dang et al. [27] © 2008 Blackwell Munksgaard, Experimental Dermatology)

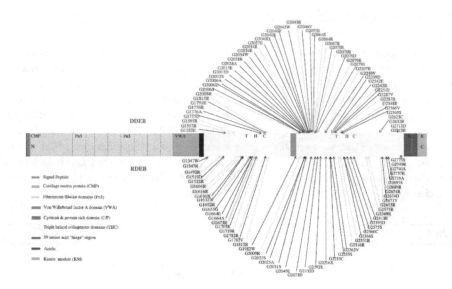

Figure 5. Glycine substitutions in DEB. These are all in the triple-helical collagenous domain; the ones above represent DDEB, the ones below RDEB. (Dang et al. [27] © 2008 Blackwell Munksgaard, Experimental Dermatology)

8. Mouse model

So far there are only two viable mouse models with defects in the *COL7A1* gene. A transgenic mouse carrying human *COL7A1* cDNA inclusive the human 7528delG mutation in exon 101, which develops the DEB phenotype gradually [45], and a collagen VII hypomorphic mouse published by Fritsch et al. 2008 [46]. In the collagen VII hypomorphic mouse reduced expression of collagen VII originates from aberrant splicing resulting from the introduction of a phosphoglycerate kinase promoter-driven neomycin phosphotransferase expression cassette (PGK-Neo cassette) in intron 2 of *COL7A1*. One out of three possible splice variants is translated into full-length type VII collagen resulting in a reduction of type VII collagen levels to about 9% of wildtype levels in *COL7A1*flNeo/flNeo mice. Hemorrhagic blisters on the soles of fore and hind paws, ears and mouth are developed by the collagen VII mice within the first 48 hours of life. Blisters of newborn *COL7A1*flNeo/flNeo mice were histopathologically classified as hemorrhagic and subepidermal. Type VII collagen immunofluorescence staining revealed weak reactivity in comparison to wildtype littermates. Ultrastructurally normal but reduced in number anchoring fibrils were detected in transmission electron microscopy of the dermal-epidermal junction of the skin. *COL7A1*flNeo/flNeo mice suffer from growth retardation due to malnutrition and subsequently have a reduced life expectancy. Moreover healing of the initial blistering on the paws with scarring results in the development of mitten deformities beginning at 2-3 weeks of age [46].

9. Therapy approaches

Due to the size of the *COL7A1* gene, a causal therapy for dystrophic epidermolysis bullosa is a great challenge. Symptomatic therapy is concentrated on prevention of skin trauma to minimize blister formation, prevention of secondary bacterial infection, treatment of infection, measures to improve wound healing, maintenance of good nutrition, treatment of correctable complications, and finally rehabilitation [3]. However, several gene and cell therapy strategies showed the potential to revert the disease-associated phenotype. Phenotypic correction of recessive DEB forms (RDEB) can be achieved by gene insertion therapy, in which the wildtype sequence of a mutated gene of interest is introduced into the target cells. Moreover alternative avenues including gene-, cell-, protein- and other systemic- therapy approaches have been tested to restore type VII collagen expression. See Table 2.

Author	Approach	Year
Woodley et al.	Type VII collagen minigene	2000
Sat et al.	Cosmid clone containing the entire *COL7A1* gene	2000
Mecklenbeck et al.	Microinjection of a *COL7A1*-PAC vector	2002
Urda et al.	ΦC31 bacteriophage integrase	2002
Chen et al.	Minimal lentiviral vectors	2002
Baldeschi et al	Canine type VII collagen	2003
Woodley et al	Targeting fibroblasts instead of keratinocytes (lentivirally)	2003
Gache et al.	Full-length cDNA (retrovirally)	2004
Woodley et al.	Intradermal injection of recombinant type VII collagen	2004
Woodley et al.	Intradermal injection of lentiviral vectors in vivo	2006
Goto et al.	Targeting fibroblasts instead of keratinocytes (retrovirally)	2006
Goto et al.	Targeted exon skipping using antisense	2006
Wong et al.	Intradermal injection of allogenic wildtype fibroblasts into a patient	2007
Fritsch et al.	Intradermal injection of murine wildtype fibroblasts in a DEB mouse model	2008
Remington et al.	Intradermal injection of human type VII collagen in mice	2009
Titeux et al.	Minimal self-inactivating retroviral vectors harbouring the full length human *COL7A1* gene	2010
Wagner et al.	Allogeneic bone marrow transplantation	2010
Siprashvili et al.	Full-length cDNA (retrovirally)	2010
Murauer et al.	3´ Trans-splicing of *COL7A1*	2011

Table 2. Therapy approaches to restore type VII collagen expression

Woodley et al. used a type VII collagen minigene, which contains the intact noncollagenous domains NC1 and NC2 and part of the central collagenous domain. This approach resulted after transduction into DEB keratinocytes in persistent synthesis and secretion of a 230kDa recombinant minicollagen VII [47]. However deletions in COL7A1 have been reported to be associated with a pathologic phenotype [5,48,49]. The same group introduced recombinant human type VII collagen into mouse and human skin equivalents transplanted onto mice, by injection. As a result the injected type VII collagen was detected within the basal membrane zone leading to a reversion of the disease associated phenotype [50]. Additionally, the group expressed type VII collagen using a self-inactivating lentiviral vector, which was injected into human skin equivalents, expanded from DEB cells, placed on nude immunodeficient mice. Experiments revealed the synthesis and insertion of the protein into the basal membrane zone [51]. Using a cosmid clone, carrying the entire COL7A1 gene, was also shown to be a promising way to direct expression of type VII collagen in skin in fetal and neonatal mice. The tested neonatal or fetal mice produced type VII collagen within the basal membrane zone of the skin showing a stable expression of the protein in vivo [52]. Microinjection of a P1-derived artificial chromosome (PAC) carrying the entire COL7A1 locus resulted in production of a procollagen VII similar to the authentic one by Mecklenbeck et al. [53]. The ΦC31 bacteriophage integrase, facilitating integration only in pseudo attP sites, was used to integrate COL7A1 stably into DEB primary epidermal progenitor cells by Urda et al. [54]. Baldeschi et al. also showed sustained and permanent expression of the transgene after transduction of canine type VII collagen into human and canine DEB keratinocytes [55]. Based on this study Gache et al. yield a full phenotypic reversion of the disease-associated phenotype of RDEB epidermal clonogenic cells after full-length human COL7A1 cDNA introduction using a retroviral system. However, the expression of COL7A1 was 50 times higher than the levels monitored in wildtype keratinocytes in monolayers, increasing the risk for an ectopic transgene expression and an abnormal accumulation in skin equivalents [56]. Chen et al. used a minimal lentiviral vector for COL7A1 expression in vitro as an alternative to the retroviral system applied by Gache et al. [57]. Goto et al. showed that COL7A1 treated fibroblasts of skin grafts provide higher amounts of type VII collagen for the dermal-epidermal junction than keratinocytes [58]. They have also demonstrated an antisense oligoribonucleotide therapy to maintain exon skipping of an exon comprising a premature stop codon. As a result a truncated type VII collagen variant was expressed [59]. Additionally, intradermal injection of untreated normal human or gene-corrected fibroblasts in mice can result in a stable production of human type VII collagen at the basal membrane zone of the skin [60]. Moreover, Wong et al. demonstrated an increased source of type VII collagen in the dermal-epidermal junction for at least three months after intradermal injection of allogeneic fibroblasts [61]. In a mouse model Fritsch et al. showed an accumulation of type VII collagen and restoration of a functional dermal-epidermal junction after injection of murine wildtype fibroblasts into a type VII collagen hypomorphic mouse [46]. In 2009 Remington et al. injected human type VII collagen into COL7A1 -/- mice, also restoring type VII collagen expression and correct generation of anchoring fibrils [62]. Titeux et al. transduced COL7A1 cDNA under the control of a human promoter using a minimal self-inactivating retroviral vector into RDEB keratinocytes and fibroblasts leading to cell correction and long lasting expression of type VII collagen. The dermal-epidermal junction in generated skin equivalents was restored [63]. A similar strategy was shown by Siprashvili et al. using an epitope-tagged *COL7A1* cDNA, providing a long term expression of the protein in skin equivalents [64]. In a clinical trial executing a bone marrow transplantation 6 RDEB patients received allogeneic stem cells to milder the RDEB phenotype. As a result, 5 patients showed an improved wound healing, but one patient died [65].

Until now, no *ex vivo* gene therapy approach passed through a phase I/II gene therapy trial. Most of these applications are focusing on the transfer of full-length *COL7A1* cDNA into the affected patient cells. The drawbacks of the insertion of the full-length 9kb cDNA of *COL7A1* are the cloning and packaging limitations of commonly used vector systems to transduce keratinocytes or fibroblasts and the instability of the *COL7A1* gene due to possible genetic rearrangements of the large repetitive cDNA sequence [47]. Additionally, the influence of *COL7A1* over- or ectopic expression in treated cells has to be clarified for a clinical application. Using the methodology of spliceosome mediated RNA *Trans*-splicing (SMaRT) can be a promising alternative to the mentioned approaches to cope with some of the suspected issues present in full-length *COL7A1* replacement strategies. Murauer et al. demonstrated the exchange of the 3′ coding *COL7A1* cDNA region spanning from exon 65 to the last exon 118 by SMaRT [66]. Thereby the risk of genetic rearrangements of the *COL7A1* cDNA sequence should be reduced significantly. Alternatively to this, we will present in this work a 5′ exon replacement strategy using SMaRT, providing the possibility to repair also relevant mutations 5′ within the *COL7A1* gene.

10. Spliceosome mediated mRNA *Trans*-splicing

10.1. General aspects

RNA *trans*-splicing is a naturally occurring event to recombine two or more mRNA molecules to a new chimeric gene product [67]. For therapeutic purposes such products can be generated by *trans*-splicing a second RNA species from a RNA *trans*-splicing molecule (RTM) into the 3′, 5′ or internal sequence of an endogenously expressed target. See Figure 6. The main advantages of this methodology are the possibility to reduce the size of the transgene, the maintained endogenous regulation of transgene expression and the feasibility to treat dominant negative diseases [68]. Undesired gene expression due to unintended delivery or misregulation is minimized as *trans*-splicing should only occur in cells expressing the target pre-mRNA [69]. Furthermore, SMaRT offers the potential for correction of dominant negative mutations into wildtype gene products [70].

10.2. Methodology of spliceosome mediated mRNA *trans*-splicing (SMaRT)

In SMaRT constructs that are engineered to bind the introns of specific pre-mRNAs – RNA *trans*-splicing molecules (RTMs) - are the key players. These RTMs effect a *trans*-

splicing event between the target pre-mRNA and the RTM which is mediated by the spliceosome. An RTM carries three domains; i) a binding domain complementary to the target intron to localize the RTM to the target pre-mRNA; ii) a splicing domain containing splicing elements for efficient *trans*-splicing; and iii) a coding domain comprising one or more wildtype exons that are *trans*-spliced to the target. The *cis*-splicing elements and the binding domain are not retained in the modified RNA product [71]. Depending on the gene portion to replace, SMaRT can be divided into 3′, 5′ or internal exon replacement [69]. See Figure 6.

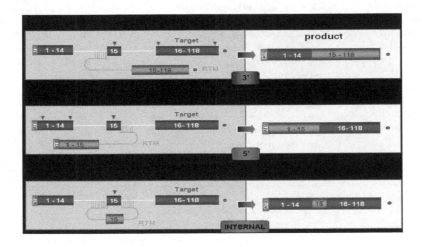

Figure 6. Schematic overview on different applications of SMaRT. **A: 3′*Trans*-splicing:** If there is a mutation in the 3′ part of the target gene a wildtype mRNA can be obtained by 3′splicing. Therefore, a 3′RTM with a binding domain situated in the intron 5′ to the first exon to be exchanged is necessary. E.g. if the mutation to be corrected is in exon 15, a binding domain for intron 14 is designed. This RTM can correct mutations more 3′ as well. After binding of the RTM the two mRNAs are *trans*-spliced and combined into a wildtype mRNA. **B: 5′*Trans*-splicing:** If correction of a mutation in the 5′ part of a gene is desired a 5′ RTM with a binding domain located in the intron 3′ to the exon to be exchanged is created. If the mutation to be corrected with 5′splicing is in exon 15, a RTM with a binding domain in intron 15 is required. This RTM can repair mutations more 5′ than exon 15 as well. **C: Internal *Trans*-splicing:** There is also a method to exchange only one exon, called internal *trans*-splicing or internal exon replacement (IER). Here an RTM with two binding domains and 5′ and 3′ splice elements is applied. Arrowheads indicate mutations.

10.3. Efficiency of SMaRT

The efficiency of *trans*-splicing to correct genetic defects and acquired disorders at pre-mRNA level has already been demonstrated for 3′ as well as for 5′ *trans*-splicing in different diseases *in vitro* and *in vivo*. See Table 3.

Author	Approach	Year
3´ trans-splicing		
Puttaraju et al.	3´ repair of lacZ in a tractable system	2001
Chao et al.	3´ repair of haemophilia A mice in vivo	2003
Dallinger et al.	3´ repair in a lacZ model system in a keratinocyte specific background	2003
Liu et al.	3´ repair of CFTR mRNA (adenovirally)	2005
Rodriguez-Martin et al.	3´ reprogramming of tau alternative splicing in a model system	2005
Zayed et al.	3´ repair of DNA-PKcs in SCID (delivery via sleeping beauty)	2007
Chen et al.	3´ repair dystrophia myotonica type 1 pre-mRNA	2008
Coady et al.	3´ SMN2 trans-splicing in combination with blocking an cis-splice sit in mice in vivo	2010
Murauer et al.	Functional 3´ repair of the COL7A1 gene	2010
Wang et al.	3´ introduction of therapeutic proteins in highly abundant albumin transcripts in mice in vivo	2009
Gruber et al.	3´ reprogramming of tumor marker genes to introduce suicide genes	2011
5´ trans-splicing		
Mansfield et al.	5´ repair of CFTR mRNA	2000
Kierlin-Duncan et al.	5´ repair of β-globin mRNA	2007
Wally et al.	5´ repair of the PLEC1 gene	2007
Wally et al.	5´ K14 mRNA reprogramming	2010
Rindt et al.	5´ trans-splicing repair of huntingtin at mRNA level	2012
Internal trans-splicing		
Lorain et al.	Exon exchange approach to repair Duchenne dystrophin transcripts in a minigene	2010
Koller et al.	A screening system for IER molecules	2011

Table 3. Overview on functional *trans*-splicing approaches so far.

RNA *trans*-splicing for gene correction is usually performed by 3' RNA *trans*-splicing to exchange 3' coding parts of a gene of interest. 3' RNA *trans*-splicing was successfully applied to restore wildtype gene expression pattern amongst others in patient cells or in animal models of epidermolysis bullosa, cystic fibrosis, X-linked immunodeficiency and hemophilia A [66,72,73]. Primarily co-transfection experiments with RTMs and artificial targets were used to give proof of principle of functionality of the *trans*-splicing process.

So a tractable lacZ model repair system, in which user defined target introns can be *trans*-spliced into a mutated lacZ gene to test target specific 3' RTMs by double transfection in 293T cells was developed by Puttaraju et al.. Functional lacZ correction was detected on mRNA and protein level by qRT-PCR and western blotting for one CFTR intron [74]. Chao et al. showed that the hemophilia A phenotype in factor VIII (FVIII) knockout mice can be repaired by the introduction of a 3' RTM. After delivery of the DNA through the portal vein, the FVIII protein was detected by western blot analysis of cryoprecipitated murine plasma. Long-term correction was shown via adenoviral tail vein transduction of the specific RTM. In the classical tail-clip test all naive knockout mice died, whereas eight out of ten treated mice survived, indicating that 3' *trans*-splicing is suitable to correct the bleeding disorder in hemophilia A [73]. Liu et al. used a recombinant adeno-associated viral vector system to target the human cystic fibrosis (CF) polarized airway epithelia from the apical membrane. The measurement of the cAMP-sensitive short circuit currents levels confirmed the CFTR correction by SMaRT [75]. Dallinger et al. showed as a proof of principle in the skin the correction of the EB-associated gene *COL17A1* by 3' *trans*-splicing. Using a lacZ model repair system, an intron specific target molecule and a rationally designed RTM, the feasibility of SMaRT was shown by co-transfection experiments in keratinocytes [76]. Using a minigene Rodriguez-Martin et al. published functional 3' *trans*-splicing on mRNA level after double transfection of the minigene and specific 3'RTM in COS-7 and SH-SY5Y cells for tau mRNA [77]. Zayed et al. demonstrated 3' correction of the DNA protein kinase catalytic subunit (DNA-PKcs) gene, which is responsible for severe combined immune deficiency (SCID). Specific 3'RTMs were transfected into scid.adh cells using the Sleeping Beauty transposon system. After this treatment irradiated cells showed an 4.3 fold increase of surviving cells over irradiated untreated scid.adh cells. Correction of the mutation was shown via QRT-PCR and sequencing on mRNA level. Additionally, functional 3'*trans*-splicing was detected on mRNA level via sequencing and on protein level via western blotting in SCID multipotent adult progenitor cells [78]. Chen et al. corrected the dystrophia myotica protein kinase gene responsible for the most common muscular dystrophy in adults by 3' *trans*-splicing on mRNA level [79]. Coady et al. showed *in vivo* correction of spinal muscular atrophy (SMA) by 3'*trans*-splicing in mice recently. A single injection of a repair construct *trans*-splicing *SMN2* carried by a PMU3 vector into the intracerebral-ventricular space of SMA neonates lessens the severity of the SMA phenotype in a severe mouse model and extends survival by around 70% [80]. Murauer et al. corrected mutations in *COL7A1* by 3'*trans*-splicing. RDEB keratinocytes retrovirally transduced with a 3'*trans*-splicing molecule showed an increase of *COL7A1* mRNA sqRT-PCR and recovery of full-length type VII collagen expression on protein level in western blot and immunofluorescent staining. Moreover normal morphology and reduced invasive capacity was achieved in transduced cells. Correct localization of type VII collagen at the basement membrane zone in skin equivalents, where it assembles into anchoring fibril like structures, showed the potential of trans-splicing to correct an RDEB phenotype in vitro [66]. There are also alternative approaches in which therapeutic proteins are produced after specific 3'trans-splicing events into highly abundant albumin transcripts using 3 'RTMs [81]. Another area of application of SMaRT was performed by Gruber et al. to treat malignant SCC tumors, which are life-threatening issues for RDEB patients. The transfection of RDEB SCC cells with a designed 3' RTM lead to the fusion of the toxin streptolysin O, carried by a 3' RTM, to MMP-9 pre-mRNA molecules, resulting in the expression of the toxin and subsequently to the cell death of transfected tumor cells [82].

5' trans-splicing to correct upstream coding sequences of an mRNA of interest was first shown by a double transfection model to repair mutations in the cystic fibrosis transmembrane receptor (CFTR) pre-mRNA. Functionality tests were performed by anion efflux transport measurements. RTMs were designed capable to repair the 5' portion of CFTR transcripts [83]. 5' trans-splicing was also applied for the substitution of exon 1 of b-globin in cells co-transfected with a target molecule and an RTM in 293T cells and lead specific trans-splicing detected by one step RT-PCR [84]. Endogenous 5' trans-splicing induced gene correction was first demonstrated by Wally et al. on the basis of the PLEC gene involved in the disease epidermolysis bullosa simplex (EBS). Restoration of wild-type plectin expression patterns was shown by immunofluorescence microscopy of patient fibroblasts after RTM treatment [61]. Additionally, exons 1–7 of the keratin 14 gene (KRT14) were replaced in an autosomal dominant model of EBS resulting in recovery of K14 on RNA and protein level, detected by SQRT-PCR, western blotting and immunofluorescence staining by transient transfection of specific 5' RTMs chosen in a screening procedure [85]. Recently 5'trans-splicing correction of a disease causing huntingtin allele on mRNA level was reported by Rindt et al. [86].

Lorain et al. primarily published the methodology of internal exon replacement (IER) to correct a dystrophin minigene on mRNA level [87]. Recently, Koller et al. developed a new RTM screening system to improve double RNA trans-splicing for the correction of the EB associated gene COL17A1 [88].

10.4. RTM screening systems

So far, there are no general rules for the design of highly efficient trans-splicing RTMs. However, recent studies revealed the influence of minor differences in length, composition and localization of the binding domain (BD) on RTM efficiency and specificity [85,88]. Due to the fact that an RTM can't be predicted rationally, we established a fluorescence-based screening system to select an efficient RTM from a pool of randomly designed RTMs. This screening system is composed of fluorescence-based RTM backbones, in which randomly created binding domains are cloned, and a gene specific target molecule. The target binding region (exon/intron sequence of a gene of interest) is PCR amplified, randomly fragmented and cloned into the RTM vector. The coding region consists of a fluorescence reporter, divided into two (5' or 3' *trans*-splicing) or three parts (internal exon replacement) and distributed to both screening molecules (target molecule and RTM). The RTM library is composed of individual RTMs with various binding domains. Their efficiency can be evaluated by fluorescence microscopy and flow cytometry. For flow cytometric analysis, individual selected RTMs of the RTM library are co-transfected with the designed target molecule, including the full-length target binding region, and the missing sequence of the split fluorescence reporter into HEK293FT cells. Co-transfection of RTM and target molecule into HEK293FT cells results in the restoration of expression of the fluorescence reporter. The intensity of the fluorescence signal of the reporter molecule gives information on the functionality of the binding domain. The most efficient BDs can be tested for endogenous experiments in patient cells. After transfection of the screening-RTM, the fusion of the splitted *trans*-splicing reporter and the endogenous target is detected by RT-PCR. To develop an mRNA based gene therapy an RTM, carrying the wildtype sequence instead of the coding sequence of the fluorescence molecule, is constructed. After RTM treatment of patient cells a mutated gene part is exchanged by *trans*-splicing and wildtype transcripts are restored.

11. RTMs for the murine COL7A1 gene

We started to establish 5' *trans*-splicing for murine *COL7A1* in order to analyze the functionality of RNA *trans*-splicing *in vivo*, due to the existence of a mouse model carrying a neo cassette in intron 2 of *COL7A1* generating aberrant splice variants, which lead to a reduction of type VII collagen expression [46]. By close similarity of this mouse model to the human RDEB phenotype and location of the defect in the 5' part of *COL7A1*, this mouse model exhibits obviously an ideal system to test our 5' repair molecules and investigate different application strategies.

Intron 15 was chosen as target intron because its size of about 1,5kb allows to create a large number of different binding domains. To generate a large amount of different RTMs, containing binding domains with different binding affinities to the target intron, the target exon/intron was digested out of the artificial target used in the screen with HindIII and BamHI and digested with CviJI*. The resulting fragments with a length of 50-750bp were cloned into the RTM backbone. Binding domains were identified by colony PCR using a forward primer situated in the 5' half of the split GFP and a vector specific reverse primer. Possible binding domains with different lengths were detected on a 2% agarose gel after gel electrophoresis. To check orientation and location of the binding domain, clones with inserts were sequenced. To evaluate the created RTM library the artificial target containing the target intron (intron15) and the 3' half of the split AcGFP instead of the 3' part of murine *COL7A1* was cotransfected with the RTM library respectively individual RTMs into HEK293FT. The RTMs contain a transfection reporter (DsRED), the 5' half of the split AcGFP instead of the first 15 exons of *COL7A1* and variable binding domains. The cotransfected cells were analyzed concerning their AcGFP/DsRED expression ratios by fluorescence microscopy and flow cytometry, whereby a higher ratio indicates the presence of a more functional binding domain in the RTM. See Figures 7+8.

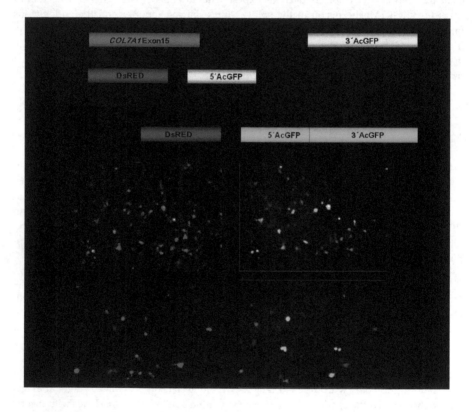

Figure 7. Fluorescence microscopy of with RTM library and target double transfected HEK293 cells. **A:** Functional binding domains lead to specific *trans*-splicing of the two pre mRNAs which are then combined into one mRNA containing DsRED and full-length AcGFP. Red fluorescence indicates the transfection of a RTM in the cells whereas red and green fluorescence indicates functional *trans*-splicing. **B:** Double transfection of an artificial target containing exon/intron 15 of murine *COL7A1* and an RTM library for this exon/intron in HEK293FT. **C:** Double transfection of an artificial target containing exon/intron 15 of murine *COL7A1* and the best RTM for this intron.

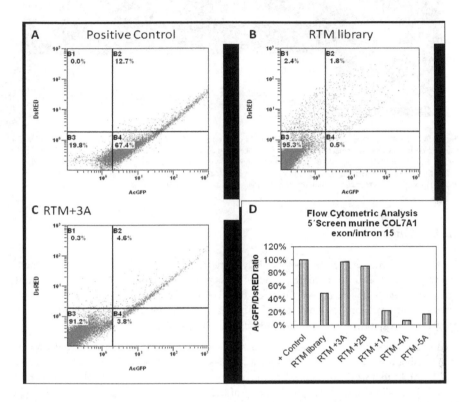

Figure 8. Flow cytometric analysis: 5′ screen for murine *COL7A1* exon/intron 15. Red fluorescence (shown on Y-axis) indicates transfection of RTMs in the cells; green fluorescence (shown on X-axis) indicates specific *trans*-splicing. **A:** The positive control is a vector containing a DsRED linker AcGFP construct. This FACS plot mimics the AcGFP and DsRED ratios expected from the product of optimal *trans*-splicing. **B:** The RTM library shows a *trans*-splicing efficiency (AcGFP/DsRED ratio) of 48,94% calculated from *trans*-splicing positive cells/all transfected cells.(B2 1,8% + B4 0,5%)/ (B1 2,4% + B2 1,8% + B4 0,5%) The fact, that several cells seem to be exclusively green can be explained by the intense AcGFP fluorescence, which tends to override the weaker DsRED fluorescence. **C:** The most efficient RTM analyzed, with a *trans*-splicing efficiency of 96,55%, (B2 4,6% + B4 3,8%)/(B1 0,3% + B2 4,6% + B4 3,8%) shows a dot plot pattern similar to the positive control. Therefore the binding domain of RTM +3A was chosen to be used in further endogenous experiments. **D:** A Comparison of AcGFP/DsRED ratios of single RTMs containing different binding domains, shows a wide variability of AcGFP/DsRED ration spanning less than 10% to nearly 100%.

The RTM with the highest AcGFP/DsRED ratio (RTM+3A) was chosen for further endogenous experiments. To check endogenous functionality of the RTM was transiently transfected into an immortalized murine keratinocyte cell line [46]. The 5′ part of the split AcGFP contained by the screening RTM was specifically *trans*-spliced with its endogenous target – the murine *COL7A1* mRNA – resulting in a AcGFP-*COL7A1* fusion mRNA detected by RT-PCR analysis and subsequent sequencing. See Figure 9.

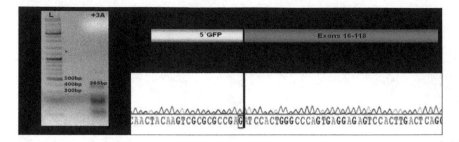

Figure 9. Endogenous *trans*-splicing into exon/intron 15 of murine *COL7A1*. **A:** RT-PCR analysis of transiently RTM+3A transfected spontaneously immortalized mouse wildtype keratinocytes [46] using primers in the 5´ part of split AcGFP and in exon 18 of *COL7A1* resulted in detection of a 365bp band after agarose gel-electrophoresis. B: The fragment was verified to be an AcGFP-*COL7A1* fusion by sequencing. **+3A** cDNA analysis of spontaneously immortalized mouse wildtype keratinocytes transiently transfected with RTM +3A **L** Ladder Mix DNA marker

12. Conclusion

RNA *trans*-splicing is a useful methodology to reprogram genes for diagnostic and thera-peutic purposes. Due to a variety of advantages over traditional gene-replacement strat-egies, RNA *trans*-splicing is used to correct the phenotype of many genetic diseases *in vitro*, ranging from epidermolysis bullosa to neurodegenerative diseases. *In vivo* studies are in progress to accelerate the way to the medical use of this RNA-based application.

We have established all three modes of *trans*-splicing (5′, 3′ and internal exon replacement) in our laboratory on the basis of several EB-associated genes (*KRT14, PLEC, COL7A1, COL17A1*). In this work we focused on the methodology of 5′ RNA *trans*-splicing to correct mutations localized within the first 15 exons of the murine *COL7A1* gene encoding for type VII collagen. *COL7A1* is a large gene with over 9kb and is therefore suitable for this ap-proach, in which only a short RTM has to be designed, harbouring only the first 15 exons of the gene. Using an RTM screening system, described by Wally et al 2011 [89], it should be possible to increase the *trans*-splicing efficiency of designed RTMs to a level where the phe-notype of *COL7A1* deficient cells can be converted into wildtype. We analyzed the binding properties of randomly designed RTMs specific for intron 15 of murine *COL7A1* and tested the most efficient RTM in *COL7A1* deficient keratinocytes for endogenous functionality. The RTM was able to induce endogenous 5′*trans*-splicing into murine *COL7A1* pre-mRNA mole-cules, manifested in the fusion of the 5′ GFP part of the RTM with exon 16 of *COL7A1*. Next steps are the exchange of the 5′ GFP part by the 5′sequence of murine *COL7A1* (exons1-15) and to investigate if our RTMs are able to increase the level of full-length *COL7A1* mRNA leading to the recovery of functional type VII collagen in *COL7A1* deficient cells and in skin equivalents. In summary we demonstrated a novel RNA-based strategy to correct disease-associated mutations within *COL7A1*, thereby avoiding or minimizing many problems present in standard cDNA gene therapies including fragmentation of the large *COL7A1* gene, the size limitation of the transgene and over- and ectopic expression of the transgene.

The development of a gene therapy for type VII collagen deficiency would increase the chance to find a cure for dystrophic EB. Additionally, the improvement of the methodology of 5' RNA *trans*-splicing will help us to move closer to the treatment of other genetic diseases caused by mutations in especially large genes.

Acknowledgements

We want to thank Prof. Leena Bruckner-Tuderman for providing the murine keratinocytes. Moreover we thank the Austrian Science Fund (FWF) for financing the project "Development of a 5'*trans*-splicing Gene Therapy" [P22039-B12] and DEBRA Austria, DEBRA Alto Adige and the Paracelsus Private Medical University for additional financial support.

Author details

E. Mayr*, U. Koller and J.W. Bauer

*Address all correspondence to: el.mayr@salk.at

EB House Austria, Dept Dermatol, Paracelsus Med Univ, Salzburg, Austria

References

[1] Laimer M, Lanschuetzer CM, B, Pohla-Gubo G, Klausegger A, Diem A, Riedl R, Bauer JW, and Hintner H. Epidermolysis Bullosa. Pädiatrie&Pädologie 2006;6 30-38.

[2] Kanitakis J. Anatomy, Histology and Immunohistochemistry of Normal Human Skin. European Journal of Dermatology 2002;12(4) 390-400.

[3] Fine JD and Hintner H. Life With Epidermolysis Bullosa .Wien: Springer Wien;

[4] Fine JD, Eady RA, Bauer EA, Bauer JW, Bruckner-Tuderman L, Heagerty A, Hintner H, Hovnanian A, Jonkman MF, Leigh I, McGrath JA, Mellerio JE, Murrell DF, Shimizu H, Uitto J, Vahlquist A, Woodley D, and Zambruno G. The Classification of Inherited Epidermolysis Bullosa (EB): Report of the Third International Consensus Meeting on Diagnosis and Classification of EB. J Am Acad Dermatol 2008;58(6) 931-950.

[5] Pulkkinen L and Uitto J. Mutation Analysis and Molecular Genetics of Epidermolysis Bullosa. Matrix Biol 1999;18(1) 29-42.

[6] Sakai LY, Keene DR, Morris NP, and Burgeson RE. Type VII Collagen Is a Major Structural Component of Anchoring Fibrils. J Cell Biol 1986;103(4) 1577-1586.

[7] Chung HJ and Uitto J. Type VII Collagen: the Anchoring Fibril Protein at Fault in Dystrophic Epidermolysis Bullosa. Dermatol Clin 2010;28(1) 93-105.

[8] Fine JD, Eady RA, Bauer EA, Briggaman RA, Bruckner-Tuderman L, Christiano A, Heagerty A, Hintner H, Jonkman MF, McGrath J, McGuire J, Moshell A, Shimizu H, Tadini G, and Uitto J. Revised Classification System for Inherited Epidermolysis Bullosa: Report of the Second International Consensus Meeting on Diagnosis and Classification of Epidermolysis Bullosa. J Am Acad Dermatol 2000;42(6) 1051-1066.

[9] Fine JD, Johnson LB, Weiner M, and Suchindran C. Gastrointestinal Complications of Inherited Epidermolysis Bullosa: Cumulative Experience of the National Epidermolysis Bullosa Registry. J Pediatr Gastroenterol Nutr 2008;46(2) 147-158.

[10] Fine JD, Johnson LB, Weiner M, Stein A, Cash S, Deleoz J, Devries DT, and Suchindran C. Eye Involvement in Inherited Epidermolysis Bullosa: Experience of the National Epidermolysis Bullosa Registry. Am J Ophthalmol 2004;138(2) 254-262.

[11] Fine JD, Johnson LB, Weiner M, and Suchindran C. Tracheolaryngeal Complications of Inherited Epidermolysis Bullosa: Cumulative Experience of the National Epidermolysis Bullosa Registry. Laryngoscope 2007;117(9) 1652-1660.

[12] Fine JD, Johnson LB, Weiner M, Stein A, Cash S, Deleoz J, Devries DT, and Suchindran C. Pseudosyndactyly and Musculoskeletal Contractures in Inherited Epidermolysis Bullosa: Experience of the National Epidermolysis Bullosa Registry, 1986-2002. J Hand Surg Br 2005;30(1) 14-22.

[13] Fine JD, Johnson LB, Weiner M, Stein A, Cash S, Deleoz J, Devries DT, and Suchindran C. Genitourinary Complications of Inherited Epidermolysis Bullosa: Experience of the National Epidermylosis Bullosa Registry and Review of the Literature. J Urol 2004;172(5 Pt 1) 2040-2044.

[14] Fine JD, Johnson LB, Weiner M, Stein A, Cash S, Deleoz J, Devries DT, and Suchindran C. Inherited Epidermolysis Bullosa and the Risk of Death From Renal Disease: Experience of the National Epidermolysis Bullosa Registry. Am J Kidney Dis 2004;44(4) 651-660.

[15] Christiano AM, Rosenbaum LM, Chung-Honet LC, Parente MG, Woodley DT, Pan TC, Zhang RZ, Chu ML, Burgeson RE, and Uitto J. The Large Non-Collagenous Domain (NC-1) of Type VII Collagen Is Amino-Terminal and Chimeric. Homology to Cartilage Matrix Protein, the Type III Domains of Fibronectin and the A Domains of Von Willebrand Factor. Hum Mol Genet 1992;1(7) 475-481.

[16] Christiano AM, Greenspan DS, Lee S, and Uitto J. Cloning of Human Type VII Collagen. Complete Primary Sequence of the Alpha 1(VII) Chain and Identification of Intragenic Polymorphisms. J Biol Chem 1994;269(32) 20256-20262.

[17] Greenspan DS, Byers MG, Eddy RL, Hoffman GG, and Shows TB. Localization of the Human Collagen Gene COL7A1 to 3p21.3 by Fluorescence in Situ Hybridization. Cytogenet Cell Genet 1993;62(1) 35-36.

[18] Parente MG, Chung LC, Ryynanen J, Woodley DT, Wynn KC, Bauer EA, Mattei MG, Chu ML, and Uitto J. Human Type VII Collagen: CDNA Cloning and Chromosomal Mapping of the Gene. Proc Natl Acad Sci U S A 1991;88(16) 6931-6935.

[19] Kivirikko S, Li K, Christiano AM, and Uitto J. Cloning of Mouse Type VII Collagen Reveals Evolutionary Conservation of Functional Protein Domains and Genomic Organization. J Invest Dermatol 1996;106(6) 1300-1306.

[20] Ryynanen J, Sollberg S, Olsen DR, and Uitto J. Transforming Growth Factor-Beta Up-Regulates Type VII Collagen Gene Expression in Normal and Transformed Epidermal Keratinocytes in Culture. Biochem Biophys Res Commun 1991;180(2) 673-680.

[21] Vindevoghel L, Kon A, Lechleider RJ, Uitto J, Roberts AB, and Mauviel A. Smad-Dependent Transcriptional Activation of Human Type VII Collagen Gene (COL7A1) Promoter by Transforming Growth Factor-Beta. J Biol Chem 1998;273(21) 13053-13057.

[22] Ryynanen J, Sollberg S, Parente MG, Chung LC, Christiano AM, and Uitto J. Type VII Collagen Gene Expression by Cultured Human Cells and in Fetal Skin. Abundant MRNA and Protein Levels in Epidermal Keratinocytes. J Clin Invest 1992;89(1) 163-168.

[23] Colombo M, Brittingham RJ, Klement JF, Majsterek I, Birk DE, Uitto J, and Fertala A. Procollagen VII Self-Assembly Depends on Site-Specific Interactions and Is Promoted by Cleavage of the NC2 Domain With Procollagen C-Proteinase. Biochemistry 2003;42(39) 11434-11442.

[24] Chen M, Marinkovich MP, Veis A, Cai X, Rao CN, O'toole EA, and Woodley DT. Interactions of the Amino-Terminal Noncollagenous (NC1) Domain of Type VII Collagen With Extracellular Matrix Components. A Potential Role in Epidermal-Dermal Adherence in Human Skin. J Biol Chem 1997;272(23) 14516-14522.

[25] Brittingham R, Uitto J, and Fertala A. High-Affinity Binding of the NC1 Domain of Collagen VII to Laminin 5 and Collagen IV. Biochem Biophys Res Commun 2006;343(3) 692-699.

[26] Ruoslahti E and Pierschbacher MD. New Perspectives in Cell Adhesion: RGD and Integrins. Science 1987;238(4826) 491-497.

[27] Dang N and Murrell DF. Mutation Analysis and Characterization of COL7A1 Mutations in Dystrophic Epidermolysis Bullosa. Exp Dermatol 2008;17(7) 553-568.

[28] Mecklenbeck S, Hammami-Hauasli N, Hopfner B, Schumann H, Kramer A, Kuster W, and Bruckner-Tuderman L. Clustering of COL7A1 Mutations in Exon 73: Implications for Mutation Analysis in Dystrophic Epidermolysis Bullosa. J Invest Dermatol 1999;112(3) 398-400.

[29] Whittock NV, Ashton GH, Mohammedi R, Mellerio JE, Mathew CG, Abbs SJ, Eady RA, and McGrath JA. Comparative Mutation Detection Screening of the Type VII

Collagen Gene (COL7A1) Using the Protein Truncation Test, Fluorescent Chemical Cleavage of Mismatch, and Conformation Sensitive Gel Electrophoresis. J Invest Dermatol 1999;113(4) 673-686.

[30] Christiano AM, Anhalt G, Gibbons S, Bauer EA, and Uitto J. Premature Termination Codons in the Type VII Collagen Gene (COL7A1) Underlie Severe, Mutilating Recessive Dystrophic Epidermolysis Bullosa. Genomics 1994;21(1) 160-168.

[31] Christiano AM, McGrath JA, Tan KC, and Uitto J. Glycine Substitutions in the Triple-Helical Region of Type VII Collagen Result in a Spectrum of Dystrophic Epidermolysis Bullosa Phenotypes and Patterns of Inheritance. Am J Hum Genet 1996;58(4) 671-681.

[32] Bruckner-Tuderman L, Nilssen O, Zimmermann DR, Dours-Zimmermann MT, Kalinke DU, Gedde-Dahl T, Jr., and Winberg JO. Immunohistochemical and Mutation Analyses Demonstrate That Procollagen VII Is Processed to Collagen VII Through Removal of the NC-2 Domain. J Cell Biol 1995;131(2) 551-559.

[33] Sawamura D, Goto M, Yasukawa K, Sato-Matsumura K, Nakamura H, Ito K, Nakamura H, Tomita Y, and Shimizu H. Genetic Studies of 20 Japanese Families of Dystrophic Epidermolysis Bullosa. J Hum Genet 2005;50(10) 543-546.

[34] Dunnill MG, McGrath JA, Richards AJ, Christiano AM, Uitto J, Pope FM, and Eady RA. Clinicopathological Correlations of Compound Heterozygous COL7A1 Mutations in Recessive Dystrophic Epidermolysis Bullosa. J Invest Dermatol 1996;107(2) 171-177.

[35] Kern JS, Kohlhase J, Bruckner-Tuderman L, and Has C. Expanding the COL7A1 Mutation Database: Novel and Recurrent Mutations and Unusual Genotype-Phenotype Constellations in 41 Patients With Dystrophic Epidermolysis Bullosa. J Invest Dermatol 2006;126(5) 1006-1012.

[36] Christiano AM, McGrath JA, and Uitto J. Influence of the Second COL7A1 Mutation in Determining the Phenotypic Severity of Recessive Dystrophic Epidermolysis Bullosa. J Invest Dermatol 1996;106(4) 766-770.

[37] Hovnanian A, Rochat A, Bodemer C, Petit E, Rivers CA, Prost C, Fraitag S, Christiano AM, Uitto J, Lathrop M, Barrandon Y, and de Prost Y. Characterization of 18 New Mutations in COL7A1 in Recessive Dystrophic Epidermolysis Bullosa Provides Evidence for Distinct Molecular Mechanisms Underlying Defective Anchoring Fibril Formation. Am J Hum Genet 1997;61(3) 599-610.

[38] Ryoo YW, Kim BC, and Lee KS. Characterization of Mutations of the Type VII Collagen Gene (COL7A1) in Recessive Dystrophic Epidermolysis Bullosa Mitis (M-RDEB) From Three Korean Patients. J Dermatol Sci 2001;26(2) 125-132.

[39] Jarvikallio A, Pulkkinen L, and Uitto J. Molecular Basis of Dystrophic Epidermolysis Bullosa: Mutations in the Type VII Collagen Gene (COL7A1). Hum Mutat 1997;10(5) 338-347.

[40] Sakuntabhai A, Hammami-Hauasli N, Bodemer C, Rochat A, Prost C, Barrandon Y, de Prost Y, Lathrop M, Wojnarowska F, Bruckner-Tuderman L, and Hovnanian A. Deletions Within COL7A1 Exons Distant From Consensus Splice Sites Alter Splicing and Produce Shortened Polypeptides in Dominant Dystrophic Epidermolysis Bullosa. Am J Hum Genet 1998;63(3) 737-748.

[41] Cserhalmi-Friedman PB, McGrath JA, Mellerio JE, Romero R, Salas-Alanis JC, Paller AS, Dietz HC, and Christiano AM. Restoration of Open Reading Frame Resulting From Skipping of an Exon With an Internal Deletion in the COL7A1 Gene. Lab Invest 1998;78(12) 1483-1492.

[42] Posteraro P, Pascucci M, Colombi M, Barlati S, Giannetti A, Paradisi M, Mustonen A, Zambruno G, and Castiglia D. Denaturing HPLC-Based Approach for Detection of COL7A1 Gene Mutations Causing Dystrophic Epidermolysis Bullosa. Biochem Biophys Res Commun 2005;338(3) 1391-1401.

[43] Christiano AM, Fine JD, and Uitto J. Genetic Basis of Dominantly Inherited Transient Bullous Dermolysis of the Newborn: a Splice Site Mutation in the Type VII Collagen Gene. J Invest Dermatol 1997;109(6) 811-814.

[44] Jiang W, Bu D, Yang Y, and Zhu X. A Novel Splice Site Mutation in Collagen Type VII Gene in a Chinese Family With Dominant Dystrophic Epidermolysis Bullosa Pruriginosa. Acta Derm Venereol 2002;82(3) 187-191.

[45] Ito K, Sawamura D, Goto M, Nakamura H, Nishie W, Sakai K, Natsuga K, Shinkuma S, Shibaki A, Uitto J, Denton CP, Nakajima O, Akiyama M, and Shimizu H. Keratinocyte-/Fibroblast-Targeted Rescue of Col7a1-Disrupted Mice and Generation of an Exact Dystrophic Epidermolysis Bullosa Model Using a Human COL7A1 Mutation. Am J Pathol 2009;175(6) 2508-2517.

[46] Fritsch A, Loeckermann S, Kern JS, Braun A, Bosl MR, Bley TA, Schumann H, von Elverfeldt D, Paul D, Erlacher M, von Rautenfeld DB, Hausser I, Fassler R, and Bruckner-Tuderman L. A Hypomorphic Mouse Model of Dystrophic Epidermolysis Bullosa Reveals Mechanisms of Disease and Response to Fibroblast Therapy. Journal of Clinical Investigation 2008;118(5) 1669-1679.

[47] Chen M, O'Toole EA, Muellenhoff M, Medina E, Kasahara N, and Woodley DT. Development and Characterization of a Recombinant Truncated Type VII Collagen "Minigene". Implication for Gene Therapy of Dystrophic Epidermolysis Bullosa. J Biol Chem 2000;275(32) 24429-24435.

[48] Bruckner-Tuderman L. Hereditary Skin Diseases of Anchoring Fibrils. J Dermatol Sci 1999;20(2) 122-133.

[49] Bruckner-Tuderman L, Hopfner B, and Hammami-Hauasli N. Biology of Anchoring Fibrils: Lessons From Dystrophic Epidermolysis Bullosa. Matrix Biol 1999;18(1) 43-54.

[50] Woodley DT, Keene DR, Atha T, Huang Y, Lipman K, Li W, and Chen M. Injection of Recombinant Human Type VII Collagen Restores Collagen Function in Dystrophic Epidermolysis Bullosa. Nat Med 2004;10(7) 693-695.

[51] Woodley DT, Keene DR, Atha T, Huang Y, Ram R, Kasahara N, and Chen M. Intradermal Injection of Lentiviral Vectors Corrects Regenerated Human Dystrophic Epidermolysis Bullosa Skin Tissue in Vivo. Molecular Therapy 2004;10(2) 318-326.

[52] Sat E, Leung KH, Bruckner-Tuderman L, and Cheah KS. Tissue-Specific Expression and Long-Term Deposition of Human Collagen VII in the Skin of Transgenic Mice: Implications for Gene Therapy. Gene Ther 2000;7(19) 1631-1639.

[53] Mecklenbeck S, Compton SH, Mejia JE, Cervini R, Hovnanian A, Bruckner-Tuderman L, and Barrandon Y. A Microinjected COL7A1-PAC Vector Restores Synthesis of Intact Procollagen VII in a Dystrophic Epidermolysis Bullosa Keratinocyte Cell Line. Hum Gene Ther 2002;13(13) 1655-1662.

[54] Ortiz-Urda S, Thyagarajan B, Keene DR, Lin Q, Fang M, Calos MP, and Khavari PA. Stable Nonviral Genetic Correction of Inherited Human Skin Disease. Nat Med 2002;8(10) 1166-1170.

[55] Baldeschi C, Gache Y, Rattenholl A, Bouille P, Danos O, Ortonne JP, Bruckner-Tuderman L, and Meneguzzi G. Genetic Correction of Canine Dystrophic Epidermolysis Bullosa Mediated by Retroviral Vectors. Hum Mol Genet 2003;12(15) 1897-1905.

[56] Gache Y, Baldeschi C, Del Rio M, Gagnoux-Palacios L, Larcher F, Lacour JP, and Meneguzzi G. Construction of Skin Equivalents for Gene Therapy of Recessive Dystrophic Epidermolysis Bullosa. Human Gene Therapy 2004;15(10) 921-933.

[57] Chen M, Kasahara N, Keene DR, Chan L, Hoeffler WK, Finlay D, Barcova M, Cannon PM, Mazurek C, and Woodley DT. Restoration of Type VII Collagen Expression and Function in Dystrophic Epidermolysis Bullosa. Nat Genet 2002;32(4) 670-675.

[58] Goto M, Sawamura D, Ito K, Abe M, Nishie W, Sakai K, Shibaki A, Akiyama M, and Shimizu H. Fibroblasts Show More Potential As Target Cells Than Keratinocytes in COL7A1 Gene Therapy of Dystrophic Epidermolysis Bullosa. J Invest Dermatol 2006;126(4) 766-772.

[59] Goto M, Sawamura D, Nishie W, Sakai K, McMillan JR, Akiyama M, and Shimizu H. Targeted Skipping of a Single Exon Harboring a Premature Termination Codon Mutation: Implications and Potential for Gene Correction Therapy for Selective Dystrophic Epidermolysis Bullosa Patients. Journal of Investigative Dermatology 2006;126(12) 2614-2620.

[60] Woodley DT, Krueger GG, Jorgensen CM, Fairley JA, Atha T, Huang Y, Chan L, Keene DR, and Chen M. Normal and Gene-Corrected Dystrophic Epidermolysis Bullosa Fibroblasts Alone Can Produce Type VII Collagen at the Basement Membrane Zone. J Invest Dermatol 2003;121(5) 1021-1028.

[61] Wally V, Klausegger A, Koller U, Lochmuller H, Krause S, Wiche G, Mitchell LG, Hintner H, and Bauer JW. 5' Trans-Splicing Repair of the PLEC1 Gene. J Invest Dermatol 2008;128(3) 568-574.

[62] Remington J, Wang XY, Hou YP, Zhou H, Burnett J, Muirhead T, Uitto J, Keene DR, Woodley DT, and Chen M. Injection of Recombinant Human Type VII Collagen Corrects the Disease Phenotype in a Murine Model of Dystrophic Epidermolysis Bullosa. Molecular Therapy 2009;17(1) 26-33.

[63] Titeux M, Pendaries V, Zanta-Boussif MA, Decha A, Pironon N, Tonasso L, Mejia JE, Brice A, Danos O, and Hovnanian A. SIN Retroviral Vectors Expressing COL7A1 Under Human Promoters for Ex Vivo Gene Therapy of Recessive Dystrophic Epidermolysis Bullosa. Mol Ther 2010

[64] Siprashvili Z, Nguyen NT, Bezchinsky MY, Marinkovich PM, Lane AT, and Khavari PA. Long-Term Type VII Collagen Restoration to Human Epidermolysis Bullosa Skin Tissue. Hum Gene Ther 2010

[65] Wagner JE, Ishida-Yamamoto A, McGrath JA, Hordinsky M, Keene DR, Woodley DT, Chen M, Riddle MJ, Osborn MJ, Lund T, Dolan M, Blazar BR, and Tolar J. Bone Marrow Transplantation for Recessive Dystrophic Epidermolysis Bullosa. N Engl J Med 2010;363(7) 629-639.

[66] Murauer EM, Gache Y, Gratz IK, Klausegger A, Muss W, Gruber C, Meneguzzi G, Hintner H, and Bauer JW. Functional Correction of Type VII Collagen Expression in Dystrophic Epidermolysis Bullosa. J Invest Dermatol 2011;131(1) 74-83.

[67] Horiuchi T and Aigaki T. Alternative Trans-Splicing: a Novel Mode of Pre-MRNA Processing. Biol Cell 2006;98(2) 135-140.

[68] Mitchell LG and McGarrity GJ. Gene Therapy Progress and Prospects: Reprograming Gene Expression by Trans-Splicing. Gene Ther 2005;12(20) 1477-1485.

[69] Wally V, Murauer EM, and Bauer JW. Spliceosome-Mediated Trans-Splicing: The Therapeutic Cut and Paste. J Invest Dermatol 2012

[70] Wally V, Koller U, Murauer EM, Mayr E, Klausegger A, Hintner H, and Bauer JW. Gene Therapy for Autosomal Dominant Diseases. Experimental Dermatology 2009;18(3) 283-283.

[71] Mansfield SG, Chao H, and Walsh CE. RNA Repair Using Spliceosome-Mediated RNA Trans-Splicing. Trends Mol Med 2004;10(6) 263-268.

[72] Tahara M, Pergolizzi RG, Kobayashi H, Krause A, Luettich K, Lesser ML, and Crystal RG. Trans-Splicing Repair of CD40 Ligand Deficiency Results in Naturally Regulated Correction of a Mouse Model of Hyper-IgM X-Linked Immunodeficiency. Nat Med 2004;10(8) 835-841.

[73] Chao H, Mansfield SG, Bartel RC, Hiriyanna S, Mitchell LG, Garcia-Blanco MA, and Walsh CE. Phenotype Correction of Hemophilia A Mice by Spliceosome-Mediated RNA Trans-Splicing. Nat Med 2003;9(8) 1015-1019.

[74] Puttaraju M, DiPasquale J, Baker CC, Mitchell LG, and Garcia-Blanco MA. Messenger RNA Repair and Restoration of Protein Function by Spliceosome-Mediated RNA Trans-Splicing. Molecular Therapy 2001;4(2) 105-114.

[75] Liu X, Luo M, Zhang LN, Yan Z, Zak R, Ding W, Mansfield SG, Mitchell LG, and Engelhardt JF. Spliceosome-Mediated RNA Trans-Splicing With Recombinant Adeno-Associated Virus Partially Restores Cystic Fibrosis Transmembrane Conductance Regulator Function to Polarized Human Cystic Fibrosis Airway Epithelial Cells. Hum Gene Ther 2005;16(9) 1116-1123.

[76] Dallinger G, Puttaraju M, Mitchell LG, Yancey KB, Yee C, Klausegger A, Hintner H, and Bauer JW. Development of Spliceosome-Mediated RNA Trans-Splicing (SMaRT (TM)) for the Correction of Inherited Skin Diseases. Experimental Dermatology 2003;12(1) 37-46.

[77] Rodriguez-Martin T, Garcia-Blanco MA, Mansfield SG, Grover AC, Hutton M, Yu Q, Zhou J, Anderton BH, and Gallo JM. Reprogramming of Tau Alternative Splicing by Spliceosome-Mediated RNA Trans-Splicing: Implications for Tauopathies. Proc Natl Acad Sci U S A 2005;102(43) 15659-15664.

[78] Zayed H, Xia L, Yerich A, Yant SR, Kay MA, Puttaraju M, McGarrity GJ, Wiest DL, McIvor RS, Tolar J, and Blazar BR. Correction of DNA Protein Kinase Deficiency by Spliceosome-Mediated RNA Trans-Splicing and Sleeping Beauty Transposon Delivery. Mol Ther 2007;15(7) 1273-1279.

[79] Chen HY, Kathirvel P, Yee WC, and Lai PS. Correction of Dystrophia Myotonica Type 1 Pre-MRNA Transcripts by Artificial Trans-Splicing. Gene Ther 2009;16(2) 211-217.

[80] Coady TH and Lorson CL. Trans-Splicing-Mediated Improvement in a Severe Mouse Model of Spinal Muscular Atrophy. J Neurosci 2010;30(1) 126-130.

[81] Wang J, Mansfield SG, Cote CA, Du Jiang P, Weng K, Amar MJA, Brewer BH, Remaley AT, McGarrity GJ, Garcia-Blanco MA, and Puttaraju M. Trans-Splicing Into Highly Abundant Albumin Transcripts for Production of Therapeutic Proteins In Vivo. Molecular Therapy 2009;17(2) 343-351.

[82] Gruber C, Gratz IK, Murauer EM, Mayr E, Koller U, Bruckner-Tuderman L, Meneguzzi G, Hintner H, and Bauer JW. Spliceosome-Mediated RNA Trans-Splicing Facilitates Targeted Delivery of Suicide Genes to Cancer Cells. Mol Cancer Ther 2011

[83] Mansfield SG, Clark RH, Puttaraju M, Kole J, Cohn JA, Mitchell LG, and Garcia-Blanco MA. 5' Exon Replacement and Repair by Spliceosome-Mediated RNA Trans-Splicing. RNA 2003;9(10) 1290-1297.

[84] Kierlin-Duncan MN and Sullenger BA. Using 5'-PTMs to Repair Mutant Beta-Globin Transcripts. RNA 2007

[85] Wally V, Brunner M, Lettner T, Wagner M, Koller U, Trost A, Murauer EM, Hainzl S, Hintner H, and Bauer JW. K14 MRNA Reprogramming for Dominant Epidermolysis Bullosa Simplex. Hum Mol Genet 2010;19(23) 4715-4725.

[86] Rindt H, Yen PF, Thebeau CN, Peterson TS, Weisman GA, and Lorson CL. Replacement of Huntingtin Exon 1 by Trans-Splicing. Cell Mol Life Sci 2012

[87] Lorain S, Peccate C, Le Hir M, and Garcia L. Exon Exchange Approach to Repair Duchenne Dystrophin Transcripts. PLoS One 2010;5(5) e10894-

[88] Koller U, Wally V, Mitchell LG, Klausegger A, Murauer EM, Mayr E, Gruber C, Hainzl S, Hintner H, and Bauer JW. A Novel Screening System Improves Genetic Correction by Internal Exon Replacement. Nucleic Acids Res 2011;39(16) e108-

[89] Wally V, Koller U, Bauer JW. High-Throughput Screening for Highly Functional RNA-Trans-Splicing Molecules: Correction of Plectin in Epidermolysis Bullosa Simplex. In: Plaseska-Karanfilska D (ed.) Human Genetic Diseases. Rijeka: InTech; 2011. p223-240 Available from: http://www.intechopen.com/books/human-genetic-diseases (Accessed 3 October 2011)

Chapter 5

Gene Therapy for Erythroid Metabolic Inherited Diseases

Maria Garcia-Gomez, Oscar Quintana-Bustamante,
Maria Garcia-Bravo, S. Navarro, Zita Garate and
Jose C. Segovia

Additional information is available at the end of the chapter

1. Introduction

Gene therapy is becoming a powerful tool to treat genetic diseases. Clinical trials performed during last two decades have demonstrated its usefulness in the treatment of several genetic diseases [1] but also the need to improve vector delivery, expression and safety [2]. New vectors should reduce genotoxicity (genomic alteration due to vector integration), immunogenicity (immune response to gene delivery vectors and/or trangenes) and cytotoxicity (induced by ectopic expression and/or overexpression of the transgene).

In mature erythrocytes, most metabolic needs are covered by glycolysis, oxidative pentose phosphate pathway and glutathione cycle. Hereditary enzyme deficiencies of all these pathways have been identified, being most of them associated with chronic non-spherocytic hemolitic anemia (CNSHA). Hereditary hemolytic anemia exhibits a high molecular heterogeneity with a wide number of different mutations involved in the structural genes of nearly all affected enzymes. Deficiency in metabolic enzymes impairs energy balance in the erythrocytes, with or without changes in oxygen affinity of hemoglobin and delivery to the tissues. Despite of having a better understanding of their molecular basis, definitive curative therapy for Red Blood Cells (RBC) enzyme defects still remains undeveloped.

Conventional bone marrow transplantation allows the generation of donor-derived functional hematopoietic cells of all lineages in the host, and represents the standard of care or at least a valid therapeutic option for many inherited diseases [3]. However, complications associated to allogeneic transplantation can be as severe as the enzymatic deficiency. The recessive inheriting trait of most of these metabolic diseases and the confined enzymatic defect to the hematopoietic/

erythropoietic system, make them suitable diseases to be treated by gene therapy. Correction by gene therapy requires the stable transfer of a functional gene into the autologous self-renewing Hematopoietic stem cells (HSCs) and their mature progeny. Autologous BM transplantation of genetically corrected cells shows several advantages over the allogeneic procedure. First, it overcomes the limitation of human leukocyte antigen (HLA)-compatible donor availability, so it can be applied to every patient. Second, the reduction of morbidity and mortality associated with the transplant procedure, as there is no risk of graft versus host disease (GvHD) and consequently no need for post-transplant immunosuppression.

To date, gene therapy approaches for the treatment of inherited metabolic deficiencies are still limited, mainly because of the frequent lack of selective advantage of genetically corrected cells. This implies that high levels of transgene expression are required, as well as an efficient transduction of HSCs. This requirement have already been described in different RBC diseases as in the erytropoietic protoporphyria (EPP) [4] caused by the deficiency of the last enzyme of the heme biosintesis pathway or in the piruvate kinase deficiency (PKD) [3], where there is an impairment in the final yield of ATP in RBC. Additionally, some RBC pathologies require switching on expression of the transgene at only the proper stage of differentiation, which represents another challenge in the development of new gene therapy protocols.

2. Gene therapy attempts for inherited metabolic diseases of erythrocytes

Although more than 14 metabolic deficiencies have been identified causing CNSHA, approaches of gene therapy have been done only in a few of them (Table 1). Below, we are including a short description of the different diseases and the attempts addressed.

Among glycolytic defects causing CNSHA, Glucose 6-phosphate dehydrogenase (G6PD) deficiency is the most common genetic disease. More than 400 million people are affected world wide, showing a vast variability of clinical features. G6PD catalyzes the first reaction of the pentose phosphate pathway, in which Glucose 6-phosphate (G6P) is oxidized and Nicotinamide adenine dinucleotide phosphate is reduced (NADPH) resulting in decarboxylation of CO_2 and pentose phosphate. G6PD plays a central role in the cellular physiology as it is the major source of NADPH, required by many essential cellular systems including the antioxidant pathways, nitric oxide synthase, NADPH oxidase, cytochrome p450 system and others. Indeed, G6PD is essential for cell survival. *G6PD* is a 20 kb X-linked gene that maps to the Xq28 region, consisting of 13 exons and 12 introns, which encode a 514 amino acids protein with ubiquitous expression. More than 100 missense mutations in the *G6PD* gene have been identified [14], being most of them single-point mutations causing an amino acid substitution. Frequently, these mutations cause mild symptoms or no disease, except when patients are challenged by increased oxidative stress or fava beans. However, some mutations provoke severe instability of the G6PD and, as a result, lifelong CNSHA with a variable severity [15,16]. Through genetic studies it has been observed that severe clinical manifestations appear preferentially in exons 7, 10 and 11. As *G6PD* is X-linked, the defect is fully expressed in affected males (hemizygotes who inherit the mutation only from the mother), whereas in homozygous females the mutations are transmitted from both parents. Thereby, female heterozygotes represent a red blood cell mosaic population, causing a wide range clinical picture.

Disease	Gene	Chrom.	Inheritance	Other sympthoms	Bone Marrow Transplantation	Gene Therapy
Glucose-6 Phosphate Dehydrogenase Deficiency (G6PD)	G6PD	Xq28	X-linked	jaundice, spleno- and hepatomegaly, hemoglobinuria, leukocyte disfunction, and susceptibility to infections		D: C57BL/6 mice P: Transduction of 5-FU treated BM cells with MMLV-hG6PD or MPSV-hG6PD vectors and subsequent transplantation. R: lethally irradiated C57BL/6 mice [5]
Pyruvate Kinase Deficiency (PKD)	PKLR	1q21	A.R	Reticulocytosis, splenomegaly, hidrops foetalis, and death in neonatal period	D: normal CBA/N$^{+/+}$ mice + 5FU R: CBA Pk-1^{slc}/ PK-1^{slc} mice C: minimal (100 or 400 cGy) [6]	D: WT mice P: Transduction of 5-FU treated BM cells with pMNSM-hLPK retroviral vector and subsequent transplantation R: lethally irradiated mice [7]
					D: normal CBA/N$^{+/+}$ mice R: CBA Pk-1^{slc}/ PK-1^{slc} mice C: no conditioning [8]	D: CBA PK-1^{slc}/PK-1^{slc} mice P: Transgenic rescue using the µLCR-PKLR-hRPK construct [9]
					D: normal Basenji dogs R: PKD Basenji dogs C: sublethal dose (200 cGy) + mycophenolate memofetil + cyclosporine [10]	D: WT mice P: Transduction of Lin⁻Sca1⁺ BM cells with a MSFV-hRPK retroviral vector and subsequent transplantation R: lethally irradiated WT mice [11]
					D: HLA-identical sister R: PKD severe patient C: busulfan + cyclophosphamide [12]	D: AcB55 mice P: Transduction of Lin⁻Sca1⁺ BM cells with a MSFV-hRPK retroviral vector and subsequent transplantation R: lethally irradiated AcB55 mice [13]
Glucose Phosphate Isomerase Deficiency (GPI)	GPI	19q13.1	A.R	neuromuscular disturbances		
Triose Phosphate Isomerase Deficiency (TPI)	TPI1	12p13	A.R	neuromuscular disorders, mental retardation, frecuent infections and death in utero		
Hexokinase Deficiency (HK)	HK1	10q22	A.R	defects in platelets		
Phosphofructokinase Deficiency (PFK)	PFKL	21q22.3	A.R	myopathy, storage disease type VII		
Bisphosphoglycerate Mutase Deficiency (BPGM)	BPGM	7q31-q34	A.R	erythrocytosis		
Glutathion Synthetase Deficiency (GSD)	GSS	20q11.2	A.R	5-oxoprolinuria, metabolic acidosis, central nervous system impairment		

A.R, autosomic recessive; D, donor; R, receptor; C, conditioning; P, protocol

Table 1. Most Common Erythroid Metabolic Inherited Diseases. BM transplantation and gene therapy approaches

Patients with CNSHA suffer anemia and jaundice, but often tolerate their condition well. However, G6PD variants with low activity are related with alterations in the erythrocyte membrane facilitating its breakdown and causing intravasal hemolysis. These symptoms are often accompanied by spleno- and hepatomegaly and hemoglobinuria. Besides, leukocyte dysfunctions caused by lower concentration of NADPH appear when G6PD activity is below 5% of the normal activity, leading to an immune depression [17]. Vives *et al.* and other groups have also observed an increased susceptibility to infections [18,19].

Preclinical work from Rovira et al demonstrates that *hG6PD* gene transfer into HSCs may be a viable strategy for the treatment of severe G6PD deficiency [5]. Through the transplantation of pluripotent hematopetic stem cells transduced with γ-retroviral vectors carrying the wild type human G6PD cDNA, they achieved a stable and lifelong expression of hG6PD in all the hematopoietic tissues of primary and secondary receptor mice. In this study, transgene expression was driven by the 3' LTR from either the Moloney murine leukemia virus (MMLV) or the myeloproliferative sarcoma virus (MPSV), obtaining an efficient transduction in murine hematopoietic progenitors. The corrected cells were then injected into lethally irradiated syngeneic mice, increasing 2-fold the enzyme activity in peripheral blood cells in comparison with non-transplanted control mice. Long-term hG6PD expression derived from the vector was also observed, which was similar to that of the endogenous enzyme activity. Similar expression was detected in RBC and in White Blood Cells (WBC) in different hematopoietic organs, as expected due to the use of a viral ubiquitous promoter. These results support gene therapy as a suitable strategy for the treatment of severe CNSHA due to G6PD deficiency. Additionally, they also demonstrated the efficacy of this gene therapy vector in human embryonic stem cells (hESC) in which the *G6PD* gene had been inactivated by targeted homologous recombination, which implies the potential application of gene therapy to G6PD hESCs. Moreover, although a selective advantage in favor of G6PD corrected cells has not been reported because the mice used showed normal G6PD activity, Rovira et al observed a strong selection after transduction of G6PD-deficient ES cells with their vectors. In this regard, the development of G6PD deficient mouse models would be a valuable tool to test new protocols. Furthermore, the mouse strain recently developed by Hay Ko et al may be useful, although it does not reproduce all the features of the human G6PD-deficiency [20].

Pyruvate kinase deficiency (PKD), the second most frequent abnormality of glycolysis causing CNSHA, has also been proposed as a potential disease to be treated by gene therapy. Pyruvate kinase (PK) catalyzes the second ATP generation reaction of the glycolysis pathway by converting phosphoenolpyruvate (PEP) into pyruvate, yielding nearly 50% of the total ATP production in red blood cells. PK plays a crucial role in erythrocyte metabolism, since mature RBC are absolutely dependent on the ATP generated by glycolysis, giving the loss of mitochondria, nucleus and endoplasmic reticulum in their mature state. RPK is therefore necessary for maintaining cell integrity and function. Reduced levels of erythrocyte Pyruvate kinase (RPK) lead to an accumulation of glycolytic intermediates that ultimately shortens the life span of mature RBC by metabolic block [21]. Four tissue-specific isoenzymes of PK (M1, M2, R and L) encoded by two different genes (*PK-M* and *PK-LR*) have been identified in humans [22]. The *PK-LR* gene, located on chromosome 1 (1q21) [23] encodes for both LPK (expressed in liver, renal cortex and small intestine) and RPK (restricted to erythrocytes) through the use of alternative promoters [24]. PK-M1 is expressed in adult nomal tissue, like brain or muscle. The PK-M2 isoform is typically expressed in proliferating tissues like fetal, tumoral and several other adult tissues [25] and during the maturation of the erythroblasts, gradually decreases, giving rise to the RPK isoform.

The codifying region of *PK-LR* gene is split into twelve exons, ten of which are shared by the two isoforms, while exons 1 and 2 are specific for the erythrocyte and the hepatic isoenzyme respectively [26]. However, clinical symptoms caused by *PK-LR* mutations are confined to RBC because the hepatic deficiency is usually compensated by the persistent enzyme synthesis in hepatocytes [27]. To date, more than 150 different mutations in the *PK-LR* have been associated with CNSHA, being most of them missense mutations, splicing and codon stop. Only two variants, -72 G and -83 C, have been identified in the promoter regions so far [26,27]. Molecular studies indicate that severe syndrome is commonly associated with disruptive mutations and missense mutations involving the active site or protein stability [28].

PK deficiency is transmitted as an autosomal recessive trait and although its global incidence is still unknown, it has been estimated in 1:20000 in the general caucasian population [29]. Clinical symptoms appear in homozygous and compound heterozygous patients, which lead to a very variable clinical picture, ranging from mild or fully compensated forms to life-treating neonatal anemia necessitating exchange transfusions and subsequent continuous support [28]. Pathological manifestations are usually observed when enzyme activity falls below 25% of normal PK activity [30], and severe disease has been associated with a high degree of reticulocytosis [31]. *Hydrops foetalis* and death in the neonatal period have also been reported in rare cases [32,33]. PK deficiency treatment is based on supportive measures since no specific therapy for severe cases is available to date. Periodic cell transfusions may be required in severe anemic cases, often impairing their quality of life. Splenectomy can be clinically useful in some patients increasing the hemoglobin levels, as well as iron chelation to decrease the common iron overload observed in PKD patients [34]. However, in some severe cases, allogeneic bone marrow transplantation is required and it has been successfully performed in one severe affected child [12].

The feasibility of gene therapy in PKD was first reported by the group of Asano, who introduced the human LPK cDNA into C57BL/6 mouse bone marrow cells using a retroviral vector [7]. They demonstrated the expression of the LPK transgene mRNA in both peripheral blood and hematopoietic organs after bone marrow transplantation. However, viral-derived expression in peripheral blood was detectable no longer than 30 days post-transplantation, indicating an insufficient transduction efficacy of the retroviral vector used or transduction of non-pluripotent BM cells. In a hemolytic anemia dog model, bone marrow transplantation of minimal conditioned receptors failed to correct the hematological symptoms [10]. Other approaches to rescue RPK phenotype through a gene addition strategy have been also addressed using a PKD transgenic mouse model (*CBA/N PK-1^{SLC}/PK-1^{SLC}*) [9]. In this assay, the hemolytic anemia and reticulocytosis was fully corrected when the human gene was highly expressed by means of pronuclear injection, although splenomegaly was still present. Interestingly, the authors observed a negative correlation between RBC PK activity and the number of apoptotic erythroid progenitors in the spleen, providing evidence that the metabolic alteration in PK deficiency affects not only the survival of RBC, but also the maturation of erythroid progenitors, resulting in ineffective erythropoiesis [35]. Further studies from this group indicate that RPK plays an important role as an antioxidant during erythrocyte differentiation, since glycolytic inhibition by mutations in *Pklr* gene increased the oxidative stress in SLC3 cells (established from *Pk-1*^{slc} mouse) and led to the activation of hypoxia-inducible factor-1 (HIF1), as well as the expression of downstream proapoptotic genes [36].

In addition, our work carried out in mouse models supported the therapeutic potential of viral vectors for the gene therapy of PK deficiency. Throughout the transduction of bone marrow cells using γ-retroviral vectors that carry the human RPK cDNA and subsequent transplantation, we reported a long-term expression of the human protein in RBC obtained from primary and secondary receptor mice, without detectable adverse effects [11]. Recently, we have also reported a successful gene therapy approach using the same retroviral vectors in the congenital mouse strain AcB55, identified by Min-Oo in studies of alleles involved in malaria susceptibility [37]. These mice carry a loss-of-function mutation (269T-> A) resulting in the amino acid substitution I90N in the *Pklr* gene, which yields a similar RBC phenotype to that observed in PKD patients, including splenomegaly and constitutive reticulocytosis. Retroviral-derived expression was capable of fully resolving the pathological phenotype in terms of hematological parameters, anemia, reticulocytosis and splenomegaly, together with normalization of bone marrow and spleen erythroid progenitors, erythropoietin (EPO), PK activity and ATP levels. Interestingly, despite a strong viral promoter was used to drive the expression of the transgene, metabolic energy balance was no modified in white blood cells. Moreover, we observed that values above 25% of genetically corrected cells were needed to fully rescue the deficiency [3], suggesting that RPK transfer protocols will always require a significant extent of gene-complemented HSC. Nevertheless, other experiments performed in the *CBA/N PK-1*^{SLC}/*PK-1*^{SLC} mouse model of PKD have reveled that 10% of normal BM renders RBC expressing nearly normal RPK protein levels [5]. Differences in the genetic defect of the mouse models used could account for these discrepancies, reinforcing the need for high transduction efficiencies to address the disease in the heterogeneous human population. Additionally, we have proposed the *in utero* transplantation of gene corrected cells as an alternative option for the treatment of PKD. The transplantation of RPK deficient lineage negative fetal liver cells transduced with lentiviruses (LVs) expressing the human wild type version of the RPK in 14.5 day-old fetuses partially restored the anemic phenotype, mainly due to a low engraftment of corrected cells [13]. Improved *in utero* cell transfer would allow therapeutic levels, thus offering an alternative therapeutic option for prenatally diagnosed severe PKD. Following our results in the AcB55 mouse model of PKD, phenotype correction could be reached if the percentage of engraftment of corrected cells is significant. We are currently developing improved lentiviral vectors that could be applied in future clinical settings.

Glucose phosphate isomerase (GPI) deficiency is the third most common hereditary cause of CNSHA, due to mutations in *GPI* gene located on the long arm of chromosome 19. The prevalence of this disease is still unknown, with no more than 50 cases reported so far, and with a higher incidence in the black population. The enzyme catalyzes the reversible isomerization from glucose 6-phosphate to fructose 6-phosphate, an equilibrium reaction of the glycolysis pathway. Glucose turnover is affected only in deficiencies below a very low critical residual GPI activity, but with a drastic decline of lactate formation. As no isoenzyme does exist, patients suffer not only from CNSHA and tissue hypoxia, but also from neuromuscular disturbances. In some cases, GPI deficiency has been found in PKD patients, increasing the severity of the clinical scenario and reflecting the degree of the perturbation of glycolysis. The lack of ATP leads to a destabilization of the erythrocyte membrane causing earlier lysis of the RBC and hemolytic anemia of variable degrees [38]. Animal models of GPI deficiency have been described, showing similar symptoms to the human disease [39]. Until now, no gene therapy attempt has been applied to this deficiency.

Other enzyme deficiencies causing CNSHA are Triose phosphate isomerase (TPI) deficiency, associated with neuromuscular disorders, mental retardation and frequent infections, Hexokinase deficiency (HK), affecting also platelet metabolism, phosphofructokinase (PFK) deficiency, 2,3-bisphosphoglycerate mutase (BPGM) deficiency and Glutathione synthetase (GS) deficiency (reviewed in [17,40,41]). Although the incidence of these diseases can be high (ie. TPI is considered as a frequent enzymopathy affecting 0.1% for caucasian populations and even 4.6% for black populations), they are considered rare or very rare diseases, because only few cases (~25 patients in the case of TPI) are diagnosed due to the severity of the clinical manifestations. No gene therapy approaches have been addressed up to now to treat these enzymopaties. However, due to their common characteristics, strategies developed in the other enzyme deficiencies could be applied directly to the treatment of all of them.

3. Optimization of vectors for the gene therapy of metabolic erythroid diseases: Erythroid specific expression vectors

The introduction of a cDNA, encoding for the correct version of the target mutated gene into patient cells using retroviral vectors has been successful for several inherited diseases. The initial integrative vectors for gene therapy design and used in clinical trials were based on Gamma(γ)-retroviral vectors in which the transgene expression was driven by the viral LTR promoter. γ-retroviruses preferably integrate in regions adjacent to the transcription initiation site [42]. The expression of the transgene is promoted by the viral LTR, which drives a high expression that can affect gene regulation of the surrounding genes. Although a high efficiency of transduction and therapeutic effects have been described with these vectors in various monogenic disorders such as immunodeficiencies, adverse effects associated with insertional mutagenesis have also been observed. This has led to the development of the next generation of integrative vectors using self-inactivating-LTR lentiviral backbones. SIN-Lentiviral vectors tend to integrate in intergenic transcribing areas, which represent a safer integrative pattern than γ-retroviral vectors. Aditionally, the expression of the transgene is driven by internal promoters, offering a more physiological expression and a less genotoxic profile when using weak promoters [43]. Current efforts to reduce the mutagenic potential of gene therapy vectors are focussed on not only the use of new viral backbones [44] but also on tissue-specific promoters to restrict the transgene expression to target cells [45] and insulators to confer position-independent expression [46]. Additional regulatory DNA elements such as locus control regions (LCR), enhancers, or silencers have also been used to increase lineage specificity.

Gene therapy for RBC disorders requires, ideally, high erythroid-specific transgene expression in order to avoid side effects in progenitors or hematopoietic lineages other than the erythroid one. In inherited enzymophaties, the overexpression of metabolic enzymes in non-erythroid cells could provide these cells with a potential energetic advantage, with the consequent risk of disturbing the physiological generation of ATP in WBC. Also, the restriction of transcriptional activity to target cells with the use of either tissue-specific or physiologically regulated vectors decreasees the effect of the integrative vectors in the host genome. This goal is particularly important for erythrocyte metabolic deficiencies, as all the affected enzymes are highly regulated and connected with central metabolic pathways. Indeed, an expression limited to the erythroid progeny would reduce the genotoxic risk, as RBC become transcriptionally inactive during differentiation, and finally extrude their nucleus. To study tissue-specific gene therapy strategies for RBC diseases, hemoglobinophaties have been the most widely used.

Erythroid regulatory elements have been extensively used to manage targeted expression to RBC using reporter genes (Table 2). The Locus Control Regions (LCR), defined by their ability to enhance the expression of linked genes to physiological levels in a tissue-specific and copy number-dependent manner at ectopic chromatin sites are commonly used. The components of the LCR normally colocalize to sites of DNase I hypersensitivity (HS) in the chromatin of expressing cells. Individual HS are composed of arrays of multiple ubiquitous and lineage-specific transcription factor-binding sites. In early experiments performed with retroviral backbones, the group of Ferrari developed an erythroid-specific vector by the replacement of the constitutive retroviral enhancer in the U3 region of the 3′ LTR with the HS2 autoregulatory enhancer of the erythroid GATA-1 transcription factor gene. The expression of this vector was restricted to the erythroblastic progeny of both human progenitors and mouse-repopulating stem cells [47,48]. Later, they showed that the addition of the HS1 enhancer to HS2, both from the GATA-1 gene, within the LTR of the retroviral vector significantly improved the expression of the reporter gene. Another enhancer element that has been used to achieve erythroid-specific expression is HS40, located upstream of the ζ-globin gene, since it is able to enhance the activity of heterologous promoters in a tissue-specific manner [49]. It has been shown to be genetically stable in MMLV vectors and enhances expression comparable to that of a single -globin gene [50], although HS40 lacks some of the properties of the LCR, like position independence [51] or copy number dependence [52].

An additional improvement to provide safer vectors for RBC gene therapy was provided by the use of insulators elements, which have been shown to reduce position effects in transgenic animals [60]. Insulators are genomic elements that can shelter genes from their surrounding chromosomal environment, by either blocking the action of a distal enhancer on a promoter [60,61], or by acting as barriers that protect the gene from the silencing effect of heterochromatin [61]. The most well studied element is the chicken hypersensit (cHS4), an insulator sequence of the chicken -like globin cluster. Studies performed by Chung et al with the γ-globin promoter and the neo reporter gene on selected cells lines, demonstrated the ability of cHS4 to insulate the expression cassette from the effects of a strong -globin LCR element [63] and therefore reducing its genotoxicity. Experiments from Arumugam et al showed a two-fold reduction in transforming activity with insulated LCR-containing lentiviral vectors comparing with vectors lacking the cHS4 element [68].

Erythroid tissue-specific vectors			
Promoter / enhancer	**transgene**	**Vector type**	**Reference**
HS2 GATA-1 enhancer within the LTR	ΔLNGFR and Neo^R / EGFP	SFCM retroviral vector	[47]
HS1 to HS2 GATA-1 enhancer within the LTR	EGFP and hΔLNGFR	SFCM retroviral vector	[48]
Ankyrin-1 and α-spectrin promoters combined or not with HS40, GATA-1, ARE and intron 8 enhancers	EGFP	HIV-1 based vectors	[53]
α-globin HS40 enhancer and Ankyrin-1 promoter	GFP / *FECH*cDNA	HIV-1 based vectors	[4]
IHK, IHβp and HS3βp chimeric enhancers/ promoters	hβ-globin cDNA	Sleeping beauty transposon	[54]
Physiologically regulated vectors			
Promoter / enhancer	**transgene**	**Vector type**	**Reference**
HSFE and β-globin promoter	hβ-globin cDNA	MSCV retroviral vector	[55]
LCR and β-globin promoter	hβ-globin cDNA or EGFP	HIV-1 based vectors	[56,57]
β-globin and θ-globin promoters combined or not with HS40, GATA-1, ARE and intron 8 enhancers	EGFP	HIV-1 based vectors	[53]
LCR HS4, HS3, HS2, β-globin promoter and truncated β-globin intron 2	EGFP	HIV-1 based vectors	[58]
LCR, cHS4 and β-globin promoter	hβ-globin cDNA	HIV-1 based vectors	[46]
β-globin promoter, LCR HS2, HS3, HS4	hβ-globin cDNA	AAV2	[59]

LTR, long terminal repeats; HS: hypersensitive site; IHK, human *ALAS2* intron 8 enhancer, HS40 from αLCR and ankyrin-1 promoter; IhΒp, human *ALAS2* intron 8 enhancer, HS40 from αLCR and β-globin promoter; HS3βp, HS3 core element form human βLCR and β-globin promoter; LCR, locus control region. Modified from Toscano *et al.*, 2011

Table 2. Specific vectors for gene therapy of erythroid inherited diseases.

Tissue-specific expression using alternative human promoters can be convenient or more efficient for some diseases, but driving the expression of the therapeutic genes using own promoters is still the most physiological approach to reduce the genotoxic risk of integrating gene vectors [62]. The use of physiologically regulated vectors has been limited mainly because the promoter and the enhancer elements have to be obtained from the affected genes and they are often too large to be included in a lentiviral backbone, and also because the gene expression pattern depends partially on chromatin positioning [63]. -globin LCR has been widely used when attempting to solve this limitation. The -globin LCR consists of 5 HS regions located upstream of the entire cluster of human -like globin genes, each containing a high density of erythroid-specific and ubiquitous transcription binding elements [64]. Much of the transcriptional activity of the -globin LCR resides in HS2 and HS3 sites, but site 4 is important in adult globin expression [65]. Previous studies *in vitro* and *in vivo* have shown that -globin LCR can enhance erythroid-specific expression from heterologous non-erythroid promoters [66,67]. First approaches using -globin LCR and 3′ enhancers were based on murine γretroviral vectors [74,75], but the limited packaging capacity of these vectors (up to 8 kb) did not allow the presence of such as large regulatory sequences. Several vector designs including different combinations of regulatory sequences and a deletion of a cryptic polyadenylation site within intron 2 of -globin gene [68], flanked by an extended promoter sequence and the -globin 3′ proximal enhancer were developed. The combination of the LCR elements (3′2 kb) spanning HS2, 3 and 4, were the best amongst several possibilities [69] to achieve a high titer retroviral vector capable of expressing high levels of the transgene.

Other approaches to achieve consistent long-term expression of a transgene have been based on the use of HSFE element, an erythroid-specific chromatin remodelling element derived from the human β-globin LCR which contains binding sites for the erythroid-specific factors NF-E2, GATA-1, EKLF and the ubiquitous factor Sp-1, all of which are necessary to establish a hypersensitive chromatin domain. Work by Nemeth *et al.*, demonstrated that the HSFE can mediate functional tissue-specific "opening" of a minimal human β-globin promoter and increases expression of a human β-globin gene in both MEL cell clones and in transgenic mice. Their results indicated that the most effective vector included tandem copies of the HSFE and produced a 5-fold increase in expression compared to the promoter alone [55] in the context of an integrated retroviral vector.

Gene therapy for RBC metabolic diseases can also benefit from the new technologies based on the modification in mRNA stability or translation efficacy of the transgenes. The use of the post-transcriptional regulatory element (Wpre) from the woodchuck hepatitis virus (WHV) has significantly increased transgene expression in target cells [64,65], even in HSC [70] by stabilization of mRNA at post-transcriptional level. However, it may raise safety concerns, since it contains a truncated form of the WHV X gene, which has been implicated in animal liver cancer [71]. Therefore, Wpre has subsequently been improved by a mutation of the open reading frame of the X gene [72]. Combination of erythroid promoters like ankyrin-1 or -spectrin with Wpre sequence increased 2-fold the expression in unilineage erythroid cultures [53], and when combined also with erythroid enhancers inserted in tandem: HS40 and GATA-1 or HS40 and I8 enhancers [53]. RNA targeting strategies have mainly been used to down regulate expression of cellular genes using vectors expressing interference RNAs (iRNAs). They can be also used to control the expression of integrating vectors knocking down the transgene by the endogenous microRNA cellular machinery. Following this strategy, engineered microRNA target sequences in the vector (miRTs-vector) are recognized by a cell specific microRNA (miR-NA), avoiding the expression of the therapeutic gene in undesired cell populations [63]. Several miRNAs are differentially expressed during hematopoiesis and their specific expression regulates key functional proteins involved in hematopoietic lineage differentiation. Particularly, miR-223 has been proposed as a myeloid-specific regulator that negatively regulates progenitor proliferation and granulocyte differentiation and activation [73]. Moreover, Felli et al observed that hematopoietic progenitor cells transduced with miR-223 showed a significant reduction of their erythroid clonogenic capacity, suggesting that down-modulation of this miRNA is required for erythroid progenitor recruitment and commitment [79]. Further studies may determine if the use of miRNA-223 target in lentiviral vectors could be useful to achieve a desirable erythroid-specific expression for gene therapy of red blood cell diseases.

In addition, the erythroid-specificity of short segments of the -globin LCR element has been documented in adeno-associated virus 2 (AAV2) system. Their efficacy to mediate an erythroid-restricted expression has been proved by Tan *et al.*, who reported a successful AAV2-mediated high and stable transduction of the human -globin gene in HSCs from -thalassemia mouse model, which were then transplanted into recipient and rescued them of the disease [59]. These vectors have gained attention as potential useful vectors for human gene therapy, mainly because of their non-pathogenic nature in humans and their relativly easy production. Besides, AAV2 vectors are easily purified to high titers and are able to transduce dividing and non-dividing cells. However, most of proviral AAV2 genomes remain episomal and the insert size is restricted to just over 4kb. Further studies are still needed to know whether they would be a better option than current lentiviral vectors. Also, long-term genotoxic risk of recombinant AAV2 therapy in human is not known up to the date.

In addition, the efficacy of some of these erythroid-specific elements and promoters has also been tested in non-viral vectors, such as transposons. Zhu et al, for instance, studied several hybrid promoters driving the expression of the human -globin gene using the sleeping beauty transposon (SB-Tn). They combined several erythroid elements to develop different chimeric promoters. Their results indicated that the ankyrin-1 minimum promoter was stronger than -globin's, and the hALAS I8 enhancer (IH) was significantly more powerful that HS3 core element from -LCR and -globin promoter [54]. SB-Tn system is a promising non-viral vector for efficient genomic insertion, even with erythroid-specificity. However, its efficiency for delivering transgenes into HSCs is still much lower than other engineering viral vectors.

4. Overcoming conventional gene therapy pitfalls: gene editing in induced plutipotent stem cells

4.1. Human induced pluripotent stem cells and reprogramming platforms

Since Yamanaka et al first reported the generation of mouse induced Pluripotent Stem Cells (iPSC) in 2006 by the ectopic expression of four transcription factors (Oct4, Sox2, Klf4 and cMyc) [74] and one year later in human cells together with Thompson's group [75,76], many laboratories around the world have been able to reprogram a large range of somatic cells into pluripotent stem cells, from neural stem cells [77] to terminally differentiated B-lymphocytes [78]. The reproducibility and potentiality (unlimited self-renewal and ability to differentiate into any cell type) of this technology has made the iPSC field to advance very rapidly. The human iPSC (hiPSC) technology brings together all the potential of hESC in terms of pluripotency without any ethical issue and the immunotolerance of the autologous cell treatment. Therefore, hiPSC technology is one of the most promising fields for future therapies for many human diseases. Safer reprogramming approaches have been designed and many patient specific hiPSC have been generated both to model human diseases and to correct by gene therapy approaches. Depending on the cell type to be reprogrammed, the number of factors used could be reduced and, what is more important, oncogenes or tumor related proteins included in the reprogramming cocktail, like c-MYC or KLF4 [79] could be removed from the original reprogramming cocktail [80-82]. Several groups developed excisable polycistronic lentiviral vectors [83,84] or transposon-based reprogramming systems [85,86], which could be removed after getting the hiPSC clones. Similar results have been obtained using recombinant proteins [82], synthetic mRNAs [87], and non integrating RNA Sendai Virus vectors [88]. Except for Sendai viruses, non integrating methods show a reduced reprogramming efficiency and the range of cells reprogrammed is not as large as with lentiviral or retroviral vectors.

iPSC technology makes feasible the availability of patient specific cells to study the biology of the disease and develop advanced tools to cure the phenotype and could potentially be used as a therapeutic option (Figure 1). Focussing on metabolic diseases, the first reported metabolic disease patient specific hiPSC line was obtained one year after the first generation of hiPSCs. It was from a 42-year old female that suffered from Type I Diabetes mellitus [89] and it showed no differences compared to a wild type hiPSC line in terms of pluripotency. Next report in which liver metabolic disease patient samples were reprogrammed was carried out by the group of Ludovic Vallier [90], and showed the potential of this kind of approaches for disease modelling and new drug discovery. They reprogrammed fibroblast obtained from α-1 Antitrypsin deficiency (A1ATD), Familiar Hypercholesterolemia (FH), Glucose-6-Phosphate deficiency (G6PD), Crigler-Najjar Syndrome and hereditary Tyrosinemia Type 1 patients, and generated hepatocytes that showed characteristics of mature hepatic cells, like albumin secretion or cytocrome p450 metabolism. Three of the five cell lines (A1ATD, FH, and GSD1a hiPSCs) were capable of recapitulating the disease phenotype in vitro. Disease modelling in erythroid diseased induced pluripotent cell lines has been performed for -Thalassemia [91,92] and sickle cell anemia [93,94]. In these reports the phenotype was corrected by LVs integrated in areas of the genome that were considered safe for viral integration [83] or by gene editing using homologous recombination of the affected locus [91,93,94].

The future therapeutic application of hiPSC will not only require non-integrative reprogramming system, but also a more precise gene correction. During last years, the cooperation between hiPSC technology and gene editing is being explored. Human iPSC technology has

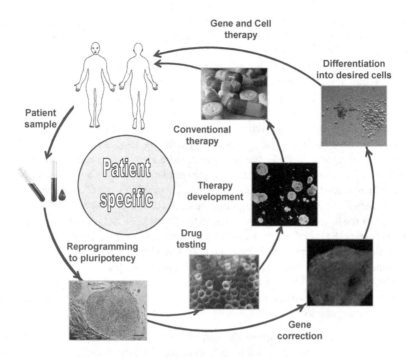

Figure 1. Potential utilities of hiPSC and iPS technology

led to the opportunity to control the integration of viral vectors at a clonal level. As we have mentioned before, the analysis of lentiviral integration sites in β-thalassemia hiPSC allowed the identification of corrected hiPSC clones expressing β-globin transgene from a safe genomic site (also called Safe harbour), a site in which integration does not disturb the expression of any neighbouring genes during their erythroid differentiation [83]. The therapeutic use of patient-specific hiPSC emerges then from the combination of gene and cell therapy. From this new research field, future gene therapy protocols will emerge.

4.2. Gene editing based on homologous recombination

Gene editing is a process in which a DNA sequence is introduced into a specific locus or a chromosomal sequence is replaced. This site-specific precise introduction requires an accurate recognition mechanism of the target site on the genome. Under normal conditions, the maintenance of the integrity of the genome requires that the cells repair DNA damage with high fidelity. One of the most harmful DNA damage is the generation of double-strand breaks (DSB). DSB are often resolved by non-homologous end joining (NHEJ), which joins the two ends of the DSB. However this DNA repair mechanism could introduce mutations. On the contrary, homologous recombination (HR) is a truly accurate DNA repair mechanism because it is basically a "copy and paste" mechanism. This process uses an undamaged homologous segment of DNA that can be exogenously provided as a template to copy the information across the DSB. The fidelity of HR gives us the specificity and accuracy that gene editing requires.

The natural HR process has been adapted by researchers to get the desirable addition of an exogenous cassette into the targeted locus. This techniques have been widely use for the generation of knock-out and knock-in transgenic animals [95]. To correct or insert and express a transgene by HR we can consider three different strategies: i) Gene correction, a base or some bases can be substituted from the original strand using an homologous sequence where this base or bases are modified; it is the way to introduce/repair point or small mutations; ii) Safe harbour integration, a complete expression cassette (promoter, transgene and regulatory signals) is inserted in a safe place of the genome, without altering the expression of the surrounding genes and without being silenced by epigenetic mechanisms; this is the case for *AASV1* and *CCR5* loci. Additionally to these well known safe harbours, there is a wide research focused on finding potential new safe harbour places. iii) Knock-in insertion, the cDNA of a gene is introduced in the same site of the endogenous gene, linked by splicing mechanisms to the endogenous gene assuring the expression of the inserted sequence by the endogenous regulatory elements of the locus where it is integrated.

Gene editing process can be separated in two different steps, generation of DSB and HR. The efficacy of gene editing in human cells depends on the generation of DSB at the specific target site and on the DNA repair mechanism that the cell uses to resolve the DSB. Unfortunately, NHEJ is the dominant pathway to solve these DNA lesions in human cells. Additionally, HR varies in different cell types and requires transit through S-G2 phase of the cell cycle [96]. These limitations make gene editing in human cells difficult to achieve. However, different approaches are being used to improve gene editing by HR, like increasing the length of the DNA sequences homologous to target site (homology arms) [97], the use of adeno-associated vectors [98], the improvement of selection methods for edited cells or the stimulation of HR by inducing DSB using DNA nucleases.

Recently, engineered DNA nucleases have been developed to specifically induce DSB at a unique and defined sequence in the cell genome. These proteins are formed by a nuclease domain and a DNA binding domain whose sequence specificity can be engineered. The most widely used DNA nucleases are Zinc finger nucleases (ZFN), homing meganucleases (MN) and transcription activator-like effector nucleases (TALEN). They identify a potentially unique sequence in the genome and generate DSBs in the desired genomic site, aiming to promote the repair of the DSB by the cell machinery and, ideally by HR. The DNA binding domain of a ZFNs is derived from zinc-finger proteins and is linked to the nuclease domain of the restriction enzyme Fok-I. DNA-biding domain is a tandem repeat of Cys_2His_2 zinc fingers, each of which recognizes three nucleotides. ZFNs work as pairs of two monomers of ZFN, one in reverse orientation. This ZFN dimer can be designed to bind to genomic sequences of 18-36 nucleotides long. TALENs have a similar structure to ZFNs, but the DNA-binding domain comes from transcription activator-like effector proteins. The DNA-binding domain in TALENs is a tandem array of amino acid repeats. Each of these units is able to bind to one of the four possible nucleotides and this makes that the DNA binding domain can be designed to recognize any desired genomic sequence. TALENs also cleave as dimers. Contrary to these synthetic DNA-nucleases, MNs are a subset of homing endonucleases which recognize a DNA sequence from 14 to 40 nucleotides. Current MNs have been engineered from natural homing endonucleases to increase the number of target DNA sequences.

ZNFs have been widely used for gene editing in hESC and hiPSC. In 2007, Dr. Naldini's laboratory showed the insertion of GFP into the CCR5 safe harbour in human stem cells (HSC and hESC) after inducing HR by ZFN expression. The CCR5-ZFN and donor DNAs were delivered into hESC by intergrative deficient lentiviruses. More interestingly, targeted hESC were able to differentiate into neurons keeping GFP expression [99]. Soon, the proof of principle for the clinical application of ZFN-mediated gene editing was tested in hiPSC from patients affected by different genetic diseases. The first pre-clinical use of ZFN for gene therapy of a metabolic disease was performed by Yusa *et al.* In this report, gene correction was performed at the α1-antitrypsin (*A1AT*) locus to revert A1AT deficiency in hiPSC derived from a patient with a point mutation. This group included a Puromycin resistence cassette flanked by piggyBac sites, so that the Puromycin selection facilitated the isolation of corrected A1ATD-iPSC clones. Afterwards, the selection cassette was removed by piggyBac transposon, obtaining corrected hiPS clones without any additional sequence. These corrected hiPS clones were then differentiated into hepatocyte-like cells to confirm the complete correction of the A1ATD [101]. Other hiPSC gene editing approaches and functional correction of erithroid diseases include gene correction of Sickle Cell Anemia [94] and -Thalassemia [91].

One of the major limitations of ZFN is the generation of "off-target" DSB, due to unspecific sequence recognition. Different studies have highlighted this as a possible limitation in the clinical use of ZFN-mediated HR [100,101]. Recent works have explored the potential of other types of DNA-nucleases in order to prevent the "off-target" cleave limitations of the ZFN, being TALEN and MN the most promising ones. The feasibility of TALEN to mediate HR in hESC and hiPSC was assess by Jaenisch's group when they designed TALEN targeting the *PPP1R12C* (at *AAVS1* locus), *POU5F1* and *PITX3* genes at precisely the same positions as the one targeted by ZFN in their previous work [102]. The authors described a gene editing efficiency similar to the one achieved by ZFN with a low level of "off-targets" [103]. A strategy to minimize the potential number of "off-targets" is to design TALEN to work as obligatory heterodimers, which has beeing already done in the engineered MNs. The application of the TALEN and MN as tools to improve HR is still on going. We are exploring the pre-clinical use of TALEN and MN to correct erythroid metabolic genetic diseases, such as PKD.

5. Complementary developments for the application of gene therapy to erythroid metabolic diseases

5.1. *In vivo* transduction using engineered envelopes

Another challenge for the clinical application of gene therapy relates to vector targeting. To achieve successful gene therapy, the appropriate gene must be delivered to target cells and specifically expressed in them, without harming non-targeted cells. The most common and easiest way to target specific cells is by *ex vivo* infection of the desired cell population. Therefore, cells can be directly exposed to the viral vectors facilitating viral-cell interaction. These interactions are driven by the envelope protein which can be adapted from other viruses redirecting the tropism of the vector. The most widely used vectors are lentiviral vectors pseudotyped with the attachment glycoprotein of the vesicular stomatitis virus (VSV-G), which allows the production of high-titre vectors and confers a broad host range [104]. In comparison with them, engineered LVs capable of delivering genes of interest to predetermined cells, can reduce the targeting of undesirable cell types and improve the safety profile, which will further enhance the use of this vector system for gene therapy applications [105,106]. As we have mentioned above, the use of promoters and regulatory sequences that are only active in target cells adds lineage specific expression, although integration of the viruses in non desired cells is still possible. *Ex vivo*-targeted gene delivery, as commonly used in HSCs transduction, is associated with a risk of inducing cell differentiation and loss of the engraftment potential of these cells [107]. On the contrary, *in vivo* gene transfer could target HSCs in their stem cell niche, a microenvironment that regulates HSC survival and maintenance [105]. To accomplish this, the vector must display a suitable system to selectively infect the desired population, for example the introduction of a specific ligand to bind a target-cell receptor [106].

Many attempts have been made to develop targeted transduction systems using retroviral and lentiviral vectors by altering the envelope glycoprotein (Env), which is responsible for the binding of the virus to the cell surface receptors and for mediating viral entry into the cell. The plasticity of the surface domain of Env allows insertion of ligands, peptides or single-chain antibodies that can direct the vectors to specific cell types [108]. However, this type of manipulation negatively affects the fusion domain of Env, resulting in low viral titers. To overcome this downside, a method to engineer lentiviral vectors has been developed. These vectors transduce specific cell types by breaking up the binding and fusion functions of the envelope protein into two distinct proteins [108]. Instead of pseudotyping lentiviral vectors with a modified viral envelope protein, these lentiviral vectors co-display a targeting antibody and a fusogenic molecule on the same viral vector surface. Based on molecular recognition, the targeting antibody should direct lentiviral vectors to the specific cell type. The binding between the antibody and the corresponding cellular antigen should induce endocytosis resulting in the transport of lentiviral vectors into the endosomal compartment. Once inside the endosome, the fusogenic molecule should undergo a conformational change in response to the decrease in pH, thereby releasing the viral core into the cytosol [109]. The use of fusion domain of the binding defective Sindbis virus glycoprotein together with an anti-CD20 antibody has been shown to mediate the targeted transduction of lentiviral vectors to CD20-expressing B cells [110].

However, two major challenges for *in vivo* gene delivery are LVthe exposure to the host immune/complement system and off-target cell transfer after systemic administration. For these reasons, second generation of early-acting-cytokine-displaying LVs has been developed, that circumvents these obstacles by specifically targeting hCD34$^+$ cells [111,112]. For example, RDTR/SCFHA-LV, consisting of RD114 glycoprotein and stem cell factor (SCF) fused to the *Influenza hameglutinin* env protein, is resistant to degradation by human complement and efficiently transduces very immature hCD34[+] HSCs [113]. This new generation of HSC-targeted LVs should improve current gene therapy protocols through the transduction of primitive HSCs directly in the bone marrow of patients with genetic diseases.

5.2. *In vitro* production of mature erythrocytes

Periodical blood transfusion is the previous to the last therapeutic option for severe cases of CNSHA patients. However, this clinical practice involves also adverse effects related to the immuneresponse against minor erythrocyte antigens which makes the patients refractory to additional blood transfusions in the long run. The availability of genetically corrected patient-specific iPSC would allow the possibility of generating disease free erythrocytes ready for transfusion, avoiding the adverse immune effects.

There have been numerous attempts to produce RBC *in vitro* from different sources of stem cells. To date, the most successful protocol has been developed by the group of Luc Douay [113,114]. Using peripheral blood CD34[+] cells, these authors were able to expand and generate RBC with *in vitro* and *in vivo* features of native RBC, and were also capable of transfusing a patient with *in vitro* generated erythrocytes. Notably, the same authors reported a protocol to generate RBC from hiPSC as an alternative source of HSC [114]. Other groups have described similar protocols to generate erythrocytes from hESC or hiPSC [115-118], although in all these studies the RBC generated from embryonic cells expressed embryonic and foetal hemoglobins but low levels of adult hemoglobin. Additional efforts should be done to make this possibility a therapeutic option.

6. Conclusions

Erythroid metabolic diseases are well defined and well known diseases which main symptom is CNSHA. As they are monogenic diseases that can be cured by allogeneic bone marrow transplantation, they are very good candidates to be treated by gene therapy. However, the low number of patients with poor prognosis requiring BM transplantation and the absence of an apparent selective advantage of the corrected cells over the diseased ones have made their approach for gene therapy less attractive than other erythropaties. Up to now, no gene therapy clinical trial for erythroid metabolic diseseases has been accomplished. Gene therapy attempts in animal models have been applied to G6PD and PKD with successful results, emphasizing the usefulness of a gene therapy approach for these diseases. Although adverse effects due to ectopic expression of the metabolic enzyme have not been observed, an erythroid specific expression is preferred. Many developments have been made for the specific expression of globin genes that could be adapted to vectors developed for the discussed erythroid metabolic diseases. Similarly, any attempt directed to the improvement of HSC transduction, including the possibility of *in vivo* targeted gene therapy could be applied. On the other hand, the combination of cell reprogramming and gene editing opens a new world of possibilities that could be easily applied to these diseases. hESC and hiPSC are helping in the development of the next generation of gene therapy, which implies a precise gene targeting. Gene editing by HR is the best and safest gene therapy procedure because avoids any perturbation in the targeted genome. Besides the combination of hiPSC and gene editing could be the future therapy for many genetic-based diseases. The hiPSC technology is the springboard for the development of more efficient HR protocols applicable to other types of stem cells such as hematopoietic stem cells. The combination of methods for obtaining big amounts of RBC from HSC or embryonic cells, along with the improvement of the different gene therapy approaches described in this chapter, opens up the possibility of the therapeutic application involving the infusion of RBC differentiated *in vitro* from genetically corrected patient specific stem cells.

Nomenclature

5-FU 5-fluorouracil

A1ATD-1 antitripsin deficiency

AAV Adeno-associated virus

BM Bone marrow

BPGM 2,3-bisphosphoglycerate mutase

CNSHA Chronic non spherocytic hemaolotyc anemia

DSB Double strand breaks

Env Viral envelope

FH familiar hypercholesterolemia

G6P Glucose-6-phosphate

G6PD Glucose-6-phopahate dehydrogenase

GPI Glucose phosphate isomerase

GS Glutathione synthetase

hESC human embryonic stem cell

hIF1 hypoxia-inducible factor-1

hiPSC Human induced pluripotent stem cell

HK Hexokinase

HR Homologous recombination

HS DNase I hypersensitive sites

HSC Hematopoietic stem cell

iPSC Induced pluripotent stem cell

kb kilobases

LCR Locus control region

LTR Long terminal repeats

LV Lentivirus

MN homing meganuclease

NHEJ non-homologous end joining

PFK phosphofructokinase

RBC Erythrocytes

SIN-LV Self-inactivated lentiviral vector

TALEN transcription activator-like effector nuclease

TPI Triose phosphate isomerase

WT wild-type

ZFN zinc finger nuclease

Aknowledgements

The authors thank L. Cerrato, M.A. Martín and I. Orman for their technical assistance. We would also like to thank Dr. J. Bueren for careful reading and suggestion of the manuscript. M.G.G. was partially supported by a short-term fellowship from the European Molecular Biology Organization (EMBO ASTF 188.00-2010). Z.G. is a fellowship of the PhD program of the Departamento de Educación, Universidades e Investigación del Gobierno Vasco. This work was funded by grants from the Ministerio de Economía y Competitividad (SAF2011-30526-C02-01), Fondo de Investigaciones Sanitarias (RD06/0010/0015) and the PERSIST European project. The authors also thank the Fundación Botín for promoting translational research at the Hematopoiesis and Gene Therapy Division-CIEMAT/CIBERER.

Author details

Maria Garcia-Gomez, Oscar Quintana-Bustamante, Maria Garcia-Bravo, S. Navarro, Zita Garate and Jose C. Segovia

Differentiation and Cytometry Unit, Hematopoiesis and Gene Therapy Division, Centro de Investigaciones Energéticas, Medioambientales y Tecnológicas (CIEMAT) and Centro de Investigación Biomédica en Red de Enfermedades Raras (CIBER-ER), Madrid, Spain

References

[1] Aiuti A, Bachoud-Levi AC, Blesch A, *et al.* Progress and prospects: gene therapy clinical trials (part 2). Gene Ther. 2007;14:1555-1563.

[2] Herzog RW, Cao O, Srivastava A. Two decades of clinical gene therapy success is finally mounting. Discov Med. 2010;9:105-111.

[3] Naldini L. Ex vivo gene transfer and correction for cell-based therapies. Nat Rev Genet. 2011;12:301-315.

[4] Richard E, Mendez M, Mazurier F, *et al.* Gene therapy of a mouse model of protoporphyria with a self-inactivating erythroid-specific lentiviral vector without preselection. Mol Ther. 2001;4:331-338.

[5] Rovira A, De Angioletti M, Camacho-Vanegas O, *et al.* Stable in vivo expression of glucose-6-phosphate dehydrogenase (G6PD) and rescue of G6PD deficiency in stem cells by gene transfer. Blood. 2000;96:4111-4117.

[6] Richard RE, Weinreich M, Chang KH, Ieremia J, Stevenson MM, Blau CA. Modulating erythrocyte chimerism in a mouse model of pyruvate kinase deficiency. Blood. 2004;103:4432-4439.

[7] Tani K, Yoshikubo T, Ikebuchi K, *et al.* Retrovirus-mediated gene transfer of human pyruvate kinase (PK) cDNA into murine hematopoietic cells: implications for gene therapy of human PK deficiency. Blood. 1994;83:2305-2310.

[8] Morimoto M, Kanno H, Asai H, *et al.* Pyruvate kinase deficiency of mice associated with nonspherocytic hemolytic anemia and cure of the anemia by marrow transplantation without host irradiation. Blood. 1995;86:4323-4330.

[9] Kanno H, Utsugisawa T, Aizawa S, *et al.* Transgenic rescue of hemolytic anemia due to red blood cell pyruvate kinase deficiency. Haematologica. 2007;92:731-737.

[10] Zaucha JA, Yu C, Lothrop CD, Jr., *et al.* Severe canine hereditary hemolytic anemia treated by nonmyeloablative marrow transplantation. Biol Blood Marrow Transplant. 2001;7:14-24.

[11] Meza NW, Quintana-Bustamante O, Puyet A, *et al.* In vitro and in vivo expression of human erythrocyte pyruvate kinase in erythroid cells: a gene therapy approach. Hum Gene Ther. 2007;18:502-514.

[12] Tanphaichitr VS, Suvatte V, Issaragrisil S, *et al.* Successful bone marrow transplantation in a child with red blood cell pyruvate kinase deficiency. Bone Marrow Transplant. 2000;26:689-690.

[13] Meza NW, Alonso-Ferrero ME, Navarro S, *et al.* Rescue of pyruvate kinase deficiency in mice by gene therapy using the human isoenzyme. Mol Ther. 2009;17:2000-2009.

[14] Bulliamy T, Luzzatto L, Hirono A, Beutler E. Hematologically important mutations: glucose-6-phosphate dehydrogenase. Blood Cells Mol Dis. 1997;23:302-313.

[15] Beutler E, Kuhl W, Gelbart T, Forman L. DNA sequence abnormalities of human glucose-6-phosphate dehydrogenase variants. J Biol Chem. 1991;266:4145-4150.

[16] Mason PJ, Sonati MF, MacDonald D, et al. New glucose-6-phosphate dehydrogenase mutations associated with chronic anemia. Blood. 1995;85:1377-1380.

[17] Jacobasch G, Rapoport SM. Hemolytic anemias due to erythrocyte enzyme deficiencies. Mol Aspects Med. 1996;17:143-170.

[18] Vives Corrons JL, Feliu E, Pujades MA, et al. Severe-glucose-6-phosphate dehydrogenase (G6PD) deficiency associated with chronic hemolytic anemia, granulocyte dysfunction, and increased susceptibility to infections: description of a new molecular variant (G6PD Barcelona). Blood. 1982;59:428-434.

[19] Roos D, van Zwieten R, Wijnen JT, et al. Molecular basis and enzymatic properties of glucose 6-phosphate dehydrogenase volendam, leading to chronic nonspherocytic anemia, granulocyte dysfunction, and increased susceptibility to infections. Blood. 1999;94:2955-2962.

[20] Ko CH, Li K, Li CL, et al. Development of a novel mouse model of severe glucose-6-phosphate dehydrogenase (G6PD)-deficiency for in vitro and in vivo assessment of hemolytic toxicity to red blood cells. Blood Cells Mol Dis. 2011;47:176-181.

[21] Zanella A, Fermo E, Bianchi P, Chiarelli LR, Valentini G. Pyruvate kinase deficiency: the genotype-phenotype association. Blood Rev. 2007;21:217-231.

[22] Fothergill-Gilmore LA, Michels PA. Evolution of glycolysis. Prog Biophys Mol Biol. 1993;59:105-235.

[23] Satoh H, Tani K, Yoshida MC, Sasaki M, Miwa S, Fujii H. The human liver-type pyruvate kinase (PKL) gene is on chromosome 1 at band q21. Cytogenet Cell Genet. 1988;47:132-133.

[24] Noguchi T, Yamada K, Inoue H, Matsuda T, Tanaka T. The L- and R-type isozymes of rat pyruvate kinase are produced from a single gene by use of different promoters. J Biol Chem. 1987;262:14366-14371.

[25] Guguen-Guillouzo C, Szajnert MF, Marie J, Delain D, Schapira F. Differentiation in vivo and in vitro of pyruvate kinase isozymes in rat muscle. Biochimie. 1977;59:65-71.

[26] Kanno H, Fujii H, Miwa S. Structural analysis of human pyruvate kinase L-gene and identification of the promoter activity in erythroid cells. Biochem Biophys Res Commun. 1992;188:516-523.

[27] Nakashima K, Miwa S, Fujii H, et al. Characterization of pyruvate kinase from the liver of a patient with aberrant erythrocyte pyruvate kinase, PK Nagasaki. J Lab Clin Med. 1977;90:1012-1020.

[28] Zanella A, Fermo E, Bianchi P, Valentini G. Red cell pyruvate kinase deficiency: molecular and clinical aspects. Br J Haematol. 2005;130:11-25.

[29] Beutler E, Gelbart T. Estimating the prevalence of pyruvate kinase deficiency from the gene frequency in the general white population. Blood. 2000;95:3585-3588.

[30] Diez A, Gilsanz F, Martinez J, Perez-Benavente S, Meza NW, Bautista JM. Life-threatening nonspherocytic hemolytic anemia in a patient with a null mutation in the PKLR gene and no compensatory PKM gene expression. Blood. 2005;106:1851-1856.

[31] Miwa S, Kanno H, Fujii H. Concise review: pyruvate kinase deficiency: historical perspective and recent progress of molecular genetics. Am J Hematol. 1993;42:31-35.

[32] Gilsanz F, Vega MA, Gomez-Castillo E, Ruiz-Balda JA, Omenaca F. Fetal anaemia due to pyruvate kinase deficiency. Arch Dis Child. 1993;69:523-524.

[33] Ferreira P, Morais L, Costa R, et al. Hydrops fetalis associated with erythrocyte pyruvate kinase deficiency. Eur J Pediatr. 2000;159:481-482.

[34] Zanella A, Bianchi P, Iurlo A, et al. Iron status and HFE genotype in erythrocyte pyruvate kinase deficiency: study of Italian cases. Blood Cells Mol Dis. 2001;27:653-661.

[35] Aizawa S, Kohdera U, Hiramoto M, et al. Ineffective erythropoiesis in the spleen of a patient with pyruvate kinase deficiency. Am J Hematol. 2003;74:68-72.

[36] Aisaki K, Aizawa S, Fujii H, Kanno J, Kanno H. Glycolytic inhibition by mutation of pyruvate kinase gene increases oxidative stress and causes apoptosis of a pyruvate kinase deficient cell line. Exp Hematol. 2007;35:1190-1200.

[37] Min-Oo G, Fortin A, Tam MF, Nantel A, Stevenson MM, Gros P. Pyruvate kinase deficiency in mice protects against malaria. Nat Genet. 2003;35:357-362.

[38] Lakomek M, Winkler H. Erythrocyte pyruvate kinase- and glucose phosphate isomerase deficiency: perturbation of glycolysis by structural defects and functional alterations of defective enzymes and its relation to the clinical severity of chronic hemolytic anemia. Biophys Chem. 1997;66:269-284.

[39] Merkle S, Pretsch W. Glucose-6-phosphate isomerase deficiency associated with nonspherocytic hemolytic anemia in the mouse: an animal model for the human disease. Blood. 1993;81:206-213.

[40] Hoyer JD, Allen SL, Beutler E, Kubik K, West C, Fairbanks VF. Erythrocytosis due to bisphosphoglycerate mutase deficiency with concurrent glucose-6-phosphate dehydrogenase (G-6-PD) deficiency. Am J Hematol. 2004;75:205-208.

[41] Njalsson R. Glutathione synthetase deficiency. Cell Mol Life Sci. 2005;62:1938-1945.

[42] Wu X, Li Y, Crise B, Burgess SM. Transcription start regions in the human genome are favored targets for MLV integration. Science. 2003;300:1749-1751.

[43] Modlich U, Navarro S, Zychlinski D, *et al.* Insertional transformation of hematopoietic cells by self-inactivating lentiviral and gammaretroviral vectors. Mol Ther. 2009;17:1919-1928.

[44] Montini E, Cesana D, Schmidt M, et al. Hematopoietic stem cell gene transfer in a tumor-prone mouse model uncovers low genotoxicity of lentiviral vector integration. Nat Biotechnol. 2006;24:687-696.

[45] Montini E, Cesana D, Schmidt M, *et al.* The genotoxic potential of retroviral vectors is strongly modulated by vector design and integration site selection in a mouse model of HSC gene therapy. J Clin Invest. 2009;119:964-975.

[46] Puthenveetil G, Scholes J, Carbonell D, et al. Successful correction of the human beta-thalassemia major phenotype using a lentiviral vector. Blood. 2004;104:3445-3453.

[47] Grande A, Piovani B, Aiuti A, Ottolenghi S, Mavilio F, Ferrari G. Transcriptional targeting of retroviral vectors to the erythroblastic progeny of transduced hematopoietic stem cells. Blood. 1999;93:3276-3285.

[48] Testa A, Lotti F, Cairns L, *et al.* Deletion of a negatively acting sequence in a chimeric GATA-1 enhancer-long terminal repeat greatly increases retrovirally mediated erythroid expression. J Biol Chem. 2004;279:10523-10531.

[49] Ren S, Wong BY, Li J, Luo XN, Wong PM, Atweh GF. Production of genetically stable high-titer retroviral vectors that carry a human gamma-globin gene under the control of the alpha-globin locus control region. Blood. 1996;87:2518-2524.

[50] Emery DW, Chen H, Li Q, Stamatoyannopoulos G. Development of a condensed locus control region cassette and testing in retrovirus vectors for A gamma-globin. Blood Cells Mol Dis. 1998;24:322-339.

[51] Robertson G, Garrick D, Wu W, Kearns M, Martin D, Whitelaw E. Position-dependent variegation of globin transgene expression in mice. Proc Natl Acad Sci U S A. 1995;92:5371-5375.

[52] Sharpe JA, Summerhill RJ, Vyas P, Gourdon G, Higgs DR, Wood WG. Role of upstream DNase I hypersensitive sites in the regulation of human alpha globin gene expression. Blood. 1993;82:1666-1671.

[53] Moreau-Gaudry F, Xia P, Jiang G, *et al.* High-level erythroid-specific gene expression in primary human and murine hematopoietic cells with self-inactivating lentiviral vectors. Blood. 2001;98:2664-2672.

[54] Zhu J, Kren BT, Park CW, Bilgim R, Wong PY, Steer CJ. Erythroid-specific expression of beta-globin by the sleeping beauty transposon for Sickle cell disease. Biochemistry. 2007;46:6844-6858.

[55] Nemeth MJ, Lowrey CH. An Erythroid-Specific Chromatin Opening Element Increases beta-Globin Gene Expression from Integrated Retroviral Gene Transfer Vectors. Gene Ther Mol Biol. 2004;8:475-486.

[56] May C, Rivella S, Callegari J, *et al.* Therapeutic haemoglobin synthesis in beta-thalas-
saemic mice expressing lentivirus-encoded human beta-globin. Nature.
2000;406:82-86.

[57] Pawliuk R, Westerman KA, Fabry ME, et al. Correction of sickle cell disease in transgenic mouse models by gene therapy. Science. 2001;294:2368-2371.

[58] Hanawa H, Yamamoto M, Zhao H, Shimada T, Persons DA. Optimized lentiviral
vector design improves titer and transgene expression of vectors containing the
chicken beta-globin locus HS4 insulator element. Mol Ther. 2009;17:667-674.

[59] Tan M, Qing K, Zhou S, Yoder MC, Srivastava A. Adeno-associated virus 2-mediated
transduction and erythroid lineage-restricted long-term expression of the human beta-globin gene in hematopoietic cells from homozygous beta-thalassemic mice. Mol
Ther. 2001;3:940-946.

[60] Lisowski L, Sadelain M. Current status of globin gene therapy for the treatment of
beta-thalassaemia. Br J Haematol. 2008;141:335-345.

[61] Sun FL, Elgin SC. Putting boundaries on silence. Cell. 1999;99:459-462.

[62] Zychlinski D, Schambach A, Modlich U, *et al.* Physiological promoters reduce the
genotoxic risk of integrating gene vectors. Mol Ther. 2008;16:718-725.

[63] Toscano MG, Romero Z, Munoz P, Cobo M, Benabdellah K, Martin F. Physiological
and tissue-specific vectors for treatment of inherited diseases. Gene Ther.
2011;18:117-127.

[64] Levings PP, Bungert J. The human beta-globin locus control region. Eur J Biochem.
2002;269:1589-1599.

[65] Navas PA, Peterson KR, Li Q, McArthur M, Stamatoyannopoulos G. The 5'HS4 core
element of the human beta-globin locus control region is required for high-level globin gene expression in definitive but not in primitive erythropoiesis. J Mol Biol.
2001;312:17-26.

[66] Blom van Assendelft G, Hanscombe O, Grosveld F, Greaves DR. The beta-globin
dominant control region activates homologous and heterologous promoters in a tissue-specific manner. Cell. 1989;56:969-977.

[67] Montiel-Equihua CA, Zhang L, Knight S, *et al.* The beta-Globin Locus Control Region
in Combination With the EF1alpha Short Promoter Allows Enhanced Lentiviral Vector-mediated Erythroid Gene Expression With Conserved Multilineage Activity. Mol
Ther. 2012;20:1400-1409.

[68] Sadelain M, Wang CH, Antoniou M, Grosveld F, Mulligan RC. Generation of a high-
titer retroviral vector capable of expressing high levels of the human beta-globin
gene. Proc Natl Acad Sci U S A. 1995;92:6728-6732.

[69] Sadelain M, Rivella S, Lisowski L, Samakoglu S, Riviere I. Globin gene transfer for treatment of the beta-thalassemias and sickle cell disease. Best Pract Res Clin Haematol. 2004;17:517-534.

[70] Ramezani A, Hawley TS, Hawley RG. Lentiviral vectors for enhanced gene expression in human hematopoietic cells. Mol Ther. 2000;2:458-469.

[71] Kingsman SM, Mitrophanous K, Olsen JC. Potential oncogene activity of the woodchuck hepatitis post-transcriptional regulatory element (WPRE). Gene Ther. 2005;12:3-4.

[72] Zanta-Boussif MA, Charrier S, Brice-Ouzet A, et al. Validation of a mutated PRE sequence allowing high and sustained transgene expression while abrogating WHV-X protein synthesis: application to the gene therapy of WAS. Gene Ther. 2009;16:605-619.

[73] Johnnidis JB, Harris MH, Wheeler RT, et al. Regulation of progenitor cell proliferation and granulocyte function by microRNA-223. Nature. 2008;451:1125-1129.

[74] Takahashi K, Yamanaka S. Induction of pluripotent stem cells from mouse embryonic and adult fibroblast cultures by defined factors. Cell. 2006;126:663-676.

[75] Takahashi K, Tanabe K, Ohnuki M, et al. Induction of pluripotent stem cells from adult human fibroblasts by defined factors. Cell. 2007;131:861-872.

[76] Yu J, Vodyanik MA, Smuga-Otto K, et al. Induced pluripotent stem cell lines derived from human somatic cells. Science. 2007;318:1917-1920.

[77] Kim JB, Zaehres H, Arauzo-Bravo MJ, Scholer HR. Generation of induced pluripotent stem cells from neural stem cells. Nat Protoc. 2009;4:1464-1470.

[78] Hanna J, Markoulaki S, Schorderet P, et al. Direct reprogramming of terminally differentiated mature B lymphocytes to pluripotency. Cell. 2008;133:250-264.

[79] Rowland BD, Bernards R, Peeper DS. The KLF4 tumour suppressor is a transcriptional repressor of p53 that acts as a context-dependent oncogene. Nat Cell Biol. 2005;7:1074-1082.

[80] Meng X, Neises A, Su RJ, et al. Efficient reprogramming of human cord blood CD34+ cells into induced pluripotent stem cells with OCT4 and SOX2 alone. Mol Ther. 2012;20:408-416.

[81] Liu T, Zou G, Gao Y, et al. High Efficiency of Reprogramming CD34(+) Cells Derived from Human Amniotic Fluid into Induced Pluripotent Stem Cells with Oct4. Stem Cells Dev. 2012.

[82] Kim D, Kim CH, Moon JI, et al. Generation of human induced pluripotent stem cells by direct delivery of reprogramming proteins. Cell Stem Cell. 2009;4:472-476.

[83] Papapetrou EP, Lee G, Malani N, *et al.* Genomic safe harbors permit high beta-globin transgene expression in thalassemia induced pluripotent stem cells. Nat Biotechnol. 2010;29:73-78.

[84] Sommer CA, Sommer AG, Longmire TA, *et al.* Excision of reprogramming transgenes improves the differentiation potential of iPS cells generated with a single excisable vector. Stem Cells. 2010;28:64-74.

[85] Mali P, Chou BK, Yen J, *et al.* Butyrate greatly enhances derivation of human induced pluripotent stem cells by promoting epigenetic remodeling and the expression of pluripotency-associated genes. Stem Cells. 2010;28:713-720.

[86] Woltjen K, Hamalainen R, Kibschull M, Mileikovsky M, Nagy A. Transgene-free production of pluripotent stem cells using piggyBac transposons. Methods Mol Biol. 2011;767:87-103.

[87] Warren L, Manos PD, Ahfeldt T, *et al.* Highly efficient reprogramming to pluripotency and directed differentiation of human cells with synthetic modified mRNA. Cell Stem Cell. 2010;7:618-630.

[88] Fusaki N, Ban H, Nishiyama A, Saeki K, Hasegawa M. Efficient induction of transgene-free human pluripotent stem cells using a vector based on Sendai virus, an RNA virus that does not integrate into the host genome. Proc Jpn Acad Ser B Phys Biol Sci. 2009;85:348-362.

[89] Park IH, Arora N, Huo H, *et al.* Disease-specific induced pluripotent stem cells. Cell. 2008;134:877-886.

[90] Rashid ST, Corbineau S, Hannan N, *et al.* Modeling inherited metabolic disorders of the liver using human induced pluripotent stem cells. J Clin Invest. 2010;120:3127-3136.

[91] Wang Y, Zheng CG, Jiang Y, *et al.* Genetic correction of beta-thalassemia patient-specific iPS cells and its use in improving hemoglobin production in irradiated SCID mice. Cell Res. 2012;22:637-648.

[92] Papapetrou EP, Lee G, Malani N, *et al.* Genomic safe harbors permit high beta-globin transgene expression in thalassemia induced pluripotent stem cells. Nat Biotechnol. 2011;29:73-78.

[93] Sebastiano V, Maeder ML, Angstman JF, *et al.* In situ genetic correction of the sickle cell anemia mutation in human induced pluripotent stem cells using engineered zinc finger nucleases. Stem Cells. 2011;29:1717-1726.

[94] Zou J, Mali P, Huang X, Dowey SN, Cheng L. Site-specific gene correction of a point mutation in human iPS cells derived from an adult patient with sickle cell disease. Blood. 2011;118:4599-4608.

[95] Robbins J. Gene targeting. The precise manipulation of the mammalian genome. Circ Res. 1993;73:3-9.

[96]   Delacote F, Lopez BS. Importance of the cell cycle phase for the choice of the appro-priate DSB repair pathway, for genome stability maintenance: the trans-S double-strand break repair model. Cell Cycle. 2008;7:33-38.

[97]   Song H, Chung SK, Xu Y. Modeling disease in human ESCs using an efficient BAC-based homologous recombination system. Cell Stem Cell. 2010;6:80-89.

[98]   Khan IF, Hirata RK, Wang PR, et al. Engineering of human pluripotent stem cells by AAV-mediated gene targeting. Mol Ther. 2010;18:1192-1199.

[99]   Lombardo A, Genovese P, Beausejour CM, et al. Gene editing in human stem cells us-ing zinc finger nucleases and integrase-defective lentiviral vector delivery. Nat Bio-technol. 2007;25:1298-1306.

[100] Gabriel R, Lombardo A, Arens A, et al. An unbiased genome-wide analysis of zinc-finger nuclease specificity. Nat Biotechnol. 2011;29:816-823.

[101] Pattanayak V, Ramirez CL, Joung JK, Liu DR. Revealing off-target cleavage specifici-ties of zinc-finger nucleases by in vitro selection. Nat Methods. 2011;8:765-770.

[102] Hockemeyer D, Soldner F, Beard C, et al. Efficient targeting of expressed and silent genes in human ESCs and iPSCs using zinc-finger nucleases. Nat Biotechnol. 2009;27:851-857.

[103] Hockemeyer D, Wang H, Kiani S, et al. Genetic engineering of human pluripotent cells using TALE nucleases. Nat Biotechnol. 2011;29:731-734.

[104] Zavada J. VSV pseudotype particles with the coat of avian myeloblastosis virus. Nat New Biol. 1972;240:122-124.

[105] Cronin J, Zhang XY, Reiser J. Altering the tropism of lentiviral vectors through pseu-dotyping. Curr Gene Ther. 2005;5:387-398.

[106] Waehler R, Russell SJ, Curiel DT. Engineering targeted viral vectors for gene therapy. Nat Rev Genet. 2007;8:573-587.

[107] Peled A, Petit I, Kollet O, et al. Dependence of human stem cell engraftment and re-population of NOD/SCID mice on CXCR4. Science. 1999;283:845-848.

[108] Yang L, Bailey L, Baltimore D, Wang P. Targeting lentiviral vectors to specific cell types in vivo. Proc Natl Acad Sci U S A. 2006;103:11479-11484.

[109] Joo KI, Wang P. Visualization of targeted transduction by engineered lentiviral vec-tors. Gene Ther. 2008;15:1384-1396.

[110] Lei Y, Joo KI, Wang P. Engineering fusogenic molecules to achieve targeted transduc-tion of enveloped lentiviral vectors. J Biol Eng. 2009;3:8.

[111] Relander T, Johansson M, Olsson K, et al. Gene transfer to repopulating human CD34+ cells using amphotropic-, GALV-, or RD114-pseudotyped HIV-1-based vec-tors from stable producer cells. Mol Ther. 2005;11:452-459.

[112] Di Nunzio F, Piovani B, Cosset FL, Mavilio F, Stornaiuolo A. Transduction of human hematopoietic stem cells by lentiviral vectors pseudotyped with the RD114-TR chimeric envelope glycoprotein. Hum Gene Ther. 2007;18:811-820.

[113] Frecha C, Costa C, Negre D, *et al.* A novel lentiviral vector targets gene transfer into human hematopoietic stem cells in marrow from patients with bone marrow failure syndrome and in vivo in humanized mice. Blood. 2011;119:1139-1150.

[114] Lapillonne H, Kobari L, Mazurier C, *et al.* Red blood cell generation from human induced pluripotent stem cells: perspectives for transfusion medicine. Haematologica. 2010;95:1651-1659.

[115] Lu SJ, Feng Q, Park JS, *et al.* Biologic properties and enucleation of red blood cells from human embryonic stem cells. Blood. 2008;112:4475-4484.

[116] Ma F, Ebihara Y, Umeda K, *et al.* Generation of functional erythrocytes from human embryonic stem cell-derived definitive hematopoiesis. Proc Natl Acad Sci U S A. 2008;105:13087-13092.

[117] Hatzistavrou T, Micallef SJ, Ng ES, Vadolas J, Stanley EG, Elefanty AG. ErythRED, a hESC line enabling identification of erythroid cells. Nat Methods. 2009;6:659-662.

[118] Dias J, Gumenyuk M, Kang H, *et al.* Generation of red blood cells from human induced pluripotent stem cells. Stem Cells Dev. 2011;20:1639-1647.

Targeting the Lung: Challenges in Gene Therapy for Cystic Fibrosis

George Kotzamanis, Athanassios Kotsinas,
Apostolos Papalois and Vassilis G. Gorgoulis

Additional information is available at the end of the chapter

1. Introduction

Cystic Fibrosis (CF) is the most common fatal autosomal recessive genetic disease in the Caucasians with a frequency of approximately 1 in 2500 newborns (Cystic Fibrosis Foundation, http://www.cff.org/). It affects several organs including the lungs, the liver, the pancreas, the sweat glands and the gastrointestinal and reproductive tracts [1]. The most severe complications that finally lead to death are those in the airway epithelium [2]. Continuous secretion of mucus causes blockage of the lungs by thick sputum and also makes the lungs susceptible to secondary bacterial infections. Subsequent inflammatory responses by the immune system damage the lungs and the combination of all these factors leads to cardiac failure and to death [3].

The primary defect at the biochemical level that is responsible for the symptoms in the lung was found to involve cAMP-mediated chloride ion (Cl⁻) conductance. Specifically, mutations in the gene that encodes a cAMP-regulated Cl⁻ channel in the apical membrane of epithelial cells are the cause of cystic fibrosis. This gene was identified, cloned and named the Cystic Fibrosis Transmembrane conductance Regulator (CFTR) [4, 5]. Though the exact mechanism of pathogenesis is not fully confirmed, the prevailing theory supports that absence or dramatic decrease in the amount of functional CFTR protein at the airways epithelium results in reduced chloride secretion, increased sodium reabsorption and therefore in insufficient airway luminal fluid due to osmosis [6]. These alterations in the respiratory epithelium subsequently result in deficient mucus clearance which determines chronic cycles of bacterial infections and inflammation [6]. In addition, the formation of thick stationary mucus traps neutrophils that might otherwise clear the infection [7].

For several reasons including the easy access to the respiratory tract without any intervention procedures, the cloning and the characterization of the *CFTR* gene and the expectation that even relatively low levels of expression of the gene may have a therapeutic outcome [8], Cystic Fibrosis became an ideal target for gene therapy and an example for gene therapy of other lung diseases. Indeed, the first gene therapy clinical trials for CF started in 1993 and 29 clinical trials have been conducted since then (http://www.wiley.com/legacy/wileychi/genmed/clinical/). Several trials have demonstrated gene transfer and transgene expression. In some cases, low levels of transient correction of Cl⁻ ion transport deficiency has been observed but overall, no clinical improvement has been achieved. The histological, immunological and intracellular barriers that exist in the lung have proven to be more difficult to overcome than what was initially thought. The purpose of this chapter is to analyze these barriers and to present the challenges the gene therapist is faced with when targeting the lung for the treatment of CF.

First, the basic histology of the lung will be described so that the reader can identify the potential target cells for CF gene therapy and realize the complexity of the lung structures that the gene transfer agent needs to penetrate in order to reach these target cells.

2. Basic histology of the lung

The lung is a complex organ that is divided into the air-conducting portion consisting of the trachea, the bronchi and the bronchioles and the respiratory portion consisting of the alveoli, which is the place of gas exchange (Figure 1).

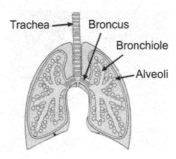

Figure 1. Schematic illustration of the lung.

The trachea and most of the bronchi are covered by pseudostratified columnar ciliated epithelium (known as the respiratory epithelium). Columnar ciliated cells are the predominant population extending from the basal lamina to the airway lumen. Other cells facing the lumen are the nonciliated Goblet cells which produce mucin polymers [9], forming a thin layer of mucus that covers the airway epithelium. The role of the airway mucus is to trap inhaled particles which are then transferred out of the lung by cilia beating and/or cough. The effectiveness of this action depends on the viscosity of the mucus which is determined by the level of its hydration [10]. Normal airway mucus consists of 97% water [11] but when luminal fluid is reduced, as in CF, the clearance of mucus by cilia and cough is also reduced. Under the basal lamina lies the lamina propria, which consists of elastic fibers and hosts the submucosal glands that together with the Goblet cells produce components of the mucus [9] (Figure 2A,B,C).

Several stem cells populations responsible for the maintenance of the respiratory epithelium have been identified in the lung. Specifically, a population of basal cells, residing at close proximity to the underlying basal lamina in the larger airways, has been shown to have a high multipotency potential allowing regulation of the epithelium homeostasis under normal circumstances or after injury [12]. Another type of cells with stem-cell-like properties is the Clara cells. These nonciliated cells are located at the terminal bronchioles and produce a solution similar to the surfactant in the alveoli. Interestingly, Clara cells can multiply and differentiate into ciliated cells to regenerate the bronchiolar epithelium [13].

The respiratory portion of each lung consists of approximately 300 million alveoli. Each alveolus has a thin wall consisting mainly of type I and type II alveolar cells (Figure 2D). Type II alveolar cells are responsible for the secretion of a thin layer of fluid that normally coats the alveolar surface in order to decrease the surface tension at the air-fluid interface, the surfactant. Surfactant turnover is mediated by the phagocytic function of alveolar macrophages, which are also located in the alveolar wall and are frequently seen in the alveolar lumen.

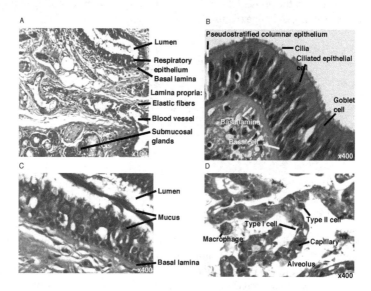

Figure 2. A) Upper respiratory tract section, B) Epithelium of upper respiratory tract, C) Mucus produced in Goblet cells and secreted in the lumen, D) Alveolar section.

It is not yet clear which of these cells are the target for gene therapy of Cystic Fibrosis. In healthy individuals there is little CFTR expression in the lung, except the submucosal glands and epithelial cells at the small airways where higher expression is observed [14]. Early studies suggested that the submucosal glands are the site of maximal CFTR expression [15], but more recent data suggested that this may be the ciliated surface epithelium of the bronchioles [16]. This uncertainty is one of the main obstacles for successful CF gene therapy. Depending on which are the cells that need to be corrected, different anatomical or immunological barriers apply and therefore different administration methods have to be used.

3. Physical barriers to gene transfer to the lung

As most formulations administered to treat CF, including gene transfer agents, are delivered directly to the airways in the form of aerosols [17], the first physical barrier that needs to be overcome before the transgene reaches the target cells is the airways mucus. Trapping in the mucus and clearance by cilia is the main factor reducing transfection efficiency in lung cells of all individuals. In Cystic Fibrosis, the lungs are progressively filled with large amounts of purulent secretions, the sputum, which consists of mucus, DNA, actin, cell debris and inflammatory cells [18]. The most commonly used in gene therapy for CF viral vectors and non-viral liposomal vectors have been proven unable to penetrate the CF sputum [19, 20], suggesting that effective treatment may be achieved only at early stages of the disease before the lungs are filled with sputum [21]. Several improvements can be made at this stage to increase transfection efficiency, such as use of methylcellulose gel formulations to inhibit mucociliary clearance [22] or of mucolytics [23, 24], but these need to be validated in clinical trials.

The second physical barrier to gene transfer to the airway epithelium is the composition of the apical surface of the cells. First, the presence of specific receptors determines the kind of viral vector to be used. For example, adenoviral vectors have low transfection efficiency due to the low abundance of the required receptors on the apical side of most human airway epithelial cells [25] and this is one of the reasons why they are not considered in clinical trials any more [21]. Making the basolateral membrane, which is more abundant in adenoviral receptors [25], accessible to the adenoviral vector has been proposed as an attractive alternative. Indeed, the use of agents such as sodium caprate that can cause transient dissociation of tight junctions, impressively increases transgene delivery and expression in animal models [26, 27] but may not have a clinical application due to the risk of systemic bacterial invasion. Second, the glycocalyx on the apical membrane seems to interfere with the interaction between adenovirus and its few receptors [28]. Removal of sialic acid residues from the glycocalyx by pretreatment with neuraminidase may be an effective way to overcome this physical barrier [28].

Although non-viral vectors are not affected by the problems described above, they are subject to possible destruction by the cell defence mechanisms against foreign DNA invasion.

These mechanisms have evolved to secure the host cell's genetic integrity but in gene therapy they constitute one more hurdle to overcome. Indeed, once the therapeutic DNA enters the target cells in the lung of CF patients, it faces a series of intra-cellular barriers that apply to gene therapy in general and not just to gene therapy for CF. These barriers include degradation by cytosolic nucleases [29, 30] and degradation inside digestive lysozomes formed by transformation of endosomes following endocytosis [31]. Several methods have been implemented so that the transgene can escape the endosomes after internalization. Cationic lipids and polycationic polymers like polyethylenimine (PEI) [32] utilised as chemical vectors in complexes with the transfected DNA, protect it from nucleases and enable it to escape the endosomes. Such complexes carrying the *CFTR* gene have been used to correct the ion transport defect in CF transgenic mice [33] and are currently being tested in clinical practice [34]. Other strategies to protect the therapeutic DNA from the endosomes and therefore to increase the transfection efficiency include the use of pharmacological endosomelytic agents such as chloroquine [35], endosome-disrupting peptides [36-38] and glycerol [39]. All these aim at destabilizing the endosomal membrane so that the contents are released intact to the cytosol but may be of limited clinical value due to safety concerns in the host cells.

The final physical barrier before the *CFTR* transgene enters the nucleus of the non-dividing airway epithelial cells and undergoes transcription is the nuclear envelope [40]. Many viral vectors can efficiently deliver their cargo in the nucleus by exploiting the nuclear transport systems of the host [41], but non-viral vectors are in most cases ineffective in front of the nuclear envelope. Strategies such as the use of chemical vectors based on PEI [42] and of Nuclear Localization Signals (NLS) which are integrated into the transfected DNA and bind to transporter proteins in order to facilitate nuclear entry [43, 44] have been implemented and found to promote nuclear delivery *in vitro*. However, these have not been validated with large therapeutic genes like the *CFTR* and in non-dividing cells *in vivo* and may not be of use for gene therapy for CF [45].

4. Immunological barriers to gene transfer to the lung

Apart from the extracellular and intracellular barriers described above, there is a second line of defence consisting of specific and non-specific immune responses that protect the lung cells against foreign particles which are present in the air. During gene therapy for CF, these immunological mechanisms can be activated by the vector carrying the transgene or the product of the transgene and therefore limit the overall efficacy [46].

Various immunological responses are directed against the carrier of the therapeutic gene before this enters the target cells. Pulmonary macrophages have been shown to ingest adenoviral vectors, but when they were removed before transfection, an increase in transgene expression was observed [47]. Furthermore, humoral immune responses mediated by helper T lymphocytes result in the production of neutralizing antibodies against the vector, which restricts the possibility of re-administration and so, the use of most viral vectors for the treatment of chronic diseases such as CF [46].

Other responses are initiated after the transgene is delivered to the lung cells. Particularly when viral vectors are used, cellular immune responses mediated by cytotoxic T lymphocytes eliminate transduced cells expressing viral proteins resulting in parallel loss of transgene expression [46]. Although in theory non-viral vectors are not associated to such problems as they are less immunogenic than viral vectors, in practice they are usually used in combination with ligands so that they overcome the physical barriers described above and this can provoke immunological reactions similar to those caused by viral vectors [46]. In addition, viral and non-viral vectors can provoke the release of host cytokines which have been shown to inhibit expression of the gene delivered if this is driven by a common viral promoter [48].

Several approaches have been developed to overcome the immunological barriers in the lung. The use of immunosuppressant drugs such as cyclophosphamide have been proved very effective in mice allowing both prolonged transgene expression and repeated administration of an adenoviral vector [49]. Similar results were obtained with corticoid steroids such as dexamethasone [50] and budesonide [51] which were found to decrease inflammation mediated by viral vectors. Other strategies include the co-administration of IL-12 [52] and blockade of CD4+ T cells [53-56]. However, all these approaches are likely to cause more damage than benefit, considering that the lungs of CF patients are colonized by pathogenic bacteria, and so they are not applicable in the clinical setting.

On the other hand, non-viral chemical vectors based on cationic lipids can be re-administered without the need to be combined with immunosuppressants [57]. From that aspect, these are safer than viral vectors for gene therapy of CF but still not absolutely harmless as they have been associated with lung toxicity due to provocation of inflammation [58]. Another mediator of inflammation in the lung can be the CpG motifs on the bacterial plasmid DNA which is usually used to clone the therapeutic gene in non-viral gene therapy [59, 60]. Unlike eukaryotic DNA, this dinucleotide is relatively unmethylated in bacteria and can be inflammatory through recognition by toll-like receptor 9 on B cells [61]. As methylation of the CpG motifs prior to gene delivery may decrease the expression of the transgene, the exclusion of any bacteria-derived DNA from the therapeutic construct is a more promising alternative.

5. Safety concerns

Immunological responses elicited by a gene therapy vector do not only pose a barrier to efficient delivery and expression of the therapeutic gene in the target cells but more importantly, they can raise very serious safety issues. This lesson has been learned from a gene therapy human trial where lethal complications were experienced [62]. In that study, an adenoviral vector containing the cDNA of the gene encoding ornithine transcarbamylase (OTC) was administered to 18 patients with partial OTC deficiency, a disease caused by a defect in urea synthesis. The adenoviral vector provoked immunologic and other side effects, such as fever, myalgia and nausea in 17 out of the 18 participants but the 18th patient developed a serious immune response to the vector that eventually led to his death 98 hours after administration [62]. This death was a setback for all gene therapy clinical studies using viral vectors, as human immune responses cannot be predicted pre-clinically. Apart from the immunological responses caused by the vector, other unfortunate events of different nature have also been found to be associated with reduced safety. Treatment of patients with X-linked severe combined immune deficiency (SCIDX1) using a retroviral vector carrying the γc gene resulted in the correction of the disease and huge enthusiasm about the future of gene therapy [63]. However, two of the cured patients developed a leukemia-like condition 2-3 years later due to disruption of an endogenous oncogene by integration of the vector [64, 65]. Since vector integration is usually random and uncontrollable, insertional mutagenesis is a general problem that all integrating vectors have. As these problems also apply to most vectors used in gene therapy for Cystic Fibrosis, avoiding unwanted immune response and insertional mutagenesis are two major challenges for the genetic treatment of CF. Strategies to respond to the second challenge of insertional mutagenesis will be discussed in the next section. To address the first problem, the solution is to use less immunogenic vectors.

Although adenoviral vectors administered systemically can cause acute and potentially life-threatening cytokine response [66] their local administration at mild doses to nose and lung tissues did not result in such unacceptable safety profile [34]. However, extensive use of these vectors during the early times of CF gene therapy has shown that cellular and humoral immune responses against the virus are generated and these limit repeated administration [67, 68]. Another approach to avoid immunologic reactions from the host is to coat the virus capsid with polyethylene glycol (PEG). Such PEGylated viruses, called "stealth viruses", are not recognised by the immune system and can significantly prolong transgene expression [69]. A less immunogenic alternative to adenoviral constructs is the use of adeno-associated virus (AAV) vectors. Indeed, several human CF trials with AAV vectors have confirmed their good safety profile albeit with low transduction efficiency [70-74].

Despite significant progress made towards the generation of safer viral vectors [75], non-viral synthetic vectors containing only human DNA sequences are the vectors of choice when safety is considered as first priority. These vectors generally consist of the therapeutic DNA either naked or mixed with chemical compounds, like cationic lipids or cationic polymers [76]. Naked DNA is in theory the safest gene therapy agent but very difficult to be introduced into the target cells. Several physical methods have been developed to facilitate DNA entry into the lung of living animals, such as the use of electrical pulses (electroporation) [77], of ultrasound waves (sonoporation) [78] and of magnetic fields (magnetofection) [79] but none of them has reached the clinical use yet. On the other hand, chemical carriers have rapidly been developed and used in 6% (n=110) of gene therapy clinical trials (http://www.wiley.com/legacy/wileychi/genmed/clinical). These act by forming complexes with the negatively charged DNA. The complexes condense the DNA, protect it from nucleases, allow its entry into the cells and protect it from the endosomes [80]. Indeed, local administration of cationic lipid/CFTR-plasmid-DNA complexes in an aerosol formulation to the lungs of cystic fibrosis transgenic mice resulted in correction of the ion transport defect [33]. Similar studies in human patients demonstrated some transgene expression, but not at sufficient levels to provide a clinical benefit [57, 81-86].

6. Duration of transgene expression

Provided that all obstacles to gene delivery to the lung are overcome and the *CFTR* transgene finally reaches the target cells, a clinical benefit for CF can only be achieved by lifelong expression of the gene. As repeated administration is in most cases restricted by immune responses generated by the patient against the vector, other strategies have been employed for efficient retention and long-term expression.

Integration into the host genome has widely been used in gene therapy to fulfil this requirement. However, the dangers of integration due to insertional mutagenesis have become a widely publicised issue as a result of the SCIDX1 clinical trial, where some patients developed leukaemia due to deregulation of the growth-promoting LIM domain only 2 (LMO2) proto-oncogene caused by integration of the vector [64, 65]. The safety concerns regarding uncontrolled integration of the therapeutic gene into the host genome have been strengthened by observations that there is a preference of integrating vectors for the regulatory regions of transcriptionally active genes [87]. Given the need for long-term expression and the problems associated with vector integration, vectors that persist in the nucleus by being maintained episomally without integrating, could be highly advantageous. Among the systems developed to achieve extra-chromosomal maintenance of the vectors carrying the therapeutic gene, two are considered safe enough for clinical application in the future: artificial chromosomes and systems based on scaffold/matrix attachment region (S/MAR).

Human Artificial Chromosomes (HACs) are vectors able to replicate and segregate in parallel with the endogenous chromosomes in human cells. To achieve this, they must contain the minimal elements required for chromosome function, namely an origin of replication, telomeres and centromeres [88]. HACs can be generated by a method similar to the one applied for YAC construction in yeast and involves assembling the functional chromosomal elements and building up a HAC *de novo* in human cells. Different strategies have been followed to generate *de novo* HACs, the most convenient of which is to transfect a BAC carrying only a large array of α-satellite (alphoid) DNA and some marker genes into HT1080 cells[89]. HACs generated this way exist as single (or low copy) chromosomes in the nucleus and have a high mitotic stability (close to 100%) in the absence of selection. The potential use of these vectors in gene therapy has been demonstrated by expression of large therapeutic genes from them [90, 91].

S/MARs are diverse sequences found in all eukaryotic genomes where they are involved in many aspects of chromatin function such as organization of chromatin into loops, which seems to be mediated by the interaction between S/MARs and the nuclear matrix [92]. Vectors containing an S/MAR element have the ability to remain episomally at low copy number for more than 100 generations in the absence of selection and with a mitotic stability of 98% [93]. This ability has been demonstrated in several cell lines and in primary cells [94] and also *in vivo* in genetically modified pigs [95] making them very attractive for use in CF clinical trials.

An alternative to the use of episomal vectors described above, that still satisfies both requirements for permanent transgene expression and elimination of genotoxic effects is the controlled integration of the therapeutic DNA at a specific site in the host genome where no active genes are present. Several vector systems have been developed to achieve this, with each one of them having its own limitations [96]. From these, vectors based on the ΦC31 integrase [97] and on transposase enzymes [98] are the most promising for use in CF gene therapy as they have a preference for specific sequences that already exist in the human genome and have been shown to work *in vivo*.

An additional problem to achieving long-term expression of the *CFTR* transgene delivered to the lung is the life span of the target cells. Depending on the rhythm of natural turnover of these cells, transgene expression can last for as long as these cells are alive. A more effective approach would be to either target putative stem cells with the capacity to differentiate to airway epithelial cells [34] or to deliver exogenous heterologous or corrected autologous stem cells to the lungs of CF patients *ex vivo* [99].

Airway basal stem cells are a candidate target for CF stem cell therapy. However, the facts that this population is estimated to represent only a minor part of the total airway epithelium [12] and that it is quite inaccessible as it is not exposed to the airway lumen make such a therapy approach very challenging.

Ex vivo gene therapy using stem cells may not only provide permanent cure without the need for re-administration, but also solve the hurdle of the low *in vivo* gene delivery efficiency. In *ex vivo* cell therapy using Embryonic Stem Cells or foetal Mesenchymal Stem Cells from a healthy embryo there is no need for transfection of a therapeutic gene. However, these stem cells are used in an allogeneic fashion which requires the parallel use of immunosuppressive drugs and are therefore not applicable for the treatment of CF. A more attractive strategy would be the transfer of the *CFTR* gene to patient-derived autologous stem cells such as Mesenchymal Stem Cells (MSCs), which can easily be isolated from the bone marrow or adipose tissue of adults [100] or Induced Pluripotent Stem Cells that can be generated by reprogramming of adult somatic cells [101, 102]. In that case, the transfection procedure would be performed *in vitro* before reimplantation of the cells back to the donor, which is far more efficient than *in vivo* delivery. Furthermore, bone marrow-derived MSCs have been shown to be able to express transgenes [103] and to differentiate to several types of cells including airway epithelial cells [104]. Nevertheless, there is little literature on how the *ex vivo* corrected MSCs can be administered and engrafted in the lung of Cystic Fibrosis patients. Both systemic and topical lung administration of bone marrow-derived cells have been applied and shown to result in some engraftment into the airways [105], but there are several challenges to be addressed, before *ex vivo* cell therapy becomes part of the CF clinical research. These challenges include the very low efficiency of engraftment (<1%) and the fact that previous damage to the surface epithelium caused by epithelia-injuring reagents seems to be required for the engraftment [75].

7. Pattern of transgene expression

For gene therapy of some diseases it is important to achieve expression of the therapeutic gene at specific levels. Expression at lower levels than normal might not be sufficient to correct the defect and at higher levels could result in undesirable effects. In other cases, tissue-specific expression may be very important. The elements responsible for controlled and tissue-specific expression of a gene usually lie within the introns and the sequences before and after the gene. Therefore, the use of genomic constructs which contain the introns and flanking DNA of the therapeutic gene is expected to be more effective than that of mini-gene/cDNA constructs in gene therapy for certain genetic diseases where precise levels of the gene product are required [88]. There is evidence that CF is such a disease.

Although some studies have shown that expression of as little as 5-10% of endogenous *CFTR* levels may suffice to observe a clinical benefit [106], other studies have shown that different functions of CFTR like Cl⁻ transport and Na⁺ absorption, when they are abnormal they can be restored by different levels of *CFTR* expression [107]. Moreover, restoration of mucus transport at normal rates requires transduction of at least 25% of target cells [108]. These data indicate that CF gene therapy may require *CFTR* expression at the right levels, at the right time and in the right population of cells, which can be achieved only if it is driven and controlled by the gene's natural promoter and regulatory elements present on a genomic therapeutic construct.

The *CFTR* gene is located on chromosome 7, is 200-250 kb long [5] and comprises 27 exons. It shows a tightly regulated temporal and spatial pattern of expression [109, 110], which was not found to be regulated by any tissue-specific regulatory elements, suggesting that other elements outside the proximal promoter are probably involved in tissue specific regulation of transcription. Several DNase I Hypersensitive Sites (DHS), usually associated with regulation of transcription, have been identified across 400 kb of DNA flanking the *CFTR* gene. These lie 5' to the gene at -79.5 and -20.9 kb with respect to the translation start site [111], in introns 1 [112], 2, 3, 10, 16, 17a, 18, 20 and 21 [113] and 3' to the gene at +5.4, +6.8, +7, +7.4 and +15.6 kb [114]. Most of these DHS have been found to be involved in tissue-specific *CFTR* expression [114-117]. Therefore, a large genomic construct spanning ~300 kb from the -79.5 kb to the +15.6 kb DHS would include all the known long-range controlling elements of the *CFTR* gene and should give full levels of tissue specific expression which would be advantageous for gene therapy of cystic fibrosis. This big in size region has recently been cloned on a single Bacterial Artificial Chromosome (BAC) vector and is currently available [118].

As the majority of recombinant viruses, commonly utilized as carriers for transfer of plasmid DNA, apart from evoking unwanted immune responses, have a maximum packaging capacity and cannot be used to deliver large genomic-DNA-containing constructs, gene therapy using genomic loci of therapeutic genes should be non-viral. This restriction raises again the issue of efficiency of delivery which is even more challenging to deal with than when using smaller constructs.

8. Clinical research for cystic fibrosis

Gene therapy clinical trials for CF started in 1993 and over 26 viral and non-viral trials have been conducted or are in progress to date. Viral trials were based on engineered adenovirus and adeno-associated virus and non-viral on various cationic lipids, with GL67 being the most predominant. The references for the published studies are listed in Table 1.

Adenoviral clinical trials	AAV clinical trials	Non-viral clinical trials using cationic lipids
Zabner et. al., 1993 [119]	Wagner et. al., 1999 [120]	Sorcher et. al., 1994 [121]
Crystal et. al., 1994 [122]	Aitken et. al., 2001 [70]	Caplen et. al., 1995 [82]
Boucher et. al., 1994 [123]	Wagner et. al., 2002 [74]	Gill et. al., 1997 [83]
Knowles et. al., 1995 [124]	Flotte et. al., 2003 [71]	Porteous et. al., 1997 [84]
Hay et. al., 1995 [125]	Moss et. al., 2004 [73]	Zabner et. al., 1997 [86]
Zabner et. al., 1996 [68]	Moss et. al., 2007 [72]	Alton et. al. 1999 [81]
Bellon et. al., 1997 [126]		Hyde et. al., 2000 [57]
Harvey et. al., 1999 [67]		Noone et. al., 2000 [127]
Zuckerman et. al., 1999 [128]		Ruiz et. al., 2001 [85]
Joseph et. al., 2001 [129]		
Perricone et. al., 2001 [130]		

Table 1. List of CF gene therapy clinical trials.

The trials have confirmed several of the safety concerns associated to the use of viral vectors. However, other challenges and questions raised pre-clinically still remain to be answered. In general, proof-of-principle for gene transfer to the airways has been demonstrated by transgene expression or partial correction of the Cl⁻ transport defect in some of the trials but clinically meaningful outcomes such as improvement in pulmonary function and decrease of bacterial colonies have not been clearly shown in any. In contrast, poor results with regards to clinical benefit, obtained so far, revealed another challenge in CF clinical research. This is the need to develop more accurate tools to assess gene transfer efficacy at the clinical level [34].

Historically, adenoviral vectors were the first to be used. However, due to the absence of adenoviral receptors on the apical side of most human airway epithelial cells [25], which results in low transduction efficiency, and due to induction of immune responses that exclude repeated administration [67, 68], adeno-associated viral vectors became an alternative. These vectors were soon found to have their own problems. First it is their small packaging capacity which barely holds the whole human *CFTR* gene and therefore restricts the use of strong promoters. Then, at least serotype 2 AAV vectors that were used in initial studies could not be re-administered due to stimulation of immune reactions [72, 73]. Suggestions made to overcome these limitations still need to be validated in humans. Non-viral vectors were found compatible with repeated administration [57], but their efficiency were variable and transgene expression was shown only in some studies. In addition, flu-like symptoms were reported [81, 85], which were associated to the presence of unmethylated CpG motifs on the plasmid DNA that was delivered. The use of genomic constructs containing only human DNA may overcome this limitation but this also needs to be shown in future clinical trials.

9. Conclusion

Almost 20 years have passed since the beginning of gene therapy trials for CF. Despite initial enthusiasm, only little progress has been made during that time. In contrast, the main conclusion was that the lung is more difficult to target than initially anticipated. Several barriers were discovered, which led to the development of respective ways to overcome them. The majority of these have not reached the level of validation in clinical trials yet. For example, the use of a non-viral vector with the ability to remain extra-chromosomally containing the whole genomic region of the *CFTR* gene or *ex vivo* stem cell therapy, are two promising approaches that need to be further explored and may be seen in clinical trials in the future.

Acknowledgements

AK and VG are financially supported from the European Commission FP7 project INsPiRE. The authors would also like to thank Dr. Ioannis Pateras for his kind gift of Figure 2.

Author details

George Kotzamanis[1], Athanassios Kotsinas[1], Apostolos Papalois[2] and Vassilis G. Gorgoulis[1]

1 University of Athens, Medical School, Greece

2 Experimental Research Center ELPEN SA, Greece

References

[1] Grubb BR, Boucher RC. Pathophysiology of gene-targeted mouse models for cystic fibrosis. Physiol Rev 1999;79(1 Suppl):S193-214.

[2] Welsh MJ, Smith JJ. cAMP stimulation of HCO3- secretion across airway epithelia. JOP 2001;2(4 Suppl):291-3.

[3]   Boucher RC. An overview of the pathogenesis of cystic fibrosis lung disease. Adv Drug Deliv Rev 2002;54(11):1359-71.

[4]   Riordan JR, Rommens JM, Kerem B, Alon N, Rozmahel R, Grzelczak Z, et al. Identification of the cystic fibrosis gene: cloning and characterization of complementary DNA. Science 1989;245(4922):1066-73.

[5]   Rommens JM, Iannuzzi MC, Kerem B, Drumm ML, Melmer G, Dean M, et al. Identification of the cystic fibrosis gene: chromosome walking and jumping. Science 1989;245(4922):1059-65.

[6]   Clunes MT, Boucher RC. Cystic Fibrosis: The Mechanisms of Pathogenesis of an Inherited Lung Disorder. Drug Discov Today Dis Mech 2007;4(2):63-72.

[7]   Lyczak JB, Cannon CL, Pier GB. Lung infections associated with cystic fibrosis. Clin Microbiol Rev 2002;15(2):194-222.

[8]   Dorin JR, Farley R, Webb S, Smith SN, Farini E, Delaney SJ, et al. A demonstration using mouse models that successful gene therapy for cystic fibrosis requires only partial gene correction. Gene Ther 1996;3(9):797-801.

[9]   Mrsny RJ. Lessons from nature: "Pathogen-Mimetic" systems for mucosal nano-medicines. Adv Drug Deliv Rev 2009;61(2):172-92.

[10] Lai SK, Wang YY, Wirtz D, Hanes J. Micro- and macrorheology of mucus. Adv Drug Deliv Rev 2009;61(2):86-100.

[11] Cu Y, Saltzman WM. Mathematical modeling of molecular diffusion through mucus. Adv Drug Deliv Rev 2009;61(2):101-14.

[12] Rock JR, Randell SH, Hogan BL. Airway basal stem cells: a perspective on their roles in epithelial homeostasis and remodeling. Dis Model Mech 2010;3(9-10):545-56.

[13] Evans MJ, Cabral-Anderson LJ, Freeman G. Role of the Clara cell in renewal of the bronchiolar epithelium. Lab Invest 1978;38(6):648-53.

[14] Engelhardt JF, Zepeda M, Cohn JA, Yankaskas JR, Wilson JM. Expression of the cystic fibrosis gene in adult human lung. J Clin Invest 1994;93(2):737-49.

[15] Engelhardt JF, Yankaskas JR, Ernst SA, Yang Y, Marino CR, Boucher RC, et al. Submucosal glands are the predominant site of CFTR expression in the human bronchus. Nat Genet 1992;2(3):240-8.

[16] Kreda SM, Mall M, Mengos A, Rochelle L, Yankaskas J, Riordan JR, et al. Characterization of wild-type and deltaF508 cystic fibrosis transmembrane regulator in human respiratory epithelia. Mol Biol Cell 2005;16(5):2154-67.

[17] Proesmans M, Vermeulen F, De Boeck K. What's new in cystic fibrosis? From treating symptoms to correction of the basic defect. Eur J Pediatr 2008 Aug;167(8):839-49.

[18] Rubin BK. Mucus, phlegm, and sputum in cystic fibrosis. Respir Care 2009;54(6): 726-32; discussion 32.

[19] Hida K, Lai SK, Suk JS, Won SY, Boyle MP, Hanes J. Common gene therapy viral vectors do not efficiently penetrate sputum from cystic fibrosis patients. PLoS One 2011;6(5):e19919.

[20] Sanders NN, Van Rompaey E, De Smedt SC, Demeester J. Structural alterations of gene complexes by cystic fibrosis sputum. Am J Respir Crit Care Med 2001;164(3): 486-93.

[21] Griesenbach U, Geddes DM, Alton EW. Gene therapy for cystic fibrosis: an example for lung gene therapy. Gene Ther 2004;11 Suppl 1:S43-50.

[22] Sinn PL, Shah AJ, Donovan MD, McCray PB, Jr. Viscoelastic gel formulations enhance airway epithelial gene transfer with viral vectors. Am J Respir Cell Mol Biol 2005;32(5):404-10.

[23] Ferrari S, Kitson C, Farley R, Steel R, Marriott C, Parkins DA, et al. Mucus altering agents as adjuncts for nonviral gene transfer to airway epithelium. Gene Ther 2001;8(18):1380-6.

[24] Kushwah R, Oliver JR, Cao H, Hu J. Nacystelyn enhances adenoviral vector-mediated gene delivery to mouse airways. Gene Ther 2007;14(16):1243-8.

[25] Walters RW, Grunst T, Bergelson JM, Finberg RW, Welsh MJ, Zabner J. Basolateral localization of fiber receptors limits adenovirus infection from the apical surface of airway epithelia. J Biol Chem 1999;274(15):10219-26.

[26] Gregory LG, Harbottle RP, Lawrence L, Knapton HJ, Themis M, Coutelle C. Enhancement of adenovirus-mediated gene transfer to the airways by DEAE dextran and sodium caprate in vivo. Mol Ther 2003;7(1):19-26.

[27] Johnson LG, Vanhook MK, Coyne CB, Haykal-Coates N, Gavett SH. Safety and efficiency of modulating paracellular permeability to enhance airway epithelial gene transfer in vivo. Hum Gene Ther 2003;14(8):729-47.

[28] Pickles RJ, Fahrner JA, Petrella JM, Boucher RC, Bergelson JM. Retargeting the coxsackievirus and adenovirus receptor to the apical surface of polarized epithelial cells reveals the glycocalyx as a barrier to adenovirus-mediated gene transfer. J Virol 2000;74(13):6050-7.

[29] Lechardeur D, Sohn KJ, Haardt M, Joshi PB, Monck M, Graham RW, et al. Metabolic instability of plasmid DNA in the cytosol: a potential barrier to gene transfer. Gene Ther 1999;6(4):482-97.

[30] Pollard H, Toumaniantz G, Amos JL, Avet-Loiseau H, Guihard G, Behr JP, et al. Ca^{2+}-sensitive cytosolic nucleases prevent efficient delivery to the nucleus of injected plasmids. J Gene Med 2001;3(2):153-64.

[31] Dean DA, Strong DD, Zimmer WE. Nuclear entry of nonviral vectors. Gene Ther 2005;12(11):881-90.

[32] Boussif O, Lezoualc'h F, Zanta MA, Mergny MD, Scherman D, Demeneix B, et al. A versatile vector for gene and oligonucleotide transfer into cells in culture and in vivo: polyethylenimine. Proc Natl Acad Sci U S A 1995;92(16):7297-301.

[33] Hyde SC, Gill DR, Higgins CF, Trezise AE, MacVinish LJ, Cuthbert AW, et al. Correction of the ion transport defect in cystic fibrosis transgenic mice by gene therapy. Nature 1993;362(6417):250-5.

[34] Davies JC, Alton EW. Gene therapy for cystic fibrosis. Proc Am Thorac Soc 2010;7(6): 408-14.

[35] Kollen WJ, Midoux P, Erbacher P, Yip A, Roche AC, Monsigny M, et al. Gluconoylated and glycosylated polylysines as vectors for gene transfer into cystic fibrosis airway epithelial cells. Hum Gene Ther 1996;7(13):1577-86.

[36] Parente RA, Nir S, Szoka FC, Jr. Mechanism of leakage of phospholipid vesicle contents induced by the peptide GALA. Biochemistry 1990;29(37):8720-8.

[37] Wagner E, Plank C, Zatloukal K, Cotten M, Birnstiel ML. Influenza virus hemagglutinin HA-2 N-terminal fusogenic peptides augment gene transfer by transferrin-polylysine-DNA complexes: toward a synthetic virus-like gene-transfer vehicle. Proc Natl Acad Sci U S A 1992;89(17):7934-8.

[38] Wyman TB, Nicol F, Zelphati O, Scaria PV, Plank C, Szoka FC, Jr. Design, synthesis, and characterization of a cationic peptide that binds to nucleic acids and permeabilizes bilayers. Biochemistry 1997;36(10):3008-17.

[39] Zauner W, Kichler A, Schmidt W, Mechtler K, Wagner E. Glycerol and polylysine synergize in their ability to rupture vesicular membranes: a mechanism for increased transferrin-polylysine-mediated gene transfer. Exp Cell Res 1997;232(1):137-45.

[40] Lam AP, Dean DA. Progress and prospects: nuclear import of nonviral vectors. Gene Ther 2010;17(4):439-47.

[41] Whittaker GR. Virus nuclear import. Adv Drug Deliv Rev 2003 Jun 16;55(6):733-47.

[42] Pollard H, Remy JS, Loussouarn G, Demolombe S, Behr JP, Escande D. Polyethylenimine but not cationic lipids promotes transgene delivery to the nucleus in mammalian cells. J Biol Chem 1998;273(13):7507-11.

[43] Escriou V, Carriere M, Scherman D, Wils P. NLS bioconjugates for targeting therapeutic genes to the nucleus. Adv Drug Deliv Rev 2003;55(2):295-306.

[44] Hebert E. Improvement of exogenous DNA nuclear importation by nuclear localization signal-bearing vectors: a promising way for non-viral gene therapy? Biol Cell 2003;95(2):59-68.

[45] Klink D, Schindelhauer D, Laner A, Tucker T, Bebok Z, Schwiebert EM, et al. Gene delivery systems--gene therapy vectors for cystic fibrosis. J Cyst Fibros 2004;3 Suppl 2:203-12.

[46] Ferrari S, Griesenbach U, Geddes DM, Alton E. Immunological hurdles to lung gene therapy. Clin Exp Immunol 2003;132(1):1-8.

[47] Worgall S, Leopold PL, Wolff G, Ferris B, Van Roijen N, Crystal RG. Role of alveolar macrophages in rapid elimination of adenovirus vectors administered to the epithelial surface of the respiratory tract. Hum Gene Ther 1997;8(14):1675-84.

[48] Qin L, Ding Y, Pahud DR, Chang E, Imperiale MJ, Bromberg JS. Promoter attenuation in gene therapy: interferon-gamma and tumor necrosis factor-alpha inhibit transgene expression. Hum Gene Ther 1997;8(17):2019-29.

[49] Jooss K, Yang Y, Wilson JM. Cyclophosphamide diminishes inflammation and prolongs transgene expression following delivery of adenoviral vectors to mouse liver and lung. Hum Gene Ther 1996;7(13):1555-66.

[50] Hazinski TA, Ladd PA, DeMatteo CA. Localization and induced expression of fusion genes in the rat lung. Am J Respir Cell Mol Biol 1991;4(3):206-9.

[51] Kolb M, Inman M, Margetts PJ, Galt T, Gauldie J. Budesonide enhances repeated gene transfer and expression in the lung with adenoviral vectors. Am J Respir Crit Care Med 2001;164(5):866-72.

[52] Yang Y, Trinchieri G, Wilson JM. Recombinant IL-12 prevents formation of blocking IgA antibodies to recombinant adenovirus and allows repeated gene therapy to mouse lung. Nat Med 1995;1(9):890-3.

[53] Chirmule N, Raper SE, Burkly L, Thomas D, Tazelaar J, Hughes JV, et al. Readministration of adenovirus vector in nonhuman primate lungs by blockade of CD40-CD40 ligand interactions. J Virol 2000;74(7):3345-52.

[54] Chirmule N, Truneh A, Haecker SE, Tazelaar J, Gao G, Raper SE, et al. Repeated administration of adenoviral vectors in lungs of human CD4 transgenic mice treated with a nondepleting CD4 antibody. J Immunol 1999;163(1):448-55.

[55] Jooss K, Turka LA, Wilson JM. Blunting of immune responses to adenoviral vectors in mouse liver and lung with CTLA4Ig. Gene Ther 1998;5(3):309-19.

[56] Scaria A, St George JA, Gregory RJ, Noelle RJ, Wadsworth SC, Smith AE, et al. Antibody to CD40 ligand inhibits both humoral and cellular immune responses to adenoviral vectors and facilitates repeated administration to mouse airway. Gene Ther 1997;4(6):611-7.

[57] Hyde SC, Southern KW, Gileadi U, Fitzjohn EM, Mofford KA, Waddell BE, et al. Repeat administration of DNA/liposomes to the nasal epithelium of patients with cystic fibrosis. Gene Ther 2000;7(13):1156-65.

[58] Scheule RK, St George JA, Bagley RG, Marshall J, Kaplan JM, Akita GY, et al. Basis of pulmonary toxicity associated with cationic lipid-mediated gene transfer to the mammalian lung. Hum Gene Ther 1997;8(6):689-707.

[59] Schwartz DA, Quinn TJ, Thorne PS, Sayeed S, Yi AK, Krieg AM. CpG motifs in bacte-
      rial DNA cause inflammation in the lower respiratory tract. J Clin Invest 1997;100(1):
      68-73.

[60] Yew NS, Wang KX, Przybylska M, Bagley RG, Stedman M, Marshall J, et al. Contri-
      bution of plasmid DNA to inflammation in the lung after administration of cationic
      lipid:pDNA complexes. Hum Gene Ther 1999;10(2):223-34.

[61] Krieg AM. CpG motifs in bacterial DNA and their immune effects. Annu Rev Immu-
      nol 2002;20:709-60.

[62] Raper SE, Chirmule N, Lee FS, Wivel NA, Bagg A, Gao GP, et al. Fatal systemic in-
      flammatory response syndrome in a ornithine transcarbamylase deficient patient fol-
      lowing adenoviral gene transfer. Mol Genet Metab 2003;80(1-2):148-58.

[63] Cavazzana-Calvo M, Hacein-Bey S, de Saint Basile G, Gross F, Yvon E, Nusbaum P,
      et al. Gene therapy of human severe combined immunodeficiency (SCID)-X1 disease.
      Science 2000;288(5466):669-72.

[64] Hacein-Bey-Abina S, von Kalle C, Schmidt M, Le Deist F, Wulffraat N, McIntyre E, et
      al. A serious adverse event after successful gene therapy for X-linked severe com-
      bined immunodeficiency. N Engl J Med 2003;348(3):255-6.

[65] Hacein-Bey-Abina S, Von Kalle C, Schmidt M, McCormack MP, Wulffraat N, Leb-
      oulch P, et al. LMO2-associated clonal T cell proliferation in two patients after gene
      therapy for SCID-X1. Science 2003;302(5644):415-9.

[66] Zhang Y, Chirmule N, Gao GP, Qian R, Croyle M, Joshi B, et al. Acute cytokine re-
      sponse to systemic adenoviral vectors in mice is mediated by dendritic cells and mac-
      rophages. Mol Ther 2001;3(5 Pt 1):697-707.

[67] Harvey BG, Leopold PL, Hackett NR, Grasso TM, Williams PM, Tucker AL, et al.
      Airway epithelial CFTR mRNA expression in cystic fibrosis patients after repetitive
      administration of a recombinant adenovirus. J Clin Invest 1999;104(9):1245-55.

[68] Zabner J, Ramsey BW, Meeker DP, Aitken ML, Balfour RP, Gibson RL, et al. Repeat
      administration of an adenovirus vector encoding cystic fibrosis transmembrane con-
      ductance regulator to the nasal epithelium of patients with cystic fibrosis. J Clin In-
      vest 1996;97(6):1504-11.

[69] Croyle MA, Chirmule N, Zhang Y, Wilson JM. "Stealth" adenoviruses blunt cell-
      mediated and humoral immune responses against the virus and allow for significant
      gene expression upon readministration in the lung. J Virol 2001;75(10):4792-801.

[70] Aitken ML, Moss RB, Waltz DA, Dovey ME, Tonelli MR, McNamara SC, et al. A
      phase I study of aerosolized administration of tgAAVCF to cystic fibrosis subjects
      with mild lung disease. Hum Gene Ther 2001;12(15):1907-16.

[71] Flotte TR, Zeitlin PL, Reynolds TC, Heald AE, Pedersen P, Beck S, et al. Phase I trial
      of intranasal and endobronchial administration of a recombinant adeno-associated

virus serotype 2 (rAAV2)-CFTR vector in adult cystic fibrosis patients: a two-part clinical study. Hum Gene Ther 2003;14(11):1079-88.

[72] Moss RB, Milla C, Colombo J, Accurso F, Zeitlin PL, Clancy JP, et al. Repeated aero-solized AAV-CFTR for treatment of cystic fibrosis: a randomized placebo-controlled phase 2B trial. Hum Gene Ther 2007;18(8):726-32.

[73] Moss RB, Rodman D, Spencer LT, Aitken ML, Zeitlin PL, Waltz D, et al. Repeated adeno-associated virus serotype 2 aerosol-mediated cystic fibrosis transmembrane regulator gene transfer to the lungs of patients with cystic fibrosis: a multicenter, double-blind, placebo-controlled trial. Chest 2004;125(2):509-21.

[74] Wagner JA, Nepomuceno IB, Messner AH, Moran ML, Batson EP, Dimiceli S, et al. A phase II, double-blind, randomized, placebo-controlled clinical trial of tgAAVCF us-ing maxillary sinus delivery in patients with cystic fibrosis with antrostomies. Hum Gene Ther 2002;13(11):1349-59.

[75] Griesenbach U, Alton EW. Gene transfer to the lung: lessons learned from more than 2 decades of CF gene therapy. Adv Drug Deliv Rev 2009 Feb 27;61(2):128-39.

[76] Al-Dosari MS, Gao X. Nonviral gene delivery: principle, limitations, and recent prog-ress. AAPS J 2009;11(4):671-81.

[77] Dean DA, Machado-Aranda D, Blair-Parks K, Yeldandi AV, Young JL. Electropora-tion as a method for high-level nonviral gene transfer to the lung. Gene Ther 2003;10(18):1608-15.

[78] Xenariou S, Liang HD, Griesenbach U, Zhu J, Farley R, Somerton L, et al. Low-fre-quency ultrasound increases non-viral gene transfer to the mouse lung. Acta Biochim Biophys Sin (Shanghai) 2010;42(1):45-51.

[79] Xenariou S, Griesenbach U, Ferrari S, Dean P, Scheule RK, Cheng SH, et al. Using magnetic forces to enhance non-viral gene transfer to airway epithelium in vivo. Gene Ther 2006;13(21):1545-52.

[80] Tros de Ilarduya C, Sun Y, Duzgunes N. Gene delivery by lipoplexes and polyplexes. Eur J Pharm Sci 2010;40(3):159-70.

[81] Alton EW, Stern M, Farley R, Jaffe A, Chadwick SL, Phillips J, et al. Cationic lipid-mediated CFTR gene transfer to the lungs and nose of patients with cystic fibrosis: a double-blind placebo-controlled trial. Lancet 1999;353(9157):947-54.

[82] Caplen NJ, Alton EW, Middleton PG, Dorin JR, Stevenson BJ, Gao X, et al. Liposome-mediated CFTR gene transfer to the nasal epithelium of patients with cystic fibrosis. Nat Med 1995;1(1):39-46.

[83] Gill DR, Southern KW, Mofford KA, Seddon T, Huang L, Sorgi F, et al. A placebo-controlled study of liposome-mediated gene transfer to the nasal epithelium of pa-tients with cystic fibrosis. Gene Ther 1997;4(3):199-209.

[84]   Porteous DJ, Dorin JR, McLachlan G, Davidson-Smith H, Davidson H, Stevenson BJ, et al. Evidence for safety and efficacy of DOTAP cationic liposome mediated CFTR gene transfer to the nasal epithelium of patients with cystic fibrosis. Gene Ther 1997;4(3):210-8.

[85]   Ruiz FE, Clancy JP, Perricone MA, Bebok Z, Hong JS, Cheng SH, et al. A clinical inflammatory syndrome attributable to aerosolized lipid-DNA administration in cystic fibrosis. Hum Gene Ther 2001;12(7):751-61.

[86]   Zabner J, Cheng SH, Meeker D, Launspach J, Balfour R, Perricone MA, et al. Comparison of DNA-lipid complexes and DNA alone for gene transfer to cystic fibrosis airway epithelia in vivo. J Clin Invest 1997;100(6):1529-37.

[87]   Bushman F, Lewinski M, Ciuffi A, Barr S, Leipzig J, Hannenhalli S, et al. Genome-wide analysis of retroviral DNA integration. Nat Rev Microbiol 2005;3(11):848-58.

[88]   Perez-Luz S, Diaz-Nido J. Prospects for the use of artificial chromosomes and mini-chromosome-like episomes in gene therapy. J Biomed Biotechnol 2010;pii:642804..

[89]   Ebersole TA, Ross A, Clark E, McGill N, Schindelhauer D, Cooke H, et al. Mammalian artificial chromosome formation from circular alphoid input DNA does not require telomere repeats. Hum Mol Genet 2000;9(11):1623-31.

[90]   Grimes BR, Schindelhauer D, McGill NI, Ross A, Ebersole TA, Cooke HJ. Stable gene expression from a mammalian artificial chromosome. EMBO Rep 2001;2(10):910-4.

[91]   Mejia JE, Larin Z. The assembly of large BACs by in vivo recombination. Genomics 2000 Dec 1;70(2):165-70.

[92]   Heng HH, Goetze S, Ye CJ, Liu G, Stevens JB, Bremer SW, et al. Chromatin loops are selectively anchored using scaffold/matrix-attachment regions. J Cell Sci 2004;117(Pt 7):999-1008.

[93]   Piechaczek C, Fetzer C, Baiker A, Bode J, Lipps HJ. A vector based on the SV40 origin of replication and chromosomal S/MARs replicates episomally in CHO cells. Nucleic Acids Res 1999;27(2):426-8.

[94]   Papapetrou EP, Ziros PG, Micheva ID, Zoumbos NC, Athanassiadou A. Gene transfer into human hematopoietic progenitor cells with an episomal vector carrying an S/MAR element. Gene Ther 2006;13(1):40-51.

[95]   Manzini S, Vargiolu A, Stehle IM, Bacci ML, Cerrito MG, Giovannoni R, et al. Genetically modified pigs produced with a nonviral episomal vector. Proc Natl Acad Sci U S A 2006;103(47):17672-7.

[96]   Voigt K, Izsvak Z, Ivics Z. Targeted gene insertion for molecular medicine. J Mol Med (Berl) 2008;86(11):1205-19.

[97]   Bertoni C, Jarrahian S, Wheeler TM, Li Y, Olivares EC, Calos MP, et al. Enhancement of plasmid-mediated gene therapy for muscular dystrophy by directed plasmid integration. Proc Natl Acad Sci U S A 2006;103(2):419-24.

[98] Ivics Z, Izsvak Z. The expanding universe of transposon technologies for gene and cell engineering. Mob DNA 2010;1(1):25.

[99] Leblond AL, Naud P, Forest V, Gourden C, Sagan C, Romefort B, et al. Developing cell therapy techniques for respiratory disease: intratracheal delivery of genetically engineered stem cells in a murine model of airway injury. Hum Gene Ther 2009;20(11):1329-43.

[100] Abdallah BM, Kassem M. Human mesenchymal stem cells: from basic biology to clinical applications. Gene Ther 2008;15(2):109-16.

[101] Takahashi K, Tanabe K, Ohnuki M, Narita M, Ichisaka T, Tomoda K, et al. Induction of pluripotent stem cells from adult human fibroblasts by defined factors. Cell 2007;131(5):861-72.

[102] Yu J, Vodyanik MA, Smuga-Otto K, Antosiewicz-Bourget J, Frane JL, Tian S, et al. Induced pluripotent stem cell lines derived from human somatic cells. Science 2007;318(5858):1917-20.

[103] Aluigi M, Fogli M, Curti A, Isidori A, Gruppioni E, Chiodoni C, et al. Nucleofection is an efficient nonviral transfection technique for human bone marrow-derived mesenchymal stem cells. Stem Cells 2006;24(2):454-61.

[104] Wang G, Bunnell BA, Painter RG, Quiniones BC, Tom S, Lanson NA, Jr., et al. Adult stem cells from bone marrow stroma differentiate into airway epithelial cells: potential therapy for cystic fibrosis. Proc Natl Acad Sci U S A 2005;102(1):186-91.

[105] Conese M, Ascenzioni F, Boyd AC, Coutelle C, De Fino I, De Smedt S, et al. Gene and cell therapy for cystic fibrosis: from bench to bedside. J Cyst Fibros 2011;10 Suppl 2:S114-28.

[106] Gan KH, Veeze HJ, van den Ouweland AM, Halley DJ, Scheffer H, van der Hout A, et al. A cystic fibrosis mutation associated with mild lung disease. N Engl J Med 1995;333(2):95-9.

[107] Johnson LG, Boyles SE, Wilson J, Boucher RC. Normalization of raised sodium absorption and raised calcium-mediated chloride secretion by adenovirus-mediated expression of cystic fibrosis transmembrane conductance regulator in primary human cystic fibrosis airway epithelial cells. J Clin Invest 1995;95(3):1377-82.

[108] Zhang L, Button B, Gabriel SE, Burkett S, Yan Y, Skiadopoulos MH, et al. CFTR delivery to 25% of surface epithelial cells restores normal rates of mucus transport to human cystic fibrosis airway epithelium. PLoS Biol 2009;7(7):e1000155.

[109] Crawford I, Maloney PC, Zeitlin PL, Guggino WB, Hyde SC, Turley H, et al. Immunocytochemical localization of the cystic fibrosis gene product CFTR. Proc Natl Acad Sci U S A 1991;88(20):9262-6.

[110] Trezise AE, Chambers JA, Wardle CJ, Gould S, Harris A. Expression of the cystic fibrosis gene in human foetal tissues. Hum Mol Genet 1993;2(3):213-8.

[111] Smith AN, Wardle CJ, Harris A. Characterization of DNASE I hypersensitive sites in the 120kb 5' to the CFTR gene. Biochem Biophys Res Commun 1995;211(1):274-81.

[112] Smith AN, Barth ML, McDowell TL, Moulin DS, Nuthall HN, Hollingsworth MA, et al. A regulatory element in intron 1 of the cystic fibrosis transmembrane conductance regulator gene. J Biol Chem 1996;271(17):9947-54.

[113] Smith DJ, Nuthall HN, Majetti ME, Harris A. Multiple potential intragenic regulatory elements in the CFTR gene. Genomics 2000;64(1):90-6.

[114] Nuthall HN, Moulin DS, Huxley C, Harris A. Analysis of DNase-I-hypersensitive sites at the 3' end of the cystic fibrosis transmembrane conductance regulator gene (CFTR). Biochem J 1999;341 (Pt 3):601-11.

[115] Nuthall HN, Vassaux G, Huxley C, Harris A. Analysis of a DNase I hypersensitive site located -20.9 kb upstream of the CFTR gene. Eur J Biochem 1999;266(2):431-43.

[116] Phylactides M, Rowntree R, Nuthall H, Ussery D, Wheeler A, Harris A. Evaluation of potential regulatory elements identified as DNase I hypersensitive sites in the CFTR gene. Eur J Biochem 2002;269(2):553-9.

[117] Rowntree RK, Vassaux G, McDowell TL, Howe S, McGuigan A, Phylactides M, et al. An element in intron 1 of the CFTR gene augments intestinal expression in vivo. Hum Mol Genet 2001;10(14):1455-64.

[118] Kotzamanis G, Abdulrazzak H, Gifford-Garner J, Haussecker PL, Cheung W, Grillot-Courvalin C, et al. CFTR expression from a BAC carrying the complete human gene and associated regulatory elements. J Cell Mol Med 2009;13(9A):2938-48.

[119] Zabner J, Couture LA, Gregory RJ, Graham SM, Smith AE, Welsh MJ. Adenovirus-mediated gene transfer transiently corrects the chloride transport defect in nasal epithelia of patients with cystic fibrosis. Cell 1993;75(2):207-16.

[120] Wagner JA, Messner AH, Moran ML, Daifuku R, Kouyama K, Desch JK, et al. Safety and biological efficacy of an adeno-associated virus vector-cystic fibrosis transmembrane regulator (AAV-CFTR) in the cystic fibrosis maxillary sinus. Laryngoscope 1999;109(2 Pt 1):266-74.

[121] Sorscher EJ, Logan JJ, Frizzell RA, Lyrene RK, Bebok Z, Dong JY, et al. Informed consent to participate in a research study -- gene therapy for cystic fibrosis using cationic liposome mediated gene transfer: a phase I trial of safety and efficacy in the nasal airway. Hum Gene Ther 1994;5(10):1271-7.

[122] Crystal RG, McElvaney NG, Rosenfeld MA, Chu CS, Mastrangeli A, Hay JG, et al. Administration of an adenovirus containing the human CFTR cDNA to the respiratory tract of individuals with cystic fibrosis. Nat Genet 1994;8(1):42-51.

[123] Boucher RC, Knowles MR, Johnson LG, Olsen JC, Pickles R, Wilson JM, et al. Gene therapy for cystic fibrosis using E1-deleted adenovirus: a phase I trial in the nasal

cavity. The University of North Carolina at Chapel Hill. Hum Gene Ther 1994;5(5): 615-39.

[124]   Knowles MR, Hohneker KW, Zhou Z, Olsen JC, Noah TL, Hu PC, et al. A controlled study of adenoviral-vector-mediated gene transfer in the nasal epithelium of patients with cystic fibrosis. N Engl J Med 1995;333(13):823-31.

[125]   Hay JG, McElvaney NG, Herena J, Crystal RG. Modification of nasal epithelial potential differences of individuals with cystic fibrosis consequent to local administration of a normal CFTR cDNA adenovirus gene transfer vector. Hum Gene Ther 1995;6(11):1487-96.

[126]   Bellon G, Michel-Calemard L, Thouvenot D, Jagneaux V, Poitevin F, Malcus C, et al. Aerosol administration of a recombinant adenovirus expressing CFTR to cystic fibrosis patients: a phase I clinical trial. Hum Gene Ther 1997;8(1):15-25.

[127]   Noone PG, Hohneker KW, Zhou Z, Johnson LG, Foy C, Gipson C, et al. Safety and biological efficacy of a lipid-CFTR complex for gene transfer in the nasal epithelium of adult patients with cystic fibrosis. Mol Ther 2000;1(1):105-14.

[128]   Zuckerman JB, Robinson CB, McCoy KS, Shell R, Sferra TJ, Chirmule N, et al. A phase I study of adenovirus-mediated transfer of the human cystic fibrosis transmembrane conductance regulator gene to a lung segment of individuals with cystic fibrosis. Hum Gene Ther 1999;10(18):2973-85.

[129]   Joseph PM, O'Sullivan BP, Lapey A, Dorkin H, Oren J, Balfour R, et al. Aerosol and lobar administration of a recombinant adenovirus to individuals with cystic fibrosis. I. Methods, safety, and clinical implications. Hum Gene Ther 2001;12(11):1369-82.

[130]   Perricone MA, Morris JE, Pavelka K, Plog MS, O'Sullivan BP, Joseph PM, et al. Aerosol and lobar administration of a recombinant adenovirus to individuals with cystic fibrosis. II. Transfection efficiency in airway epithelium. Hum Gene Ther 2001;12(11): 1383-94.

Molecular Therapy for Lysosomal Storage Diseases

Daisuke Tsuji and Kohji Itoh

Additional information is available at the end of the chapter

1. Introduction

Lysosomes are organella involving the catabolism of biomolecules extracellularly and intracellularly incorporated, which contain more than 60 distinct acidic hydrolases (lysosomal enzymes) and their co-factors. Lysosomal storage diseases (LSDs) are caused by germ-line gene mutations encoding lysosomal enzymes, their activator proteins, integral membrane proteins, cholesterol transporters and proteins concerning intracellular trafficking of lysosomal enzymes [1,2]. The LSDs associate with excessive accumulation of natural substrates, including glycoconjugates (glycosphingolipids, oligosaccharides derived from glycoproteins, and glycosaminoglycans from proteoglycans) as well as heterogeneous manifestations in both visceral and nervous systems [1,2]. LSDs comprise greater than 40 diseases, of which incidence is about 1 per 100 thousand births, and recognized as so-called 'Orphan diseases'.

In the biosynthesis of lysosomal matrix enzymes, newly synthesized enzymes are N-glycosylated in the endoplasmic reticulum (ER) and then phosphorylated in the Golgi apparatus on the 6 position of the terminal mannose residues (M6P) via two step reactions catalyzed by Golgi-localized phosphotransferase and uncovering enzyme necessary to expose the terminal M6P residues [3,4]. The M6P-carrying enzymes then bind the cation-dependent mannose 6-phosphate receptor (CD-M6PR) at physiological pH in the Golgi. The enzyme–receptor complex is then transported to late-endosomes where the M6P-carrying enzymes dissociate from the receptor at acidic pH, while the CD-M6PR then traffics back to the Golgi as a shuttle. M6P-carrying enzymes are delivered to lysosomes via fusion with late-endosomes. A small percentage of lysosomal enzymes is known secreted from the cell. The secreted M6P-carrying enzymes or the dephosphorylated enzyme with terminal mannose residues can then bind either cation-independent M6P/IGFII receptor (CI-M6PR) or mannose receptor (MR) on the plasma membrane [4,5]. Thus, the extracellular lysosomal enzymes can be endocytosed via both glycan receptors to be delivered to the lysosomes where the captured enzymes can exhibit their normal catabolic functions.

Many therapeutic approaches developed for LSDs, including bone marrow transplantation (BMT), stem cell-based therapy (SCT), enzyme replacement therapy (ERT) and *ex vivo* gene therapy, are based on this physiologic secretion/uptake system (cross-correction). In successful intravenous ERT for LSDs involving mainly visceral symptoms, including type 1 Gaucher disease [6,7] and mucopolysaccharidosis I (MPS I) [8], MPS VI [9], Fabry [10,11], and Pompe diseases [12,13], either MR or CI-M6PR have been utilized as delivery targets of the recombinant lysosomal enzyme drugs produced by mammalian cell lines including CHO cells and human fibrosarcoma cells. However, intravenous ERT has several disadvantages: i) long-life therapy, ii) requirement of large amounts of recombinant human enzymes, iii) high cost, iv) immune response to the exogenous enzymes [14], and v) ineffectiveness towards LSDs involving neurological signs because of the blood–brain barrier (BBB), although clinical trials are under-going of intrathecal ERT for MPS type I [15], II and IIIB patients. SCT using hematopoietic stem cell (HSC), hematopoietic precursor cell (HPC) and mesenchymal stem cell (MSC) derived from bone marrows has also been utilized as a treatment for LSDs animal models and patients [16-20]. BMT and SCT are based on that stem cells distribute widely *in vivo* as sources continuously producing the deficient enzymes. However, application of BMT is generally limited to LSDs that show a clear beneficial response and for which ERT is not available.

On the other hand, the gene replacement therapy (GT) [21-24] has advantages, including i) long-lasting therapy by a single transduction utilizing recombinant viral gene transfer vectors [25-29], ii) cross-correction effects, and iii) possible CNS-directed application to LSDs involving neurological symptoms [23,24,30-33], whereas GT has disadvantages, including i) low levels and persistence of expression in all tissues of patients, ii) incomplete response to therapy dependent on clinical phenotypes, and iii) insertional mutagenesis resulting in neoplasia. GT is one of the promising therapeutic approaches, especially toward LSDs involving CNS symptoms. In this review, we focus on the challenges to develop the CNS-directed GT for LSDs including GM2 gangliosidoses.

2. GM2 gangliosidoses

Lysosomal β-hexosaminidase (Hex, EC 3.2.1.52) is a glycosidase that catalyzes the hydrolysis of terminal N-acetylhexosamine residues at the non-reducing ends of oligosaccharides of glycoconjugates [34,35]. There are two major Hex isozymes in mammals including man, HexA (αβ, a heterodimer of α- and β-subunits) and HexB (ββ, a homodimer of β-subunit), and a minor unstable isozyme, HexS (αα, a homodimer of α-subunit). All these Hex isozymes can degrade terminal β-1,4 linked N-acetylglucosamine (GlcNAc) and N-acetylgalactosamine (GalNAc) residues, while only HexA and HexS prefer negatively charged substrates and cleave off the terminal N-acetylglucosamine 6-sulfate residues in keratan sulfate. Hex A is essential for cleavage of the GalNAc residue from GM2 ganglioside (GM2) in co-operation with GM2 activator protein (GM2A) [34,35].

Tay-Sachs disease (TSD) (MIM 272800) and Sandhoff disease (SD) (MIM 268800) are autosomal recessive GM2 gangliosidoses caused by germ-line mutations of *HEXA* (locus 15q23-24) encoding the Hex α-subunit, and *HEXB* (locus 5q13) encoding the Hex β-subunit, respectively [34,35]. The genes exhibit sequence homology, and the gene products exhibit 57% similarity in amino acid sequence. In TSD, the genetic defect of *HEXA* causes a deficiency of HexA (αβ with excessive accumulation of GM2 in the central nervous system (CNS), resulting in neurological disorders, including weakness, startle reaction, early blindness, progressive cerebellar ataxia, psychomotor retardation, and cherry red spots, and macrocephaly. In SD, the inherited defect of *HEXB* leads to simultaneous deficiencies of HexA and HexB with accumulation of GM2 in the CNS and of oligosaccharides carrying the terminal N-acetylhexosaminyl residues at their non-reducing ends, resulting in involvement of the visceral organs including cardiomegaly and minimal hepatosplenomegaly as well as the neurological symptoms. GM2 gangliosidosis AB variant (MIM 272750) is very rare autosomal recessive LSD caused by the gene mutation of GM2 activator protein (*GM2A* locus 5q31.3-q33.1) [34,36]. The gene product GM2A specifically binds GM2 to pull up from membranes in lysosomes, and present it to HexA for degradation of GM2. The deficiency of GM2A also cause the GM2 accumulation and neurological symptoms similar to those of TSD and SD [34,36]. The pathogenic mechanisms of these GM2 ganliosidoses has not been fully elucidated, although neurodegeneration and neuroinflammation have been reported to contribute to the pathogenesis [34,35,37,38].

GM2 gangliosidoses including TSD and SD exhibit a spectrum of clinical phenotypes, which vary from the severe infantile form (classical type), which is of early onset and fatal culminating in death before the age of 4 years, to the late-onset and less severe form (atypical type), which allows survival into childhood (subacute form) or adulthood (chronic form) [34,35,37,38]. Many mutations have been identified for each gene, including missense, deletion and insertion mutations [34,39-41]. Structural information on the basis of the crystal structures of human Hex B [42,43] and HexA [44] allowed us to predict the effects of missense mutaitons identified in TSD [34,39,40] and SD [34,39,41] on the protein structures of mutated gene products. According to these reports, the β-subunit of Hex comprises two domains (domain I and II). Domain I has an α/β topology, and domain II is folded into a $(\beta/\alpha)_8$-barrel with the active site pocket at the C-termini of the β-strands. An extrahelix that follows the eighth helix of the $(\beta/\alpha)_8$-barrel is located between domain I and the barrel structure. Only the α-subunit active site can hydrolyze GM2 due to a flexible loop structure that is removed post-translationally from β, and to the presence of αN423 and αR424. The loop structure is involved in binding the GM2A, while αR424 is critical for binding the carboxylate group of the N-acetylneuraminic acid residue of GM2. The β-subunit lacks these key residues and has βD452 and βL453 in their place. The β-subunit therefore cleaves only neutral substrates efficiently. The representative amino acid substitutions have been reported in the α-subunit, including R170W, R178H, W420C, C458Y, L484P, R499C/H, and R504C/H, as well as in the β-subunit, R505Q and C534Y. The dysfunctional and destabilizing defects in Hex α- and β-subunits well reflect biochemical and phenotypic abnormalities in TSD and SD, respectively. Such structural information should be useful to develop novel therapeutic approaches for these disorders [34,45].

3. General aspects of gene therapy for LSDs

Gene therapy (GT) utilizing various vectors for gene transfer has been preclinically and clinically applied for LSDs in recent years [21-33]. Recombinant viral vectors including retroviruses [25,32], adenovirus [26-28], herpes simplex virus (HSV) [33], adeno-associated virus (AAV) [29,46-48] and lentiviruses [24,49-51] are utilized currently as the effective means of gene transfer and enzyme expression. The retroviruses have been used primarily in *ex vivo* applications to transduce the dividing cells, such as HPC, HSC and other stem cells in culture, which are then transplanted into a recipient. However, the retroviral vectors are not suitable for *in vivo* GT due to lack of ability to transduce non-dividing cells. On the other hand, the adenoviruses can infect very efficiently non-dividing cells. However, the use of the early generation adenoviral vectors has been limited due to their strong antigenicity. In contrast, lentiviruses can infect both dividing and non-dividing cells, and are applicable to both *ex vivo* and *in vivo* GT. AAV vectors are able to transduce many cell types *in vivo* effectively, and it is often used as a safer tool for gene transfer because of the lower immunogenicity.

The application of recombinant viral vectors varies dependently on several factors, including ease of vector delivery, expression level in cell types and target tissues and organs mainly affected with LSD. At initial stage of development of GT for LSDs, the *ex vivo* transduction of HPC derived from type 1 Gaucher disease [25] and fibroblasts obtained from MPS VII model mice [32] using retroviral vectors was successful to secrete high levels of the enzymes and corrected the deficiencies. The *ex vivo* GT using retroviral vector and autologous HSC or HPC (human CD34+ cells) derived from bone marrow of the patient as donor cells for transplantation was clinically applied to type 1 Gaucher disease patients, and demonstrated the production of therapeutically effective levels of enzyme activity, resulting in persistent circulating enzyme available to tissues and organs [52]. The transduced cells also migrated into many tissues, expressed high levels of enzyme and reduced lysosomal storage in several critical tissues. However, several problems had been emerged, including less efficiency in transduction of human HSC or HPC using murine-based retroviral vector and difficulty in continuous production of sufficient amounts of recombinant enzymes to maintain the effectiveness.

The lentiviral vector based on human immunodeficiency virus had been expected to overcome the limitation of early generation of murine-based retroviral vectors in *ex vivo* GT [53]. Transduction efficiency of human HPC derived from Gaucher disease patient [54] was improved by using HIV-based lentiviral vector. β-Glucuronidase (GUSB)-deficient mobilized peripheral blood CD34(+) cells from a patient with MPSVII were transduced with a third-generation lentiviral vector encoding human GUSB, and then xenotransplantation to murine model with MPSVII. The corrected cells distributed widely throughout recipient tissues, resulting in significant therapeutic effects including improvements in biochemical parameters and reduction of the lysosomal distension of several host tissues [24].

Direct *in vivo* GT using adenoviral vector have been preclinically applied to murine models with Pompe, Fabry, and Wolman diseases, resulted in sufficient expression of circulating enzymes and reduction of storage materials in the affected tissues [27,55, 56]. However, these therapeutic effects were transient because of the severe immune reactions directed against the adenoviral vector. Single intravenous administration of a modified adenoviral vector to Pompe disease mice was demonstrated to reduce glycogen storage with minimal immune response [57].

The AAV vector has been also developed as an alternative gene transfer tool for direct *in vivo* GT for LSDs. Intramuscular injection of AAV2 serotype vector [58,] in the murine models of Pompe disease, Fabry disease and MPS VII caused high level expression in the muscle tissues but lower levels of circulating enzyme activity [59-61], although the efficacy varied depending on the diseases. Intravenous injection of AAV2 vectors in young adult mice with MPS VII and Fabry disease reduced the lysosomal storage in many tissues [61,62] Significant improvement was observed in MPS VII and MPS I mice following intravenous delivery of AAV2 vector during the neonatal period [28,63]. These findings suggested the effectiveness of AAV vector delivery at early presymptomatic stage to prevent onset rather than delayed intervention for progressive LSDs.

As mentioned above, GT has therapeutic potency for LSDs involving neurological symptoms superior to that of clinically applied intravenous ERT, in which the enzyme cannot cross the BBB. Several CNS-directed *ex vivo* and *in vivo* GT have been performed for animal models of LSDs with brain involvement. Genetically modified bone marrow stromal cells using retroviral vector improved CNS pathology and cognitive function in MPS VII and GM1-gangliosidosis mice following intraventricular transplantation [64, 65]. Genetically modified human neuronal precursor cells (NPCs) differentiated into neurons and astrocytes and expressed β-glucuronidase for at least 6 months after injection into striata of adult MPS VII model mice. However, the cells did not migrate and correction was limited to regions adjacent to the transplantation site [66] *In vivo* GT of metachromatic leukodystrophy (MLD) by lentiviral vector corrected neuropathology and protected against learning impairments in the model mice [49]. CNS-directed in vivo GT using AAV vectors have been demonstrated to have therapeutic effects on the mouse model of LSDs involving neurological signs, including MPS IIIB [67], MPS VII [68], Globoid cell leukodystrophy (GLD) [69], Nieman-Pick A (NPA)[70] and α-mannosidosis [71] by intracranial administration of recombinant AAV vectors. Thus, AAV vectors exhibit a number of properties that have made this vector system an excellent choice for both CNS gene therapy and basic neurobiological investigations. In vivo, the preponderance of AAV vector transduction occurs in neurons where it is possible to obtain long-term, stable gene expression with very little accompanying toxicity. Promoter selection, however, significantly influences the pattern and longevity of neuronal transduction distinct from the tropism inherent to AAV vectors. AAV vectors have successfully manipulated CNS function using a wide variety of approaches including expression of foreign genes, expression of endogenous genes, expression of antisense RNA and expression of RNAi. With the discovery and characterization of different AAV serotypes, as well as the creation of novel chimeric serotypes, the potential patterns of in vivo vector transduction have been expanded substantially, offering alternatives to the more studied AAV 2 serotype. Furthermore, the development of specific AAV chimeras offers the potential to further refine targeting strategies. These different AAV serotypes also provide a solution to the immune silencing that proves to be a realistic likelihood given broad exposure of the human population to the AAV 2 serotype. These advantageous CNS properties of AAV vectors have fostered a wide range of clinically relevant applications including Parkinson's disease, lysosomal storage diseases, Canavan's disease, epilepsy, Huntington's disease and ALS. In many cases the proposed therapies have progressed to phase I/II clinical trials. Each individual application, however, presents a unique set of challenges that must be solved in order to attain clinically effective gene therapies [72].

4. Gene therapy for GM2 gangliosidoses

4.1. Experimental and preclinical gene therapy using animal models

GM2 gangliosidoses, including Tay-Sachs disease (TSD), Sandhoff disease (SD) and the AB variant disorder, are characterized by excessive accumulation of GM2 and neurological symptoms due to progressive neurodegeneration and gliosis, as described above. However, there is no effective therapy for GM2 gangliosidoses at present, although we have reported and proposed the clinical potential of the intrathecal ERT using recombinant modified human HexA [73] and HexB [74,75] in recent years. It is crucial for treatment of GM2 gangliosidoses to develop the CNS-directed molecular therapy including such intrathecal ERT, *ex vivo* and *in vivo* GT or the combined methods including SRT [76]. In this chapter, we would focus on the CNS-directed GT and summarize the preclinical approaches using small and large animal models with GM2 gangliosidoses.

At early stage of development of GT for GM2 gangliosidoses, gene transduction of cultured cells was performed by utilizing recombinant vectors (virus or plasmids), and examined the effect of cross correction due to the secreted Hex isozymes. Guidotti, JE. *et al.* constructed a retroviral vector encoding for the α-subunit of human HexA (*HEXA* cDNA) and transduced the HexA-deficient fibroblasts derived from Tay-Sach disease model mice (*Hexa$^{-/-}$* mice) [77]. Transduced cells overexpressed the human Hex α-subunit to produce the chimeric HexA composed of human α-subunit and murine β-subunit, which were taken up via CI-M6PR by non-transduced cells and exhibited the cross-correction effect.

On the other hand, Martino *et al.* also constructed a retroviral vector encoding for the α-subunit of human HexA (*HEXA* cDNA) and transduced NIH3T3 murine fibroblasts, resulting in production of large amount of human Hex activity. The secreted Hex was incorporated into the fibroblasts derived from TSD patient, but failed to correct intracellular GM2 storage, probably because of the absence of HexA isozyme sufficient for degrading the accumulated GM2 [78]. Akli S et al. produced a replication-deficient recombinant adenovirus (AdRSV) coding the human *HEXA* cDNA, and transduced the fibroblasts derived from TSD patients. Transdused cells restored the Hex activity ranging from 40 to 84% of the normal, and secreted the Hex a-subunit, which were delivered to lysosomes and degraded the GM2 accumulated in TSD fibroblasts [79].

We transfected an expression vector plasmid coding the human *HEXB* cDNA to fibroblasts derived from Sandhoff disease mice (*Hexb*[-/-] mice) and established a transformed murine cell line stably producing the human Hex β-subunit [80]. However, the GM2 accumulated in the transformed murine cell line was not reduced, while co-transfection of the human *HEXA* cDNA resulted in restoration of HexA activity and reduction of GM2 storage.

Yamaguchi *et al.* evaluated the systemic *in vivo* GT for *Hexb*[-/-] mice using cationic liposome-mediated plasmid using the *Hexb*[-/-] mice [81]. The mice received a single intravenous injection of two plasmids, encoding the human α and β subunits of hexosaminidase cDNAs. As a result, 10–35% of normal levels of Hex expression, theoretically therapeutic levels, were achieved in most visceral organs, but not in the brain, 3 days after injection with decreased levels by day 7. Histochemical staining confirmed widespread enzyme activity in visceral organs. Both GA2 and GM2 were reduced by almost 10% and 50%, respectively, on day 3, and by 60% and 70% on day 7 compared with untreated age-matched *Hexb*[-/-] mice.

These findings suggested that brain-directed *in vivo* GT based on direct transduction of the affected tissues by single gene transfer or *ex vivo* GT utilizing double genes (i.e. *HEXA* and *HEXB* cDNAs) for producing the homo-specific HexA should be required to achieve the therapeutic effects on TSD and SD. Since then, studies on the CNS-directed *in vivo* GT and *ex vivo* GT have been performed as two streams of development of molecular therapy for GM2 gangliosidoses.

4.2. CNS-directed *in vivo* gene therapy

Bourgoin *et al.* constructed the recombinant adenovirus coding the human *HEXB* cDNA, and transduced the fibroblasts derived from patient with SD resulting in high expression of HexA and HexB activities. They also administered the adenoviral vector intracerebrally to SD mice (*Hexb-/-* mice), and succeeded in expression of near-normal level of enzymatic activity in the entire brain. Co-injection of hyperosmotic concentrations of mannitol with low doses of the adenoviral vector enhanced the vector diffusion in the injected hemisphere without viral cytotoxicity. It was suggested that such combination will allow a high and diffuse transduction efficiency of adeno-viral vector in the brain with higher safety [82].

Martino *et al.* also constructed a non-replicating herpes simplex viral (HSV) vector encoding *Hexa* cDNA. They transplanted the encapsuled recombinant HSV into the brain of *Hexa-/-* mice. The diffusion of recombinant HSV and the secreted HexA derived from transduced neural cells corrected the GM2 storage in the brain during one month due to cross correction effects without adverse effects due to the viral vector [83].

Caillaud and co-workers reported that mono and bicistronic lentiviral vectors based on a simian immunodeficiency virus (SIV) containing the human *HEXA* or/and *HEXB* cDNAs were constructed and tested on the fibroblasts derived from the SD patient [84]. The bicistronic SIV.ASB vector encoding both *HEXA* and *HEXB* cDNAs enabled a massive restoration of Hex activity. A large reduction of GM2 accumulation in SIV.ASB transduced cells. Moreover, the Hex isozymes secreted by transduced SD fibroblasts were endocytosed in deficient cells via CI-M6PR, allowing GM2 metabolism restoration in cross-corrected cells.

Therefore, the bicistronic lentivector supplying both HexA and HexB isozymes may provide a potential therapeutic tool for the treatment of TSD and SD. A mechanistic link was demonstrated among GM2 accumulation, neuronal cell death, reduction of sarcoplasmic/endoplasmic reticulum Ca^{2+}-ATPase (SERCA) activity, and axonal outgrowth. Arfi *et al.* examined the ability of the SIV.ASB vector to reverse these pathophysiological events, hippocampal neurons derived from embryonic *Hexb*-/- mice, which were transduced with the lentival vector [85]. Normal axonal growth rates, the rate of Ca2+ uptake via the sarcoplasmic/endoplasmic reticulum Ca2+-ATPase (SERCA) activity and the sensitivity of the neurons to thapsigargin-induced cell death were restored concomitantly with a decrease in GM2 and GA2 levels. Thus, the bicistronic SIV.ASB vector was revealed to reverse the biochemical defects and down-stream consequences in SD neurons, suggesting its potential of systemic and CNS-directed *in vivo* GT. Kyrkanides S. *et al.* performed the system in vivo GT utilizing the recombinant lentiviral vector FIV coding human *HEXB* cDNA to the neonatal *Hexb*-/- mice via intrapenitoneal administration. They also demonstrated the distribution of Hex isozymes into the CNS, including periventricular areas of the cerebrum as well as in the cerebellar cortex, and reduction of GM2 accumulated in these areas [86].

Cachon-Gonzalez *et al.* has reported that the *Hexb*-/- mice treated by stereotaxic intracranial inoculation of recombinant adeno-associated viral (rAAV) vectors encoding the human *HEXA* and *HEXB* cDNAs, including an HIV tat sequence as a protein transduction domain (PTD), to enhance protein expression and distribution [87]. *Hexb*-/- mice survived for >1 year with sustained, widespread and abundant enzyme delivery in the CNS. Onset of the disease was delayed with preservation of motor function; inflammation and GM2 storage in the brain and spinal cord was reduced. Gene delivery of the human HexA (αβ) by using AAV vectors has realistic potential for treating the TS and SD patients. Sargeant TJ. *et al.* demonstrated that intracranial co -injection of rAAV serotype 2/1 (rAAV2/1) vectors encoding the human *HEXA* and *HEXB* cDNAs prevents neuronal loss in the *Hexb*-/- mice brain tissues, including thalamus, brainstem and spinal cord, and correlated with increased lifespan [88]. Moreover, they performed intracranial co-injection of rAAV2/1 vectors into 1-month-old *Hexb*-/- mice [89]. As a result, the treated mice gave unprecedented survival to 2 years and prevented disease throughout the brain and spinal cord. Classical manifestations of disease, including spasticity were resolved by localized gene transfer to the striatum or cerebellum, respectively. Abundant biosynthesis of Hex isozymes and their global distribution via axonal, perivascular, and cerebrospinal fluid (CSF) spaces, as well as diffusion, account for the sustained phenotypic rescue—long-term protein expression by transduced brain parenchyma, choroid plexus epithelium, and dorsal root ganglia neurons supplies the corrective enzyme. Prolonged survival permitted expression of cryptic disease in organs not accessed by intracranial vector delivery.

4.3. CNS-directed *ex vivo* gene therapy

Ex vivo GT for GM2 gangliosidoses is based on the results of BMT previously reported [90,91]. BMT was demonstrated to prolong life span and ameliorate neurological symptoms in *Hexb*-/- mice [90], and the synergistic effects was also shown in combination with substrate reduction therapy (SRT) utilizing deoxynojirimycin derivatives [91]. Transduction of neural cells derived from $Hexa^{-/-}$ and $Hexb^{-/-}$ mice by recombinant viral vectors was performed.

Lacorazza HD *et al.* constructed the ecotropic retrovirus encoding the human *HEXA* cDNA and transduced multipotent neural progenitor cell lines, which stably expressed and secreted high levels of active HexA and cross-corrected the metabolic defect including GM2 storage in TSD fibroblastic cell line. The genetically engineered CNS progenitors were transplanted into the brains of both normal fetal and neonatal mice, in which substantial amounts of human Hex α-subunit and activity were observed throughout the brain enough for therapeutic effect in TSD [92].

Tsuji D. *et al.* constructed a recombinant lentiviral vector encoding the murine *Hexb* cDNA, and transduced microglial cells established from the brains of $Hexb^{-/-}$ mice [50]. Transduced microglial cells produced and secreted Hex activity, in which the intracellularly accumulated GM2 and oligosaccharides with terminal N-acetylglucosamine residues were reduced. Transduced microglial cell line was expected as a donor for brain-directed *ex vivo* GT.

Mesenchymal stem cells (MSCs) derived from bone marrow stromal cells are one of the candidates for autologous donor cells for ex vivo GT, and have the multipotency to differentiate under specific culture conditions into other cell types such as osteoblasts, adipocytes, and chondrocytes [93,] as well as into neural lineages [94]. Recently, we established MSCs derived from bone marrow of adult $Hexb^{-/-}$ mice. The MSCs expressed cell-type specific markers, including CD29, CD90 and CD54, but not CD45, and exhibited the ability to differentiate into various cell types, including neuron-restricted precursor cells (NRPs) expressing N-CAM carrying polysialic acid (PSA-NCAM). We produced a bicistronic retroviral vector (MSV-*modB*) encoding for the modified human *HEXB* cDNAs (*modB*) causing six α-subunit type amino acid substitutions as well as *EGFP* gene [75]. The gene products, modified HexB (modB, a homodimer of the modified β-subunits) different from the wild-type HexB, can recognize negatively charged artificial substrates and bind to GM2A to exhibit GM2-degrading activity. We transduced the MSCs derived from $Hexb^{-/-}$ mice (SD MSCs) with the MSV-*modB*, resulting in restoration of HexA-like activity and reduction of the accumulated GM2 and GlcNAc-oligosaccharides. The modB was also secreted from the transduced SD MSCs. In addition, we performed intraventricular engraftment of the transduced SD MSCs expressing *modB* into the brain of $Hexb^{-/-}$ mice. As a result, the injected transduced SD MSCs expressing HexA-like activity and EGFP were observed in periventricular region of the brain (Figure 1). Reduction of the immunoreactivity towards natural substrates including GM2 and GlcNAc-oligosaccharides were also observed around the periventricular region of $Hexb^{-/-}$ mice brain (Figure 2). These results suggest that genetically modified MSCs can be utilized as a brain-directed donor cells for *ex vivo* GT for LSDs involving neurological manifestations, including Tay-Sachs and Sandhoff diseases.

Lee J-P. *et al.* demonstrated intracranial transplantation of neural stem cells (NSCs) delayed onset, improved motor function, reduced GM2 storage and prolonged life span in the $Hexb^{-/-}$ mice partly due to the cross correction effect of the Hex isozymes secreted from NSCs. Human NSCs derived directly from the CNS and secondarily induced from embryonic stem

(ES) cells also demonstrated a broad repertoire of potentially therapeutic actions, which are expected to be applied for the treatment of neurodegenerative diseases [95]

5. Conclusion

A number of preclinical and therapeutic approaches for GM2 gangliosidoses, including stem cell therapy, substrate deprivation therapy, gene therapy, and enzyme replacement therapy, are being examined and evaluated with disease model mice, although there is no effective therapy for treatment of the patients with GM2 gangliosidoses at present. However, according to the preclinical results obtained by using animal disease models, CNS-directed *in vivo* gene therapy utilizing recombinant viral vectors and *ex vivo* gene therapy based on the cross-correction by transduced autologous and heterologous stem cells are promising for development of novel therapies for LSDs associated with neurological abnormalities, including GM2 gangliosidoses. Improvement of these GTs and their combination with other clinical approaches will facilitate the development of efficient therapies for neurodegenerative disorders caused by neuroinflammation and gliosis.

Acknowledgements

Recent our research was supported by NIBIO (Osaka, Japan). We would appreciate Ms. Mayuko Oe for assisting us to prepare this review.

Author details

Daisuke Tsuji[1,2] and Kohji Itoh[1,2]

*Address all correspondence to: dtsuji@tokushima-u.ac.jp

1 Department of Medicinal Biotechnology, Graduate School of Pharmaceutical Sciences, Institute for Medicinal Research, The University of Tokushima, Tokushima, Japan

2 NIBIO, Ibaraki, Osaka, Japan

References

[1] Scriver CR. In The Metabolic and Molecular Bases of Inherited Disease http://www.ommbid.com ;part16: 134-154.

[2] Figura KV. Andrej H. Lysosomal Enzymes and Their Receptors. Annual Review of Biochemistry 1986;55: 167-193.

[3] Kornfeld S. Structure and Function of the Mannose 6-Phosphate/Insulin-like Growth Factor II Receptors. Annual Review of Biochemistry 1992;61: 307-330.

[4] Neufeld EF. Fratantoni, JC. Inborn Errors of Mucopolysaccharide Metabolism. Science 1970;169: 141-146.

[5] Achord DT. Human Beta-Glucuronidase: in Vivo Clearance and in Vitro Uptake by a Glycoprotein Recognition System on Reticuloendothelial Cells. Cell 1978;15: 269-278.

[6] Barton NW. Replacement Therapy for Inherited Enzyme Deficiency-Macrophage-Targeted Glucocerebrosidase for Gaucher's Disease. The New England Journal of Medicine 1991;324(21): 1464-1470.

[7] Weinreb NJ. Effectiveness of Enzyme Replacement Therapy in 1028 Patients with Type 1 Gaucher Disease After 2 to 5 Years of Treatment: a Report from the Gaucher Registry. The American Journal of Medicine 2002;113(2): 112-119.

[8] Kakkis ED. Enzyme-Replacement Therapy in Mucopolysaccharidosis I. The New England Journal of Medicine 2001;344(3): 182-188.

[9] Harmatz P. Enzyme Replacement Therapy in Mucopolysaccharidosis VI (Maroteaux-Lamy Syndrome). The Journal of Pediatrics 2004;144(5): 574-580.

[10] Schiffmann R. Enzyme Replacement Therapy in Fabry Disease A Randomized Controlled Trial. The Journal of American Medical Association 2001;285(21): 2743-2749.

[11] Eng CM. Safety and Efficacy of Recombinant Human α-Galactosidase a Replacement Therapy in Fabry's Disease. The New England Journal of Medicine 2001;345(1): 9-16.

[12] Amalfitano A. Recombinant Human Acid Alpha-Glucosidase Enzyme Therapy for Infantile Glycogen Storage Disease Type II: Results of a Phase I/II Clinical Trial. Genetics in Medicine 2001;3(2): 132-138.

[13] Winkel LP. Enzyme Replacement Therapy in Late-Onset Pompe's Disease: a Three-Year Follow-Up. Annals of Neurology 2004;55(4): 495-502.

[14] Wang J. Neutralizing Antibodies to Therapeutic Enzymes: Considerations for Testing, Prevention and Treatment. Nature Biotechnology 2008;26: 901-908.

[15] Patricia ID. Intrathecal Enzyme Replacement Therapy for Mucopolysaccharidosis I: Translating Success in Animal Models to Patients. Current Pharmaceutical Biotechnology 2011;12(6): 946-955.

[16] Shapiro EG. Neuropsychological Outcomes of Several Storage Diseases with and without Bone Marrow Transplantation. Journal of Inherited Metabolic Disease 1995;18(4): 413-429.

[17] Miranda SR. Bone Marrow Transplantation in Acid Sphingomyelinase-Deficient Mice: Engraftment and Cell Migration into The Brain as a Function of Radiation, Age, and Phenotype. Blood 1997;90(1): 444-452.

[18] Lönnqvist T. Hematopoietic Stem Cell Transplantation in Infantile Neuronal Ceroid Lipofuscinosis. Neurology 2001;57(8): 1411-1416.

[19] Jin HK. Intracerebral Transplantation of Mesenchymal Stem Cells into Acid Sphingo-myelinase-Deficient Mice Delays the Onset of Neurological Abnormalities and Extends Their Life Span. The Journal of Clinical Investigation 2002;109(9): 1183-1191.

[20] Hofling AA. Human CD34+ Hematopoietic Progenitor Cell-Directed Lentiviral-Mediated Gene Therapy in a Xenotransplantation Model of Lysosomal Storage Disease. Molecular Therapy 2004;9(6): 856-865.

[21] Mark SS. Gene Therapy for Lysosomal Storage Diseases. Molecular Therapy 2006;13: 839–849.

[22] Haskins M. Gene Therapy for Lysosomal Storage Diseases (LSDs) in Large Animal Models. The ILAR Journal 2009;50(2): 112-121.

[23] Sands MS. CNS-Directed Gene Therapy for Lysosomal Storage Diseases. ACTA PAE-DIATRICA SUPPLEMENT 2008;97(457): 22-27.

[24] Hofling A. Engrafment of Human CD34+ Cells Leads to Widespread Distribution of Donor-Derived Cells and Correction of Tissue Pathology in a Novel Murine Xeno-transplantation Model of Lysosomal Storage Disease. Blood 2003;101: 2054-2063.

[25] Fink JK. Correction of Glucocerebrosidase Deficiency after Retroviral-Mediated Gene Transfer into Hematopoietic Progenitor Cells from Patients with Gaucher Disease. Proceedings of the National Academy of Sciences of the United States of America 1990;87(6): 2334-2338.

[26] Nicolino MP. Adenovirus-Mediated Transfer of the Acid Alpha-Glucosidase Gene into Fibroblasts, Myoblasts and Myotubes From Patients with Glycogen Storage Disease Type II Leads to High Level Expression of Enzyme and Corrects Glycogen Accumulation. Human Molecular Genetics 1998;7(11): 1695-1702.

[27] Ziegler RJ. Correction of Enzymatic and Lysosomal Storage Defects in Fabry Mice by Adenovirus-Mediated Gene Transfer. Human Gene Therapy 1999;10(10): 1667-1682.

[28] Daly TM. Neonatal Intramuscular Injection with Recombinant Adeno-Associated Virus Results in Prolonged Beta-Glucuronidase Expression in Situ and Correction of Liver Pathology in Mucopolysaccharidosis Type VII Mice. Human Gene Therapy 1999;10: 85-94.

[29] Griffey M. Adeno-Associated Virus 2-Mediated Gene Therapy Decreases Autofluor-escent Storage Material and Increases Brain Mass in a Murine Model of Infantile Neuronal Ceroid Lipofuscinosis. Neurobiology of Disease 2004;16(2): 360-369.

[30] Biffi A. Gene Therapy of Metachromatic Leukodystrophy Reverses Neurological Damage and Deficits in Mice. The Journal of Clinical Investigation 2006;116(11): 3070-3082.

[31] Wang D. Reprogramming Erythroid Cells for Lysosomal Enzyme Production Leads to Visceral and CNS Cross-Correction in Mice with Hurler Syndrome. Proceedings of the National Academy of Sciences of the United States of America 2009; 106(47): 19958-19963.

[32] Taylor RM. Decreased Lysosomal Storage in the Adult MPS VII Mouse Brain in the Vicinity of Grafts of Retroviral Vector-Corrected Fibroblasts Secreting High Levels of Bold Beta-Glucuronidase. Nature Medicine 1997;3(7): 771-774.

[33] Berges BK. Widespread Correction of Lysosomal Storage in the Mucopolysaccharidosis Type VII Mouse Brain with A Herpes Simplex Virus Type 1 Vector Expressing Beta-Glucuronidase. Molecular Therapy 2006;13(5): 859-869.

[34] Gravel RA. GM2 Gangliosidoses in The Metabolic and Molecular Bases of Inherited Disease. McGraw-Hill 2001; 3827-3876.

[35] Mahuran DJ. Biochemical Consequences of Mutations Causing the GM2 Gangliosidoses. Biochimica et Biophysica Acta 1999;1455(2-3): 105-138.

[36] Kytzia HJ. Evidence for Two Different Active Sites on Human β-Hexosaminidase A. The Journal of Biological Chemistry 1985;260: 7568-7572.

[37] Sakuraba H. Molecular Pathologies of and Enzyme Replacement Therapies for Lysosomal Diseases. CNS & Neurological Disorders - Drug Targets 2006;5: 401-413.

[38] Itoh K. Neurochemical Aspects of Sandhoff Disease in Neurochemistry of Metabolic Diseases-Lysosomal Storage Diseases, Phenylketonuria and Canavan Disease 2007; 55-82.

[39] Tanaka A. A New Point Mutation in the Beta-Hexosaminidase Alpha Subunit Gene Responsible for Infantile Tay-Sachs Disease in a Non-Jewish Caucasian Patient (a Kpn Mutant). The American Journal of Human Genetics 1990;47(3): 568-574.

[40] Ohno K. Mutation in GM2-Gangliosidosis B1 Variant. Journal of Neurochemistry 1988;50(1): 316-318.

[41] Kytzia HJ. Variant of GM2-Gangliosidosis with Hexosaminidase a Having a Severely Changed Substrate Specificity. The EMBO Journal 1983;2(7): 1201–1205.

[42] Mark BL. Crystal Structure of Human Beta-Hexosaminidase B: Understanding the Molecular Basis of Sandhoff and Tay-Sachs Disease. Journal of Molecular Biology 2003;327: 1093-1109.

[43] Timm M. The X-ray Crystal Structure of Human β-Hexosaminidase B Provides New Insights into Sandhoff Disease. Journal of Molecular Biology 2003;328(3): 669-681.

[44] Lemieux MJ. Crystallographic Structure of Human Beta-Hexosaminidase A: Interpretation of Tay-Sachs Mutations and Loss of GM2 ganglioside hydrolysis. Journal of Molecular Biology 2006; 359: 913-929.

[45] Sakuraba H. Molecular and Structural Studies of the GM2 Gangliosidosis 0 Variant. Journal of Human Genetics 2002;47(4): 176-183.

[46] Liu G. Functional Correction of CNS Phenotypes in a Lysosomal Storage Disease Model using Adeno-Associated Virus Type 4 Vectors. The Journal of Neuroscience 2005;25(41): 9321-9327.

[47] Sevin C. Intracerebral Adeno-Associated Virus-Mediated Gene Transfer in Rapidly Progressive Forms of Metachromatic Leukodystrophy. Human Molecular Genetics 2006;15(1): 53-64.

[48] Spampanato C. Efficacy of a Combined Intaracerebral and Systemic Gene Delivery Approach for the Treatment of a Severe Lysosomal Storage Disorder. Molecular Therapy 2011;19(5): 860-869.

[49] Consiglio A, In Vivo Gene Therapy of Metachromatic Leukodystrophy by Lentiviral Vectors: Correction of Neuropathology and Protection Against Learning Impairments in Affected Mice. Nature Medicine 2001;7(3): 310-316.

[50] Tsuji D. Metabolic Correction in Microglia Derived from Sandhoff Disease Model Mice. Journal of Neurochemistry 2005; 94(6): 1631-1638.

[51] McIntyre C. Lentiviral-Mediated Gene Therapy for Murine Mucopolysaccharidosis Type IIIA. Molecular Genetics of Metabolism 2008;93(4): 411-418.

[52] Bahnson AB. Transduction of CD34+ Enriched Cord Blood and Gaucher Bone Marrow Cells by a Retroviral Vector Carrying the Glucocerebrosidase Gene. Gene Therapy 1994;1(3): 176-184.

[53] Fabrega S. Gene Therapy of Gaucher's and Fabry's Diseases: Current Status and Prospects. Journal of Social Biology 2002;196(2): 175-181.

[54] Dunbar CE. Retroviral Transfer of the Glucocerebrosidase Gene into CD34+ Cells from Patients with Gaucher Disease: in Vivo Detection of Transduced Cells Without Myeloablation. Human Gene Therapy 1998;9(17): 2629-2640.

[55] Amalfitano A. Systemic Correction of the Muscle Disorder Glycogen Storage Disease Type 2 after Hepatic Targeting of a Modified Adenovirus Vector Encording Human Acid-Alpha-Gulucosidase. Proceedings of the National Academy of Sciences 1999;96: 8861-8866.

[56] Du H. Lysosomal Acid Lipase Deficiency: Correction of Lipid Storage by Adenovirus-Mediated Gene Transfer in Mice. Human Gene Therapy 2002;13: 1361-1372.

[57] Xu F. Glycogen Storage in Multiple Muscles of Old GSD-II Mice can be Rapidly Cleared after a Single Intravenous Injection with a Modified Adenoviral Vector Expressing hGAA. The Journal of Gene Medicine 2005;7: 171-178.

[58] Hermonat PL. Use of Adeno-Associated Virus as a Mammalian DNA Cloning Vector: Transduction of Neomycin Resistance into Macka-Kian Tissue Culture Cells. Proceedings of the National Academy of Sciences 1984;81: 6466-6470.

[59] Fraites TJ. Correction of the Enzymatic and Functional Deficits in a Model of Pompe Disease using Adeno-Associated Virus Vectors. Molecular Therapy 2002;5: 571-578.

[60] Takahashi H. Long-Term Systemic Therapy of Fabry Disease in a Knockout Mouse by Adeno-Associated Virus-Mediated Muscle-Directed Gene Transfer. Proceedings of the National Academy of Sciences 2002;99: 13777-13782.

[61] Watson G. Intrathecal Administration of AAV Vectors for the Treatment of Lysosomal Storage in the Brains of MPS I Mice. Gene Therapy 2006;13: 917-925

[62] Jung SC. Adeno-Associated Viral Vector-Mediated Gene Transfer Results in Long-Term Enzymatic and Functional Correction in Multiple Organs of Fabry Mice. Proceedings of the National Academy of Sciences 2001;98: 2676-2681.

[63] Hartung SD. Correction of Metabolic, Craniofacial, and Neurologic Abnormalities in MPS I Mice Treated at Birth with Adeno-Associated Virus Vector Transducing the Human α-L-Iduronidase Gene. Molecular Therapy 2004;9: 866-875.

[64] Sakurai K. Brain Transplantation of Genetically Modified Bone Marrow Stromal Cells Corrects CNS Pathology and Cognitive Function in MPS VII Mice. Gene Therapy 2004;11: 1475-1481.

[65] Sano R. Chemokine-Induced Recruitment of Genetically Modified Bone Marrow Cells into the CNS of GM1-Gangliosidosis Mice Corrects Neuronal Pathology. Blood 2005;106: 2259-2268.

[66] Buchet D. Long-Term Expression of Beta-Glucuronidase by Genetically Modified Human Neural Progenitor Cells Grafted into the Mouse Central Nervous System. Molecular and Cellular Neuroscience 2002;19: 389-401.

[67] Fu H. Neurological Correction of Lysosomal Storage in a Mucopolysaccharidossis IIIB Mouse Model by Adeno-Associated Virus-Mediated Gene Delivery. Molecular Therapy 2002;5: 42-49.

[68] Frisella WA, Intracranial Injection of Recombinant Adeno-Associated Virus Improves Cognitive Function in a Murine Model of Mucopolysaccharidosis Type VII. Molecular Therapy 2001;3: 351-358.

[69] Rafi MA. AAV-Mediated Expression of Galactocerebrosidase in Brain Results in Attenuated Symptoms and Extended Life Span in Murine Models of Globoid Cell Leukodystrophy. Molecular Therapy 2005;11: 734-744.

[70] Passini MA. Distribution of a Lysosomal Enzyme in the Adult Brain by Axonal Transport and by Cells of the Rostral Migratory Stream. The Journal of Neuroscience 2002;22: 6437-6446.

[71] Vite CH. Effective Gene Therapy for an Inherited CNS Disease in a Large Animal Model. Annals of Neurology 2005;57: 355-364.

[72] McCown TJ. Adeno-Asoociated Virus (AVV) Vectors in the CNS. Current Gene Therapy 2005;5(3): 333-338.

[73] Tsuji D. Highly Phosphomannosylated Enzyme Replacement Therapy for GM2 Gangliosidosis. Annals of Neurology 2011;69(4): 691-701.

[74] Matsuoka K. Introduction of an N-Glycan Sequon into HEXA Enhances Human β-Hexosaminidase Cellular Uptake in a Model of Sandhoff Disease. Molecular Therapy 2010;18(8): 1519-1526.

[75] Matsuoka K. Therapeutic Potential of Intracerebroventricular Replacement of Modified Human β-Hexosaminidase B for GM2 Gangliosidosis. Molecular Therapy 2011;19(6): 1017-1024.

[76] Pastores GM. Miglustat: Substrate Reduction Therapy for Lysosomal Storage Disorders Associated with Primary Central Nervous System Involvement. Recent Patents on CNS Drug Discovery 2006;1(1): 77-82.

[77] Guidotti J. Retrovirus-Mediated Enzymatic Correction of Tay-Sachs Defect in Transduced and Non-Transduced Cells. Human Molecular Genetics 1998; 7(5): 831-838.

[78] Martino S. A Direct Gene Transfer Strategy via Brain Internal Capsule Reverses the Biochemical Defect in Tay-Sachs Disease. Human Molecular Genetics 2005;14(15): 2113-2123.

[79] Akli S. Restoration of Hexosaminidase A Activity in Human Tay-Sachs Fibroblasts via Adenoviral Vector-Mediated Gene Transfer. Gene Therapy 1996;3(9): 769-774.

[80] Itakura T. Inefficiency in GM2 Ganglioside Elimination by Human Lysosomal β-Hexosaminidase β-Subunit Gene Transfer to Fibroblastic Cell Line Derived from Sandhoff Disease Model Mice. Biological & Pharmaceutical Bulletin 2006;29(8): 1564-1569.

[81] Yamaguchi A. Plasmid-Based Gene Transfer Ameliorates Visceral Storage in a Mouse Model of Sandhoff Disease. Journal of Molecular Medicine 2003;81(3): 185-193.

[82] Bourgoin C. Widespread Distribution of Beta-Hexosaminidase Activity in the Brain of a Sandhoff Mouse Model After Co-injection Of Adenoviral Vector And Mannitol. Gene Therapy 2003;10(21) 1841-1849.

[83] Martino S. A Direct Gene Transfer Strategy via Brain Internal Capsule Reverses the Biochemical Defect in Tay-Sachs Disease. Human Molecular Genetics 2005;14(15) 2113-2123.

[84] Arfi A. Bicistronic Lentiviral Vector Corrects Beta-Hexosaminidase Deficiency in Transduced and Cross-Corrected Human Sandhoff Fibroblasts. Neurobiology of Disease 2005;20(2) 583-593.

[85] Arfi A. Reversion of the Biochemical Defects in Murine Embryonic Sandhoff Neurons Using a Bicistronic Lentiviral Vector Encoding Hexosaminidase Alpha and Beta. Journal of Neurochemistry 2006;96(6): 1572-1579.

[86] Kykanides S. Beta-Hexosaminidase Lentiviral Vectors: Transfer into the CNS via Systemic Administration. Molecular Brain Research 2005;133: 286-298.

[87] Cachón-González MB. Effective Gene Therapy in an Authentic Model of Tay-Sachs-related Diseases. Proceedings of the National Academy of Sciences of the United States of America 2006;103(27): 10373-10378.

[88] Sargeant TJ. Adeno-Associated Virus-Mediated Expression of β-Hexosaminidase Prevents Neuronal Loss in the Sandhoff Mouse Brain. Human Molecular Genetics 2011;20(22): 4371-4380.

[89] Cachón-González M. Gene Transfer Correct Acute GM2 Gangliosidosis – Potential Therapeutic Contribution of Perivascular Enzyme Flow. Molecular Therapy 2012;20(8): 1489-1500.

[90] Norflus F. Bone Marrow Transplantation Prolongs Life Span and Ameliorates Neurologic Manifestations in Sandhoff Disease Mice. Journal of Clinical Investigation 1998;101: 1881-1888.

[91] Jeyakumar M. Enhanced Survival in Sandhoff Disease Mice Receiving a Combination of Substrate Deprivation Therapy and Bone Marrow Transplantation. Blood 2001;97: 327-329.

[92] Lacorazza HD. Expression of Human Beta-Hexosaminidase Alpha-Subunit Gene (The Gene Defect of Tay-Sachs Disease) in Mouse Brains Upon Engraftment of Transduced Progenitor Cells. Nature Medicine 1996;2(4): 424-429.

[93] Pittenger MF. Multilineage Potential of Adult Human Mesenchymal Stem Cells. Science 1999;284(5411): 143-147.

[94] Dezawa M. Specific Induction of Neuronal Cells from Bone Marrow Stromal Cells and Application for Autologous Transplantation. The Journal of Clinical Investigation 2004;113(12): 1701-1710.

[95] Lee JP. Stem Cells Act through Multiple Mechanisms to Benefit Mice with Neurodegenerative Metabolic Disease. Nature Medicine 2007;13(4): 439-447.

Applications: Others

Chapter 8

Gene Therapy in Critical Care Medicine

Gabriel J. Moreno-González and
Angel Zarain-Herzberg

Additional information is available at the end of the chapter

1. Introduction

Critical care medicine is directed toward patients with a wide spectrum of illnesses. These have the common denominators of marked exacerbation of an existing disease, severe acute new problems, or severe complications from disease or treatments. In recent years has been an explosion of evidence based medicine with improvement in outcome, however there are several conditions in critical care patients that maintains a high morbidity and high mortality that is necessary to be addressed [1]. Of these, severe sepsis and the acute respiratory distress syndrome (ARDS), including acute lung injury (ALI) (syndromes consisting of acute respiratory failure associated with pulmonary infiltrates due to intra- or extra-pulmonary diseases) are two important conditions that have increased mortality in critical care units around the world [2, 3].

In 1991, a Consensus Conference of the American College of Chest Physicians an the Society for Critical Care (ACCP-SCCM) introduced the term systemic inflammatory response syndrome (SIRS) as the presence of at least two of four clinical criteria: body temperature more than 38°C or less than 36°C, heart rate more than 90 beats per minute, respiratory rate more than 20 breaths per minute or hyperventilation with $PaCO_2$ less than 32 mmHg, white blood cell count more than 12000/mm³, less than 4000/mm³ or with more than 10% immature neutrophils [4]. In 2001, a new consensus suggests that other signs and symptoms could reflect the clinical response to infection, including: fever/hypothermia, tachypnea/respiratory alkalosis, positive fluid balance/edema, general inflammatory reaction, altered white blood count, increased biomarkers (C-reactive protein, IL-6, pro-calcitonin), hemodynamic alterations, arterial hypotension, tachycardia, increased cardiac outflow/low systemic vascular resistance/high venous saturation O_2, altered skin perfusion, decreased urine output, hyperlactacemia, signs of organ dysfunction, hypoxemia, coagulation abnormalities, altered mental status, hyperglycemia, thrombocytopenia, disseminated intravascular coagulation, altered liver function, intolerance to feeding [5].

Systemic inflammatory response syndrome can result from diverse etiologies, including, but not limited to infectious, trauma, pancreatitis, ischemia-reperfusion injury, and burns [6]. Sepsis is defined as the presence of infection and some of the listed signs and symptoms of SIRS, whereas severe sepsis is defined as sepsis associated with organ dysfunction and shock septic as severe sepsis with hypotension, despite adequate fluid resuscitation [7].

Over 18 million cases of severe sepsis occur each year. The number of severe sepsis cases is set to grow a rate of 1.5% per year from the annual incidence of 3 cases per 1000 of the population in 2001 [8, 9]. Sepsis is a major cause of mortality throughout the world, killing approximately 1400 people every day, being as high as an additional fifty per cent as deaths are often attributed to complications from cancer or pneumonia, and not related to sepsis [10]. Death is common among sepsis patients, with around 28-50% of patients dying within the first month of diagnosis [11-13]. Sepsis impacts the lives of many people, including the patient and their families, in addition to doctors, nursing and care staff. The intense demands made on hospital staff, equipment and facilities to treat septic patients places a significant burden on healthcare resources, accounting for 40% of total ICU expenditure [10]. Each year the cost of treating septic patients increases and is as high as 7.6 billion euro in Europe [10] and 17.4 billion euro in the USA [8].

One common complication of SIRS and sepsis is acute lung injury/adult respiratory distress syndrome (ALI/ARDS). According to a Join North American European consensus committee (NAECC), ARDS is defined as an inflammatory process in the lungs with acute onset of respiratory failure, new bilateral pulmonary infiltrates on frontal chest radiograph or computed tomography, absence of left ventricular failure (clinically diagnosed or a pulmonary artery occlusion pressure <18mmHg) and hypoxemia with a ratio between the partial pressure of arterial oxygen and the fraction of inspired oxygen (PaO_2/FiO_2 ratio) of $\leq$27 kPa independent of the level of positive end-expiratory pressure (PEEP) [14]. ALI is defined by the same criteria except that the PaO_2/FiO_2 ratio is between 27 kPa and 40 kPa[14-16]. Sepsis is the most common cause of ALI/ARDS and also the most common cause of death after patients develop ALI/ARDS [17]. The incidence of ALI/ARDS is estimated to be 20 to 50 cases per 100000 person-year, with approximately 18% to 25% of cases meeting oxygenation criteria for ALI but not for ARDS [18, 19].

The reported rate of mortality from ARDS ranges from 31% to 74% depending on the characteristics of patients, with most deaths occurring as a consequence of multiple organ failure and sepsis [18, 19]. ALI has a significant lower crude hospital mortality (32%) compared with those with ARDS (57.9%) [20]. Crude estimates of the health care costs associated with ALI/ARDS may exceed 5 billion dollars per year in the United States alone [21].

2. Physiopathology of sepsis

Microorganisms express macromolecular motifs, named pathogen-associated molecular patterns (PAMs) such as lipopolysaccharide (LPS), flagellin, double-stranded RNA and CpG DNA [22]. These molecules are recognized by the immune system through a family of transmembrane or intra-cytoplasmic receptors, the pattern recognition receptors (PRRs), classified in three general families: a) Toll-like receptors (TLRs); b) NOD-like receptors (NLRs); and c) RIG-I-like receptors (RLRs) [22].

The TLRs are type I integral membrane glycoproteins characterized by the extracellular domains containing varying numbers of leucine-rich-repeat (LRR) motifs and a cytoplasmic signaling domain homologous to that of the interleukin 1 receptor (IL-1R), termed the Toll/IL-1R homology (TIR) domain [23]. Based on their primary sequences, TLRs can be divides into several subfamilies, each of which recognized related PAMPs: the subfamily of TLR1, TLR2 and TLR6 recognize lipids, whereas the highly related TLR7, TLR8, TLR9 recognize nucleic acids. TLR4 recognize a very divergent collection of ligands [24]. The NLRs proteins are implicated in the recognition of bacterial components. Proteins in this family possess LRRs that mediate ligand sensing: a nucleotide binding oligomerization domain (NOD) and a domain for the initiation of signaling such as CARDs, PYRIN of baculovirus inhibitor of apoptosis repeat (BIR) domains [25]. The retinoic-acid inducible protein-I (RIG-I) is an INF-inducible protein containing CARDs and a DExD/H box helicase domain and has been identified as a cytoplasmic detector in viral infection in the TLR3 independent manner [26]. In addition to the numerous exogenous pathogen-derived ligands that activate different TLRs, endogenous TLR ligands have been identified, including hyaluronic acid, high mobility group box-1 (HMGB1) and heat shock proteins (HSPs), termed as damaged-associated molecular patterns (DAMPs). During tissue injury or proteolysis, extracellular matrix components undergo cleavage, exposing moieties that can act as ligands for TLRs and therefore initiating TLR-induced signal transduction [27].

The PAM/PPR interaction leads to immune cell activation with initiation of microbe-killing systems, production and secretion of pro-inflammatory cytokines and chemokines, enhanced expression of co-stimulatory receptors essential for efficient T cell activation, production of arachinoid acid metabolites and initiation of extrinsic coagulation cascade [28-33]. The activation of the TLR signaling originated from the cytoplasmic Toll/IL-1 receptor (TIR) domain requires the association with the TIR domain-containing adaptor protein, MyD88. With ligands binding, MyD88 recruits IL-1 receptor-associates kinase-4 (IRAK-4) to TLRs through interaction of the death domains of both molecules. IRAK-1 activated by phosphorylation then associates with TRAF6, finally leading to activation of MAP kinases and NFκB. Additional modes of regulation for these pathways include TRIF-dependent induction of TRAF6 signaling by RIP1 and negative regulation of TIRAP mediated downstream signaling by ST2L, TRIAD3A and SOCS1. MyD88-independent pathways induce activation of IRF3 and expression of interferon-β. TIR-domain containing adaptors such as TIRAP, TRIF and TRAM regulate TLR-mediated signaling pathways by providing specificity for individual TLR signaling cascades [28-33].

The interaction of PAMs with NRL recruits the receptor-interacting protein-2 (RIP2) kinase activating NFκB and MAPK kinases. A number of the NRL molecules have been shown to form a complex with caspase-1 and the adaptor molecule apoptosis associated speck-like protein containing CARD (ASC) termed inflammasome. The central effector molecule of the inflammasome is the cysteine protease caspase-1 that, upon activation cleaves cytosolic pro-IL-1β, pro-IL-18 and pro-IL-33 to their active forms enabling them to be secreted into the extracellular/systemic compartments [34]. The important fact is that NRLs and TLRs may synergize. T-cell subgroups are modified in sepsis. Helper (CD4$^+$) T-cells can be categorized as type 1 helper (Th1) or 2 (Th2). Th1 cells generally secrete pro-inflammatory cytokines such as tumor necrosis factor-α(TNFα) and interleukin-1β (IL-1β); Th2 cells secrete anti-inflammatory cytokines such as IL-4 and IL-10, depending on the infecting organism, the burden of infection and other factors during sepsis may also induce apoptosis of lung and intestinal cells [35]. Activated helper T cells evolve from a Th1 phenotype, producing pro-inflammatory cytokines, to a Th2 phenotype producing anti-inflammatory cytokines [35]. In addition, apoptosis of circulating and tissue lymphocytes (B cells and CD4$^+$ T cells) contributes to immunosuppression [36]. The increased pro-inflammatory cytokines, activated B cells and T cells and circulating glucocorticoid levels causes apoptosis in septic patients [37]. Increased levels of TNF-α and lipopolysaccharide during sepsis may also induce apoptosis [35].

3. Physiopathology of acute respiratory distress syndrome

There are two general types of ALI/ARDS, direct and indirect. Independent of the initial insult, the final result is that alveolar-capillary barrier becomes compromised. Direct ALI/ARDS is often associated with direct mechanical, chemical or infectious stimuli, or other direct interactions capable to induce damage to lung structures [38]. Indirect pulmonary insults such as extra-pulmonary sepsis, trauma, shock, pancreatitis, brain injury or massive transfusion are the mainly causes of indirect ALI/ARDS. However, the highest incidence of indirect ALI/ARDS is seen during sepsis.

The emigration of activated PMNs and passage through the endothelium in the lungs, one of the characteristics of ALI, is regulated via adhesion molecules. Among them, L-selectin (CD62L) on PMNs appears to be involved in the initial rolling proceed on the endothelial surface, while CD11b/CD18 on PMNs mediate a tighter contact between them. CD31 of PECAM-1 is needed in the final step for the vascular diapedesis of leukocytes [38-40]. Neutrophils are able to release a variety of harmful substances, such as proteolytic enzymes, reactive oxygen/nitrogen species, cytokines and chemokynes, which may be injurious to the adjacent endothelial cell and to the alveoli [39]. PMN apoptosis is a crucial injury-limiting mechanism of inflammatory resolution. Several inflammatory agents such as LPS, TNF, IL-8, IL-6, IL-1 and granulocyte colony stimulating factor (G-CSF) can delay apoptotic response, providing PMN with a longer life, allowing accumulating at local tissues [41]. NFκB has been reported as a modulator of apoptosis in inflammatory cells [42, 43] allowing a pro-inflammatory state.

Loss of epithelial cells and endothelial cell injury are involved in pathogenesis of ALI/ARDS. The former is due to the activation of Fas related apoptosis and the secretion of cytokines and chemokines by lung epithelial cells [44]. The latter is caused by the interaction of endothelial cells with neutrophils that stimulate release of vasoactive compounds, increased pulmonary vascular resistance with pulmonary hypertension [45], but also endothelial cells can be directly stimulated by endotoxin via TLR-1 with the release of vasoactive mediators and molecules altering lung permeability, such as TNFα, thromboxane-A2 and endothelin-1 [46].

Resolution from lung injury is an actively regulated program involving a removal of apoptotic neutrophils, remodeling of matrix, clearance of protein-rich alveolar fluid [47]. Recently, has been demonstrated that CD4+ lymphocytes as well as plasmacytoid dendritic cells are active players in this process [48, 49].

4. Vectors for gene therapy

Gene therapy is defined as the introduction of nucleic acids into cells for the purpose of altering the course of a medical condition o disease [50]. In general, the advantages of gene therapy over the other treatments are the selective treatment of affected tissues, the possibility of using locally endogenous proteins in cases where its systemic application would incur in serious adverse secondary effects, and the possibility of therapeutic long term after a single application [51]. Currently, there are three categories of gene delivery methods: viral vector based, non-viral vector based and physical methods [52]. Viral-based gene delivery systems is accomplished by using replication-deficient viruses containing the gene of interest, but with the disease-causing sequences deleted from the viral genome [53] including RNA-based viral vectors [54, 55], DNA-based viral vectors such as adenoviral vectors [56], adeno-associated viruses (AAV) vectors orherpes simplex viral vector [57].The non-viral gene delivery methods use synthetic or natural compounds or physical forces to deliver a piece of DNA into a cell [58]. Two main groups of non-viral delivery methods have developed: chemical-based, including lipofection [59] and inorganic nanoparticles that are usually prepared from metals, inorganic salts or ceramics [60]; and using physical forces such as local or rapid systemic injection [61], particle impact [62, 63], electric pulse [64] or laser irradiation [65].

5. Gene therapy in sepsis

Currently, there is evidence that applying therapeutic maneuvers such as early effective antibiotic administration, intensive fluid resuscitation, mechanical ventilation in selected patients and use of C activated protein in sickest patients improve significantly the survive in these patients [66]. There are several clinical studies that are trying to validate another kind of therapies such as extra-renal depuration, levosimendan, the use of immunoglobulins, nitric oxide, statins, selenium, the use of enteral nutrition with eicosapentaenoic acid (EPA)/ψlinolenic acid (GLA) that are in progress [67]. Basic research and clinical trials have focused on alternative therapeutic approaches [68].

5.1. Pattern associated membrane receptors

Different approaches have designed trying to block the interaction between PAMs and PPRs. One is the generation of antibodies that bind TLRs. Studies conducted with anti-lipopolysaccharide binding protein or anti-CD14 in experimental models of endotoxic shock and Gram-negative bacterial sepsis, failed to show a protection when treatment was administered after LPS o simultaneously with or shortly after bacterial inoculation [69-71]. By using a recombinant chimeric fusion protein composed of the N-terminal and central domains (amino-acids 1-334) of the extracellular part of TLR4 and the Fc portion of the human IgG1, Roger et al [72] produced an anti-TLR4 antibodies that inhibited LPS-induced intracellular signaling and cytokine production and protected mice from lethal endotoxic shock and E. coli bacterial sepsis, not only in pre-treatment with the antibodies, but also even when treatment was delayed for several hours after endotoxemia of the onset of sepsis.

The RAGEs (receptor for advanced glycation end products) are part of DAMPs that may play a role in the perpetuation of inflammation that carries to severe sepsis or septic shock. RAGEs are up-regulated in acute and chronic inflammation and bind multiple endogenous mediators involved in sepsis and products of oxidative stress [73]. In a recent work, Christaki et al demonstrated that blocking RAGEs either before or after infection protected mice from lethality in sepsis due to *S. pneumoniae* pneumonia [74] probably by indirect inhibition of NFκB activation.

Exposure to Staphylococcal enterotoxin (SE) or SE plus lipopolysaccharide (LPS, endotoxin) in mice, triggers vigorous intracellular signaling that leads to hyper-inflammation and release of pro-inflammatory cytokines such as TNFα, INFγ, IL-1β, IL-1α, IL-2 and IL-6 by activation of innate immunity [75]. In order to evaluate the role of MyD88, the anchor adaptor protein that integrates and transduces intracellular signals from TLRs and IL-1 receptor superfamily, Kisssner et al evaluates a synthetic molecule, hydrocinnamoyl-L-valyl-pyrrolidine (Compd1), which mimics the BB-loop in the TIR domain of MyD88. They observed an inhibited pro-inflammatory cytokine production in human primary cells. Also, administration of Compd1 to mice inhibited pro-inflammatory cytokine response and increased survival from toxic shock induced death-limiting hyper-inflammation [76].

Recently, the knockdown or TLR2 by three different small interfering RNAs (siRNA) (A: 5'-aactatccactggtgaaacaa-3', B: 5'-aaacttgtcagtggccagaaa-3', C: 5'-aaagtcttgattgattggcca-3') reduce de tumorigenesis generated by the injection of BEL-7402 cells in an athymic mouse. Also, the levels of cytokines IL-6 and IL-8 were found to be markedly depressed [77]. In this line, Lei Ming et al have designed four siRNA:

siRNA-180, 5'-GCCUGGAAUACCUUCUAAATT-3';

siRNA-224, 5'-GGGCAGUUCACUGAUAUUATT-3';

siRNA-341, 5'-CAGGAACUGACUCUUGAAATT-3';

siRNA-987, 5'-CCCACUCGGAGAAGUUUAATT-3' against mCD14. *In vitro* experiments with RAW264.7 cells (a transformed murine macrophage cell line) shown that siRNA-224 effectively inhibited LPS-induced TNFα, MIP-2 and IL-6 release and NO production [78].

5.2. Intracellular signaling

Severely burned patients are greatly susceptible to infection with various pathogens [79]. Macrophages (MΦs) have an important role in antibacterial innate immunity. In methicillin-resistant *Staphylococcus aureus* infection (MRSA), MΦs (IL-12⁻ IL-10⁻) differentiate in two different subpopulations, M1MΦ (IL-12⁺ IL-10⁻) and M2MΦ (IL-12⁻ IL-10⁺). The former are converted by the TLRs stimulation and has the ability to kill bacteria, to produce reactive nitrogen intermediates, and to release antimicrobial peptides [80], playing a pivotal role in host microbial resistance. M2MΦ have reduced ability to kill bacteria; IL-10 and CCL7 released by M2MΦ are inhibitory molecules on the pathogen-stimulated MΦ conversion to M1MΦ. IL-10 is also a deactivator of antibacterial immunocompetent cells [81] and an inhibitory molecule on various immunocompetent cell functions. Asai et al have demonstrated that IL-10 antisense oligonucleotides in a severely burned mice prevents the burn associated conversion of MΦ to M2MΦ and infectious complications stemming for MRSA local infection did not develop [82].

CCL2 is a chemokine that attracts and activates mononuclear cells. The necessity of this chemokine for Th2-cell generation has been demonstrated. In a study Shigematsu K et al [83] tried to protect thermally injured mice orally infected with a lethal dose of *E. faecalis* by gene therapy utilizing phosphorothioate-CCL2 antisense oligodeoxynucleotides. They demonstrate that sepsis stemming from *E. faecalis* translocation in severely burned mice is controllable by the gene therapy using CCL2 antisense ODNs, through the elimination of mesenteric lymph node macrophages (MLN- MΦ)-M2aMΦs and M2cMΦs subtypes. [83].

IL-1β binds the type-1 IL-1 receptor, while LPS binds to TLR4, both activates intracellular pathways by phosphorylation of IRAK family members including IRAK-1, which involve the MyD88 adaptor protein [84]. The group of Johns RE et al developed a family of "smart" polymeric carriers, termed encrypted polymers that enhance the cytoplasmic delivery of therapeutic antisense oligonucleotides (ASONs). This group has demonstrated that these ASONs block LPS activation of the transcription factor NFκB reducing the LPS-induced expression of cytokines and chemokines. IL-6 shows a 2-fold decrease whereas TNFα expression trended to decrease. There was a 2-fold decrease in expression of several genes including MCP1, MCP3, eotaxin and IP10 [85].

5.3. Apoptosis

Caspases are pro-enzymes of the aspartate-specific cysteine protease family and its activation plays a central role in the execution of apoptosis [86]. Depending of the stimuli, two caspase-activation pathways have been described, the mitochondria-initiated caspase-8-dependent pathway and mitochondria-initiated caspase-9-mediated pathway. Activation of these pathways initiates a downstream cascade of effector caspases, such as caspase-3 tha cleaves substrates such as D4-GDI leading to cell death [87]. The group of Ayala A et al in 2005 demonstrated that suppression of Fas or caspase-8 gene expression with hydrodynamic administration of siRNA conferred a survival advantage in septic mice model after caecal ligation and perforation (CLP) [88]. In a work of Matsuda N et al, they examined the therapeutic efficacy of caspase-8 and caspase-3 gene silencing with siRNAs delivered by systemic injection in a CLP endotoxic shock mouse model. They demonstrate that *in vivo* delivery of caspase-8/caspase-3 siRNAs conferred a dramatic survival advantage to CLP mice as compared to controls. Also they demonstrated that the survival benefit was observed despite administration of siRNA as late as 10h after CLP [88].

BRCA1 is a critical regulator of DNA damage repair and cell survival. In a recent article, Teoh H et al demonstrated a reduction in 24 hours post caecal ligation and perforation and thioglycollate stimulation mortality with pretreatment with human BRCA1 adenovirus (AdBRCA1). Treatment with AdBRCA1, a human adenovirus type-5 (dE1/E3), blunted CLP-associated cardiac, pulmonary, hepatic and renal dysfunction and also reduced CLP-elicited double strand breaks and apoptosis in the liver. BRCA1 gene therapy was associated with lower CLP-evoked cardiac and hepatic superoxide generation that in the liver was in part due to improved reactive oxygen species removal. CLP also elevated mesenteric arteriolar and serum intercellular adhesion molecule-1, both of which were partially abrogated with AdBRCA1 administration. Thioglycollate-challenged AdBRCA1-treated mice displayed reduced peritoneal neutrophil recruitment and dampened cytokine elaboration relative to their Ad-null-treated counterparts [89].

6. Gene therapy in ARDS/ALI

Over the past 20 years, the feasibility of using gene transfer to treat ALI/ARDS has been demonstrated using a variety of viral and non-viral vectors to deliver various transgenes to the lung [90].

6.1. Strategies to increase pulmonary surfactant

ALI/ARDS is a surfactant-deficient state. *Pseudomonas aeruginosa* infection is a cause of pulmonary infection and ARDS with surfactant deficient phenotype. Zhou J et al have demonstrated the attenuation of the deleterious effects of *Pseudomonas aeruginosa* infection by adenoviral gene transfer overexpressing CCTpenta (a mutant form of the regulatory enzyme CCTα required for the biosynthesis of dipalmitoyl phosphatidylcholine (DPPC), the major phospholipid of surfactant) with a significant increase of the biosynthesis of surfactant. This study suggests that augmentation of DPPC synthesis via gene delivery of CCTα can attenuate impaired lung function in surfactant-deficient states such as bacterial sepsis [91].

6.2. Strategies to improve pulmonary edema

The physiological hallmark of ARDS is disruption of the alveolar-capillary membrane barrier, leading to development of non-cardiogenic pulmonary edema, in which proteinaceous exudate floods the alveolar spaces, impairs gas exchange and precipitates respiratory failure [92]. Several studies indicate that CLP (cecal ligation and puncture) sepsis model, sepsis and endotoxemia impair the expression of heat shock protein (HSP-70). Data shown that HSP-70 can limit inflammatory responses protect proteins from damage, restore function to proteins that are damaged and prevent cellular destruction, key processes of ALI/ARDS [93]. Weiss et al have demonstrated that the use of an adenoviral vector (AdHSP, an adenovirus carrying the gene for HSP-70) correcting the relative defect in HSP-70 expression prevents neutrophil accumulation, reduce protein rich edema fluid and improve the outcome in ARDS secondary to CLP [94].

Injury of the alveolo-capillary barrier alters active Na^+ transport, leading to impaired edema fluid clearance from the alveolar spaces. Failure to return to normal clearance is associated with poor prognosis [95]. The primary force driving fluid reabsorption from the alveolar space into the interstitium and the pulmonary circulation is active Na^+ transport. Sodium is taken up on the apical surface of the alveolar epithelium by amiloride-sensitive and -insensitive Na^+ channels [96] and is subsequently pumped out of the cell by the Na^+/K^+-adenosine triphosphatase (Na^+/K^+-ATPase) on the baso-lateral side [96]. Some studies have demonstrated the importance of Na^+/K^+-ATPase in ALI/ARDS. In normal adults rats, overexpression of the β1-subunit gene by utilizing a replication-incompetent human type-5 adenovirus expressing Na^+/K^+-ATPase-β1 subunit cDNA increased alveolar edema clearance over twofold compared with controls [97]. Similarly, gene transfer of the Na^+/K^+-ATPase-β1 subunit using electroporation increased alveolar fluid reabsorption [98]. Furthermore, while rats exposed to 100% oxygen develop ALI and impaired alveolar fluid clearance; overexpression of the Na^+/K^+-ATPase-β1 subunit in the alveolar epithelium of rats increased lung liquid clearance and, most importantly, overexpression of the Na^+/K^+-ATPase-β1 subunit resulted in 100% survival over 14 days of hyperoxia (compared with 25-31% survival in the non-treated or null virus-treated control groups) [99].

In this line, Stern M et al used a cationic liposome to transfer cDNA encoding both α and β subunits of Na^+/K^+-ATPase to the lung of a mouse model of pulmonary edema induced by thiourea; they observe a significant resolution of pulmonary edema *in vivo*. Also, overexpression of the β2-adrenergic receptor leads to increased alveolar fluid clearance in rats by increasing both membrane-bound amiloride-sensitive Na^+-channel expression and Na^+/K^+-ATPase function, probably enhancing responsiveness to endogenous catecholamines in the alveolar epithelium [100].

The regulation of alveolar transport proteins is vital in the maintenance of alveolar fluid balance in patients [101]. The exposure to hypoxia results in decreased Na^+/K^+-ATPase activity and protein abundance at the plasma membrane by promoting the endocytosis of the pump, which contributes to a decrease in alveolar fluid reabsorption in both *in vivo* an *ex vivo* models of hypoxia. Also, the overexpression of the reactive oxygen species scavenger, SOD2, prevents this hypoxia-mediated decrease in alveolar fluid reabsorption and Na^+/K^+-ATPase function [102].

6.3. Strategies to afford oxidant injury-related injury, apoptosis and inflammation

Keratinocyte growth factor (KGF) is an epithelial-specific growth factor secreted by fibro-blast and vascular smooth muscle cells and a main mitogen for alveolar type II cells [103]. Baba et al have demonstrated that transient over-expression of KGF in the lungs attenuate pathophysiological impairments in hyperoxia-induced acute lung injury by increasing Ki67 and surfactant protein C (Sp-C)-positive cells and proliferation of epithelial cuboidal cells [104]. There is an abundance of evidence regarding the protective effect of pre-treatment with KGF on lung injury induced by hyperoxia, acid instillation, radiation, bleomycin, α-naphthylthiourea, ventilator and bacterial pneumonia there are some studies that supports the potential clinical application of KGF-2 in the treatment of ALI/ARDS [105].

Human angiopoeitin-1 (ANGPT1), a ligand for the endothelial-restricted receptor TEK tyro-sine kinase, plays an essential role in blood vessel maturation and stabilization during em-bryonic development. In postnatal, ANGPT1 maintains the normal quiescent phenotype of vascular ECs, protecting against vascular inflammation reducing permeability and promot-ing ECs survival. In a study of Mei SH and co-workers carried out in an ALI mice model (by intra-tracheal instillation of LPS), they have demonstrated that mesenchymal stem cells (MSCs) administration alone into the pulmonary circulation partially prevents LPS-induced lung inflammation. However, cell-based gene transfer using pANGPT1-transfected MSCs resulted in further improvement in both alveolar inflammation and membrane permeability. Also, MSCs-pANGPT1 dramatically reduced cytokine levels (IFNγ, TNFα, IL-6 and IL1-β) to the baseline values observed in naïve mice, suggesting a potential therapeutic approach to ALI/ARDS [106].

Pearl M and colleagues in a 2005 study using Fas- and caspase-8 siRNA intra-tracheal ad-ministration in a CLP mice model of sepsis demonstrated that the main targets of siRNA de-livery are the epithelial cells. Also, that down-regulation of Fas but not caspase-8 reduces pulmonary apoptosis and lung inflammation, decreases neutrophil influx and attenuates ALI [107].

Overexpression of interleukin IL-10 trough recombinant adeno-associated virus type-5 (AAV5) vector expressing murine IL-10 into pulmonary, tissue proinflammatory cytokines IL-1β and TNFα, macrophage inhibitory protein-1$\alpha$and keratinocyte chemoattractant in the epithelial lining fluid and lung homogenate were decreased and neutrophil infiltration was less pronounced and more localized neutrophil infiltration in lung section [108].

Finally, Hemoxygenase-1 (HO-1) is an inducible isoform of the first and rate-controlling en-zyme of the degradation of heme into iron, carbon monoxide, and biliverdin, the latter being subsequently converted into bilirubin. Several positive biological effects exerted by this en-zyme have gained attention, as anti-inflammatory, antiapoptotic, angiogenic, and cytopro-tective functions are attributable to carbon monoxide and/or bilirubin Also, the enzyme has been involved in controlling infiltration of neutrophils into the injured lung and in the reso-lution of inflammation by modulating apoptotic cell death and cytokine expression. Several groups have delivered HO-1 expressing adenoviruses to the lungs in both pneumonia and hyperoxia models and have shown significant reductions in inflammation and subsequent lung injury [90].

7. Future directions and conclusion

Sepsis and acute lung injury/acute respiratory distress syndrome are important pathologies in critical care medicine. There are increasing evidence from relevant pre-clinical studies that support the efficacy of gene-based therapies. Multiple barriers exist to the successful use of gene therapy in critical care medicine and particularly in sepsis and ALI/ARDS. Future research approaches are necessary to overcome these barriers by developing better viral and non-viral vectors, enhanced and specific gene expression strategies, improved cellular uptake of vectors and better therapeutic targets.

Although the treatment by transference of genetic material still presents many challenges, the technology is rapidly evolving and the possible use in clinical trials could be in a near future. So, the aim of this chapter was to understand the molecular mechanisms involved in acute respiratory distress syndrome and sepsis, to review the viral and non-viral gene therapies that have been developed to improve survival and to address the challenges of gene therapy in critical care patients using these two life-threating conditions as a model.

Acknowledgments

This work was supported by CONACYT grant 164413 and PAPIIT-UNAM grant IN204410.

Author details

Gabriel J. Moreno-González[1] and Angel Zarain-Herzberg[2]

1 Intensive Care Unit, Hospital Universitari de Bellvitge, L'Hospitalet Llobregat, Barcelona, Spain

2 Biochemistry Department, School of Medicine, Universidad Nacional Autónoma de México, Mexico City, México

References

[1] Vincent JL. Evidence-based medicine in the ICU: important advances and limitations. Chest. 2004;126(2):592-600. Epub 2004/08/11.

[2]   Rubenfeld GD, Caldwell E, Peabody E, Weaver J, Martin DP, Neff M, et al. Incidence and outcomes of acute lung injury. The New England journal of medicine. 2005;353(16):1685-93. Epub 2005/10/21.

[3]   Linde-Zwirble WT, Angus DC. Severe sepsis epidemiology: sampling, selection, and society. Crit Care. 2004;8(4):222-6. Epub 2004/08/18.

[4]   American College of Chest Physicians/Society of Critical Care Medicine Consensus Conference: definitions for sepsis and organ failure and guidelines for the use of innovative therapies in sepsis. Crit Care Med. 1992;20(6):864-74. Epub 1992/06/01.

[5]   Levy MM, Fink MP, Marshall JC, Abraham E, Angus D, Cook D, et al. 2001 SCCM/ESICM/ACCP/ATS/SIS International Sepsis Definitions Conference. Intensive care medicine. 2003;29(4):530-8. Epub 2003/03/29.

[6]   Johnson SB, Lissauer M, Bochicchio GV, Moore R, Cross AS, Scalea TM. Gene expression profiles differentiate between sterile SIRS and early sepsis. Annals of surgery. 2007;245(4):611-21. Epub 2007/04/07.

[7]   Guidelines for the management of severe sepsis and septic shock. The International Sepsis Forum. Intensive care medicine. 2001;27 Suppl 1:S1-134. Epub 2001/08/25.

[8]   Angus DC, Linde-Zwirble WT, Lidicker J, Clermont G, Carcillo J, Pinsky MR. Epidemiology of severe sepsis in the United States: analysis of incidence, outcome, and associated costs of care. Crit Care Med. 2001;29(7):1303-10. Epub 2001/07/11.

[9]   Angus DC, Wax RS. Epidemiology of sepsis: an update. Crit Care Med. 2001;29(7 Suppl):S109-16. Epub 2001/07/11.

[10] Bone RC, Balk RA, Cerra FB, Dellinger RP, Fein AM, Knaus WA, et al. Definitions for sepsis and organ failure and guidelines for the use of innovative therapies in sepsis. The ACCP/SCCM Consensus Conference Committee. American College of Chest Physicians/Society of Critical Care Medicine. Chest. 1992;101(6):1644-55. Epub 1992/06/01.

[11] Rivers E, Nguyen B, Havstad S, Ressler J, Muzzin A, Knoblich B, et al. Early goal-directed therapy in the treatment of severe sepsis and septic shock. The New England journal of medicine. 2001;345(19):1368-77. Epub 2002/01/17.

[12] Bernard GR, Vincent JL, Laterre PF, LaRosa SP, Dhainaut JF, Lopez-Rodriguez A, et al. Efficacy and safety of recombinant human activated protein C for severe sepsis. The New England journal of medicine. 2001;344(10):699-709. Epub 2001/03/10.

[13] Natanson C, Esposito CJ, Banks SM. The sirens' songs of confirmatory sepsis trials: selection bias and sampling error. Crit Care Med. 1998;26(12):1927-31. Epub 1999/01/06.

[14] Phua J, Stewart TE, Ferguson ND. Acute respiratory distress syndrome 40 years later: time to revisit its definition. Crit Care Med. 2008;36(10):2912-21. Epub 2008/09/04.

[15] Villar J, Perez-Mendez L, Lopez J, Belda J, Blanco J, Saralegui I, et al. An early PEEP/ FIO2 trial identifies different degrees of lung injury in patients with acute respiratory distress syndrome. American journal of respiratory and critical care medicine. 2007;176(8):795-804. Epub 2007/06/23.

[16] Raghavendran K, Napolitano LM. Definition of ALI/ARDS. Critical care clinics. 2011;27(3):429-37. Epub 2011/07/12.

[17] Martin GS. Temporal changes in clinical outcomes with ARDS. Chest. 2005;128(2): 479-81. Epub 2005/08/16.

[18] Frutos-Vivar F, Ferguson ND, Esteban A. Epidemiology of acute lung injury and acute respiratory distress syndrome. Seminars in respiratory and critical care medicine. 2006;27(4):327-36. Epub 2006/08/16.

[19] Rubenfeld GD. Epidemiology of acute lung injury. Crit Care Med. 2003;31(4 Suppl):S276-84. Epub 2003/04/12.

[20] MacCallum NS, Evans TW. Epidemiology of acute lung injury. Current opinion in critical care. 2005;11(1):43-9. Epub 2005/01/22.

[21] Martin GS, Bernard GR. Airway and lung in sepsis. Intensive care medicine. 2001;27 Suppl 1:S63-79. Epub 2001/04/20.

[22] Mogensen TH. Pathogen recognition and inflammatory signaling in innate immune defenses. Clinical microbiology reviews. 2009;22(2):240-73, Table of Contents. Epub 2009/04/16.

[23] Bowie A, O'Neill LA. The interleukin-1 receptor/Toll-like receptor superfamily: signal generators for pro-inflammatory interleukins and microbial products. Journal of leukocyte biology. 2000;67(4):508-14. Epub 2000/04/19.

[24] Akira S, Uematsu S, Takeuchi O. Pathogen recognition and innate immunity. Cell. 2006;124(4):783-801. Epub 2006/02/25.

[25] Inohara, Chamaillard, McDonald C, Nunez G. NOD-LRR proteins: role in host-microbial interactions and inflammatory disease. Annual review of biochemistry. 2005;74:355-83. Epub 2005/06/15.

[26] Yoneyama M, Kikuchi M, Natsukawa T, Shinobu N, Imaizumi T, Miyagishi M, et al. The RNA helicase RIG-I has an essential function in double-stranded RNA-induced innate antiviral responses. Nature immunology. 2004;5(7):730-7. Epub 2004/06/23.

[27] Wagner H. Endogenous TLR ligands and autoimmunity. Advances in immunology. 2006;91:159-73. Epub 2006/08/30.

[28] Barton GM, Kagan JC. A cell biological view of Toll-like receptor function: regulation through compartmentalization. Nature reviews Immunology. 2009;9(8):535-42. Epub 2009/06/27.

[29] Blasius AL, Beutler B. Intracellular toll-like receptors. Immunity. 2010;32(3):305-15. Epub 2010/03/30.

[30] Li X, Jiang S, Tapping RI. Toll-like receptor signaling in cell proliferation and survival. Cytokine. 2010;49(1):1-9. Epub 2009/09/25.

[31] McGettrick AF, O'Neill LA. Localisation and trafficking of Toll-like receptors: an important mode of regulation. Current opinion in immunology. 2010;22(1):20-7. Epub 2010/01/12.

[32] Miggin SM, O'Neill LA. New insights into the regulation of TLR signaling. Journal of leukocyte biology. 2006;80(2):220-6. Epub 2006/05/16.

[33] Pasare C, Medzhitov R. Toll-like receptors: linking innate and adaptive immunity. Advances in experimental medicine and biology. 2005;560:11-8. Epub 2005/06/04.

[34] Martinon F, Burns K, Tschopp J. The inflammasome: a molecular platform triggering activation of inflammatory caspases and processing of proIL-beta. Molecular cell. 2002;10(2):417-26. Epub 2002/08/23.

[35] Russell JA. Management of sepsis. The New England journal of medicine. 2006;355(16):1699-713. Epub 2006/10/20.

[36] Hotchkiss RS, Swanson PE, Freeman BD, Tinsley KW, Cobb JP, Matuschak GM, et al. Apoptotic cell death in patients with sepsis, shock, and multiple organ dysfunction. Crit Care Med. 1999;27(7):1230-51. Epub 1999/08/14.

[37] Ayala A, Herdon CD, Lehman DL, DeMaso CM, Ayala CA, Chaudry IH. The induction of accelerated thymic programmed cell death during polymicrobial sepsis: control by corticosteroids but not tumor necrosis factor. Shock. 1995;3(4):259-67. Epub 1995/04/01.

[38] Perl M, Lomas-Neira J, Venet F, Chung CS, Ayala A. Pathogenesis of indirect (secondary) acute lung injury. Expert review of respiratory medicine. 2011;5(1):115-26. Epub 2011/02/26.

[39] Suzuki T, Moraes TJ, Vachon E, Ginzberg HH, Huang TT, Matthay MA, et al. Proteinase-activated receptor-1 mediates elastase-induced apoptosis of human lung epithelial cells. American journal of respiratory cell and molecular biology. 2005;33(3): 231-47. Epub 2005/05/14.

[40] Woodfin A, Voisin MB, Nourshargh S. PECAM-1: a multi-functional molecule in inflammation and vascular biology. Arteriosclerosis, thrombosis, and vascular biology. 2007;27(12):2514-23. Epub 2007/09/18.

[41] Dunican AL, Leuenroth SJ, Grutkoski P, Ayala A, Simms HH. TNFalpha-induced suppression of PMN apoptosis is mediated through interleukin-8 production. Shock. 2000;14(3):284-8; discussion 8-9. Epub 2000/10/12.

[42] Nakanishi C, Toi M. Nuclear factor-kappaB inhibitors as sensitizers to anticancer drugs. Nature reviews Cancer. 2005;5(4):297-309. Epub 2005/04/02.

[43] Liu G, Park YJ, Tsuruta Y, Lorne E, Abraham E. p53 Attenuates lipopolysaccharide-induced NF-kappaB activation and acute lung injury. J Immunol. 2009;182(8): 5063-71. Epub 2009/04/04.

[44] Albertine KH, Soulier MF, Wang Z, Ishizaka A, Hashimoto S, Zimmerman GA, et al. Fas and fas ligand are up-regulated in pulmonary edema fluid and lung tissue of patients with acute lung injury and the acute respiratory distress syndrome. The American journal of pathology. 2002;161(5):1783-96. Epub 2002/11/05.

[45] Gropper MA, Wiener-Kronish J. The epithelium in acute lung injury/acute respiratory distress syndrome. Current opinion in critical care. 2008;14(1):11-5. Epub 2008/01/16.

[46] Maniatis NA, Kotanidou A, Catravas JD, Orfanos SE. Endothelial pathomechanisms in acute lung injury. Vascular pharmacology. 2008;49(4-6):119-33. Epub 2008/08/30.

[47] Tsushima K, King LS, Aggarwal NR, De Gorordo A, D'Alessio FR, Kubo K. Acute lung injury review. Intern Med. 2009;48(9):621-30. Epub 2009/05/08.

[48] Pene F, Zuber B, Courtine E, Rousseau C, Ouaaz F, Toubiana J, et al. Dendritic cells modulate lung response to Pseudomonas aeruginosa in a murine model of sepsis-induced immune dysfunction. J Immunol. 2008;181(12):8513-20. Epub 2008/12/04.

[49] Benjamim CF, Lundy SK, Lukacs NW, Hogaboam CM, Kunkel SL. Reversal of long-term sepsis-induced immunosuppression by dendritic cells. Blood. 2005;105(9): 3588-95. Epub 2004/12/18.

[50] Kay MA, Liu D, Hoogerbrugge PM. Gene therapy. Proc Natl Acad Sci U S A. 1997;94(24):12744-6. Epub 1997/12/05.

[51] Yla-Herttuala S, Alitalo K. Gene transfer as a tool to induce therapeutic vascular growth. Nature medicine. 2003;9(6):694-701. Epub 2003/06/05.

[52] Kamimura K, Suda T, Zhang G, Liu D. Advances in Gene Delivery Systems. Pharmaceut Med. 2011;25(5):293-306. Epub 2011/12/28.

[53] Thomas CE, Ehrhardt A, Kay MA. Progress and problems with the use of viral vectors for gene therapy. Nature reviews Genetics. 2003;4(5):346-58. Epub 2003/05/03.

[54] Barquinero J, Eixarch H, Perez-Melgosa M. Retroviral vectors: new applications for an old tool. Gene therapy. 2004;11 Suppl 1:S3-9. Epub 2004/09/30.

[55] Daniel R, Smith JA. Integration site selection by retroviral vectors: molecular mechanism and clinical consequences. Human gene therapy. 2008;19(6):557-68. Epub 2008/06/07.

[56] Khare R, Chen CY, Weaver EA, Barry MA. Advances and future challenges in adenoviral vector pharmacology and targeting. Current gene therapy. 2011;11(4):241-58. Epub 2011/04/02.

[57] Friedman GK, Pressey JG, Reddy AT, Markert JM, Gillespie GY. Herpes simplex vi-
      rus oncolytic therapy for pediatric malignancies. Molecular therapy : the journal of
      the American Society of Gene Therapy. 2009;17(7):1125-35. Epub 2009/04/16.

[58] Al-Dosari MS, Gao X. Nonviral gene delivery: principle, limitations, and recent prog-
      ress. The AAPS journal. 2009;11(4):671-81. Epub 2009/10/17.

[59] Wasungu L, Hoekstra D. Cationic lipids, lipoplexes and intracellular delivery of
      genes. Journal of controlled release : official journal of the Controlled Release Society.
      2006;116(2):255-64. Epub 2006/08/18.

[60] Sokolova V, Epple M. Inorganic nanoparticles as carriers of nucleic acids into cells.
      Angew Chem Int Ed Engl. 2008;47(8):1382-95. Epub 2007/12/22.

[61] Wolff JA, Malone RW, Williams P, Chong W, Acsadi G, Jani A, et al. Direct gene
      transfer into mouse muscle in vivo. Science. 1990;247(4949 Pt 1):1465-8. Epub
      1990/03/23.

[62] Liu F, Song Y, Liu D. Hydrodynamics-based transfection in animals by systemic ad-
      ministration of plasmid DNA. Gene therapy. 1999;6(7):1258-66. Epub 1999/08/24.

[63] O'Brien J, Lummis SC. An improved method of preparing microcarriers for biolistic
      transfection. Brain research Brain research protocols. 2002;10(1):12-5. Epub
      2002/10/16.

[64] Titomirov AV, Sukharev S, Kistanova E. In vivo electroporation and stable transfor-
      mation of skin cells of newborn mice by plasmid DNA. Biochimica et biophysica ac-
      ta. 1991;1088(1):131-4. Epub 1991/01/17.

[65] Kim HJ, Greenleaf JF, Kinnick RR, Bronk JT, Bolander ME. Ultrasound-mediated
      transfection of mammalian cells. Human gene therapy. 1996;7(11):1339-46. Epub
      1996/07/10.

[66] Dellinger RP, Levy MM, Carlet JM, Bion J, Parker MM, Jaeschke R, et al. Surviving
      Sepsis Campaign: international guidelines for management of severe sepsis and sep-
      tic shock: 2008. Crit Care Med. 2008;36(1):296-327. Epub 2007/12/26.

[67] Loza Vazquez A, Leon Gil C, Leon Regidor A. [New therapeutic alternatives for se-
      vere sepsis in the critical patient. A review]. Medicina intensiva / Sociedad Espanola
      de Medicina Intensiva y Unidades Coronarias. 2011;35(4):236-45. Epub 2011/01/07.
      Nuevas alternativas terapeuticas para la sepsis grave en el paciente critico. Revision.

[68] Matsuda A, Jacob A, Wu R, Aziz M, Yang WL, Matsutani T, et al. Novel therapeutic
      targets for sepsis: regulation of exaggerated inflammatory responses. Journal of Ni-
      hon Medical School = Nihon Ika Daigaku zasshi. 2012;79(1):4-18. Epub 2012/03/09.

[69] Frevert CW, Matute-Bello G, Skerrett SJ, Goodman RB, Kajikawa O, Sittipunt C, et al.
      Effect of CD14 blockade in rabbits with Escherichia coli pneumonia and sepsis. J Im-
      munol. 2000;164(10):5439-45. Epub 2000/05/09.

[70] Gallay P, Heumann D, Le Roy D, Barras C, Glauser MP. Lipopolysaccharide-binding protein as a major plasma protein responsible for endotoxemic shock. Proc Natl Acad Sci U S A. 1993;90(21):9935-8. Epub 1993/11/01.

[71] Le Roy D, Di Padova F, Adachi Y, Glauser MP, Calandra T, Heumann D. Critical role of lipopolysaccharide-binding protein and CD14 in immune responses against gram-negative bacteria. J Immunol. 2001;167(5):2759-65. Epub 2001/08/18.

[72] Roger T, Froidevaux C, Le Roy D, Reymond MK, Chanson AL, Mauri D, et al. Protection from lethal gram-negative bacterial sepsis by targeting Toll-like receptor 4. Proc Natl Acad Sci U S A. 2009;106(7):2348-52. Epub 2009/02/03.

[73] Schmidt AM, Yan SD, Yan SF, Stern DM. The multiligand receptor RAGE as a progression factor amplifying immune and inflammatory responses. J Clin Invest. 2001;108(7):949-55. Epub 2001/10/03.

[74] Christaki E, Opal SM, Keith JC, Jr., Kessimian N, Palardy JE, Parejo NA, et al. A monoclonal antibody against RAGE alters gene expression and is protective in experimental models of sepsis and pneumococcal pneumonia. Shock. 2011;35(5):492-8. Epub 2011/01/26.

[75] Beno DW, Uhing MR, Goto M, Chen Y, Jiyamapa-Serna VA, Kimura RE. Staphylococcal enterotoxin B potentiates LPS-induced hepatic dysfunction in chronically catheterized rats. American journal of physiology Gastrointestinal and liver physiology. 2001;280(5):G866-72. Epub 2001/04/09.

[76] Kissner TL, Moisan L, Mann E, Alam S, Ruthel G, Ulrich RG, et al. A small molecule that mimics the BB-loop in the Toll interleukin-1 (IL-1) receptor domain of MyD88 attenuates staphylococcal enterotoxin B-induced pro-inflammatory cytokine production and toxicity in mice. The Journal of biological chemistry. 2011;286(36):31385-96. Epub 2011/06/23.

[77] Huang Y, Cai B, Xu M, Qiu Z, Tao Y, Zhang Y, et al. Gene silencing of toll-like receptor 2 inhibits proliferation of human liver cancer cells and secretion of inflammatory cytokines. PloS one. 2012;7(7):e38890. Epub 2012/07/21.

[78] Lei M, Jiao H, Liu T, Du L, Cheng Y, Zhang D, et al. siRNA targeting mCD14 inhibits TNF-alpha, MIP-2, and IL-6 secretion and NO production from LPS-induced RAW264.7 cells. Applied microbiology and biotechnology. 2011;92(1):115-24. Epub 2011/06/28.

[79] Vostrugina K, Gudaviciene D, Vitkauskiene A. Bacteremias in patients with severe burn trauma. Medicina (Kaunas). 2006;42(7):576-9. Epub 2006/07/25.

[80] Houghton AM, Hartzell WO, Robbins CS, Gomis-Ruth FX, Shapiro SD. Macrophage elastase kills bacteria within murine macrophages. Nature. 2009;460(7255):637-41. Epub 2009/06/19.

[81] Katakura T, Miyazaki M, Kobayashi M, Herndon DN, Suzuki F. CCL17 and IL-10 as effectors that enable alternatively activated macrophages to inhibit the generation of classically activated macrophages. J Immunol. 2004;172(3):1407-13. Epub 2004/01/22.

[82] Asai A, Kogiso M, Kobayashi M, Herndon DN, Suzuki F. Effect of IL-10 antisense gene therapy in severely burned mice intradermally infected with MRSA. Immunobiology. 2012;217(7):711-8. Epub 2012/01/03.

[83] Shigematsu K, Kogiso M, Kobayashi M, Herndon DN, Suzuki F. Effect of CCL2 antisense oligodeoxynucleotides on bacterial translocation and subsequent sepsis in severely burned mice orally infected with Enterococcus faecalis. European journal of immunology. 2012;42(1):158-64. Epub 2011/10/18.

[84] Dunne A, O'Neill LA. The interleukin-1 receptor/Toll-like receptor superfamily: signal transduction during inflammation and host defense. Science's STKE : signal transduction knowledge environment. 2003;2003(171):re3. Epub 2003/02/28.

[85] Johns RE, El-Sayed ME, Bulmus V, Cuschieri J, Maier R, Hoffman AS, et al. Mechanistic analysis of macrophage response to IRAK-1 gene knockdown by a smart polymer-antisense oligonucleotide therapeutic. Journal of biomaterials science Polymer edition. 2008;19(10):1333-46. Epub 2008/10/16.

[86] Cohen GM. Caspases: the executioners of apoptosis. The Biochemical journal. 1997;326 (Pt 1):1-16. Epub 1997/08/15.

[87] Goyal L. Cell death inhibition: keeping caspases in check. Cell. 2001;104(6):805-8. Epub 2001/04/06.

[88] Wesche-Soldato DE, Chung CS, Lomas-Neira J, Doughty LA, Gregory SH, Ayala A. In vivo delivery of caspase-8 or Fas siRNA improves the survival of septic mice. Blood. 2005;106(7):2295-301. Epub 2005/06/09.

[89] Teoh H, Quan A, Creighton AK, Annie Bang KW, Singh KK, Shukla PC, et al. BRCA1 gene therapy reduces systemic inflammatory response and multiple organ failure and improves survival in experimental sepsis. Gene therapy. 2012. Epub 2012/01/20.

[90] Lin X, Dean DA. Gene therapy for ALI/ARDS. Critical care clinics. 2011;27(3):705-18. Epub 2011/07/12.

[91] Zhou J, Wu Y, Henderson F, McCoy DM, Salome RG, McGowan SE, et al. Adenoviral gene transfer of a mutant surfactant enzyme ameliorates pseudomonas-induced lung injury. Gene therapy. 2006;13(12):974-85. Epub 2006/03/03.

[92] Ware LB, Matthay MA. The acute respiratory distress syndrome. The New England journal of medicine. 2000;342(18):1334-49. Epub 2000/05/04.

[93] Ryter SW, Alam J, Choi AM. Heme oxygenase-1/carbon monoxide: from basic science to therapeutic applications. Physiological reviews. 2006;86(2):583-650. Epub 2006/04/08.

[94] Weiss YG, Maloyan A, Tazelaar J, Raj N, Deutschman CS. Adenoviral transfer of HSP-70 into pulmonary epithelium ameliorates experimental acute respiratory distress syndrome. J Clin Invest. 2002;110(6):801-6. Epub 2002/09/18.

[95] Comellas AP, Briva A. Role of endothelin-1 in acute lung injury. Translational research : the journal of laboratory and clinical medicine. 2009;153(6):263-71. Epub 2009/05/19.

[96] Matthay MA, Robriquet L, Fang X. Alveolar epithelium: role in lung fluid balance and acute lung injury. Proceedings of the American Thoracic Society. 2005;2(3): 206-13. Epub 2005/10/14.

[97] Factor P, Saldias F, Ridge K, Dumasius V, Zabner J, Jaffe HA, et al. Augmentation of lung liquid clearance via adenovirus-mediated transfer of a Na,K-ATPase beta1 subunit gene. J Clin Invest. 1998;102(7):1421-30. Epub 1998/10/14.

[98] Machado-Aranda D, Adir Y, Young JL, Briva A, Budinger GR, Yeldandi AV, et al. Gene transfer of the Na+,K+-ATPase beta1 subunit using electroporation increases lung liquid clearance. American journal of respiratory and critical care medicine. 2005;171(3):204-11. Epub 2004/11/02.

[99] Factor P, Dumasius V, Saldias F, Brown LA, Sznajder JI. Adenovirus-mediated transfer of an Na+/K+-ATPase beta1 subunit gene improves alveolar fluid clearance and survival in hyperoxic rats. Human gene therapy. 2000;11(16):2231-42. Epub 2000/11/21.

[100] Dumasius V, Sznajder JI, Azzam ZS, Boja J, Mutlu GM, Maron MB, et al. beta(2)-adrenergic receptor overexpression increases alveolar fluid clearance and responsiveness to endogenous catecholamines in rats. Circulation research. 2001;89(10): 907-14. Epub 2001/11/10.

[101] Ware LB, Matthay MA. Alveolar fluid clearance is impaired in the majority of patients with acute lung injury and the acute respiratory distress syndrome. American journal of respiratory and critical care medicine. 2001;163(6):1376-83. Epub 2001/05/24.

[102] Litvan J, Briva A, Wilson MS, Budinger GR, Sznajder JI, Ridge KM. Beta-adrenergic receptor stimulation and adenoviral overexpression of superoxide dismutase prevent the hypoxia-mediated decrease in Na,K-ATPase and alveolar fluid reabsorption. The Journal of biological chemistry. 2006;281(29):19892-8. Epub 2006/04/26.

[103] Ware LB, Matthay MA. Keratinocyte and hepatocyte growth factors in the lung: roles in lung development, inflammation, and repair. American journal of physiology Lung cellular and molecular physiology. 2002;282(5):L924-40. Epub 2002/04/12.

[104] Baba Y, Yazawa T, Kanegae Y, Sakamoto S, Saito I, Morimura N, et al. Keratinocyte growth factor gene transduction ameliorates acute lung injury and mortality in mice. Human gene therapy. 2007;18(2):130-41. Epub 2007/03/03.

[105] Fang X, Bai C, Wang X. Potential clinical application of KGF-2 (FGF-10) for acute lung injury/acute respiratory distress syndrome. Expert review of clinical pharmacology. 2010;3(6):797-805. Epub 2011/11/25.

[106] Mei SH, McCarter SD, Deng Y, Parker CH, Liles WC, Stewart DJ. Prevention of LPS-induced acute lung injury in mice by mesenchymal stem cells overexpressing angiopoietin 1. PLoS medicine. 2007;4(9):e269. Epub 2007/09/07.

[107] Perl M, Chung CS, Lomas-Neira J, Rachel TM, Biffl WL, Cioffi WG, et al. Silencing of Fas, but not caspase-8, in lung epithelial cells ameliorates pulmonary apoptosis, inflammation, and neutrophil influx after hemorrhagic shock and sepsis. The American journal of pathology. 2005;167(6):1545-59. Epub 2005/11/30.

[108] Buff SM, Yu H, McCall JN, Caldwell SM, Ferkol TW, Flotte TR, et al. IL-10 delivery by AAV5 vector attenuates inflammation in mice with *Pseudomonas pneumonia*. Gene therapy. 2010;17(5):567-76. Epub 2010/04/02.

Chapter 9

Gene Therapy for Chronic Pain Management

Isaura Tavares and Isabel Martins

Additional information is available at the end of the chapter

1. Introduction

This chapter provides an overview of the main current applications of gene therapy for chronic pain in what concerns animal studies and putative clinical applications. The value of gene therapy in unravelling neuronal brain circuits involved in pain modulation is also analysed. After alerting to the huge socioeconomic impact of chronic pain in modern societies and justifying the need to develop new avenues in pain management, we review the most common animal studies using gene therapy, which consisted on deliveries of replication-defective viral vectors at the periphery with the aim to block nociceptive transmission at the spinal cord. Departing from the data of these animal studies, we present the latest results of clinical trials using gene therapy for pain management in cancer patients. The animal studies dealing with gene delivery in pain control centres of the brain are analysed in what concerns their complexity and interest in unravelling the neurobiological mechanisms of descending pain modulation. The chapter will finish by analysing possible futures of gene therapy for chronic pain management based on the development of vectors which are safer and more specific for the different types of chronic pain.

2. Chronic pain: A burden for modern societies

Pain is not easy to define since it is a highly subjective experience. The more consensual definition of pain was provided by the International Association for the Study of Pain (IASP) and states that *"Pain is an unpleasant sensory and emotional experience associated with actual or potential tissue damage, or described in terms of such damage"* [1]. Acute pain is important as an alert signal to potentially threaten situations (internal or external to the organism) and it is important for survival. Acute pain may progress to chronic pain which, according to IASP, is the pain that lasts more than 3 months and persists beyond the normal tissue healing time [2].

Chronic pain may be divided into "nociceptive" and "neuropathic" [3]. Nociceptive pain is caused by activation of nociceptors, the thin nerve fibers which convey nociceptive input from the periphery to the spinal cord. Neuropathic pain is caused by malfunction or damage of the nervous system. Neuropathic pain is frequently difficult to treat being associated to spontaneous pain, exaggerated responses to nociceptive stimuli (*hyperalgesia*) and nociceptive responses to stimuli which are usually non-nociceptive (*allodynia*).

The number of people affected by chronic pain is increasing due to multifactorial causes such as increasing aging of the population. In Europe, about 20% of people suffer from moderate to severe chronic pain [4]. In the United States the prevalence of chronic pain ranges from 2% to 40%, with a median of 15% [5], which cost the country 560 to 635 million dollars [6]. People suffering from chronic pain are less able to walk, sleep normally, perform social activities, exercise or have sexual relations. Chronic pain strongly affects the productivity. About 60% of chronic pain patients are unable or less able to work, 19% lost their jobs and 13% change jobs due to their pain [6]. Chronic pain is associated to several co-morbidities, namely depression and anxiety [6]. Besides all of these indirect costs, chronic pain is a burden due to direct costs of pain management. Despite major investments in basic and clinical pain research, the available analgesics remain considerably unchanged during the last decades. Opioids are useful to manage several pain types but they have a modest efficacy in several pain conditions (e.g. neuropathic pain). Furthermore, long term treatments with opioids frequently induce severe off-target effects, like nausea, constipation and addiction [7]. Intractable pain remains a clinical problem and a drama for the patients and their families [8]. During the last decade, pain clinicians and pain researchers were challenged to search for alternatives to conventional pain treatment, which should be more specific and sustained than conventional analgesics. Gene therapy outstands as a powerful technique to overcome some current problems of chronic pain treatments.

Neurobiological research in the pain field provided solid information regarding the transmission and modulation of nociceptive information from the periphery to the brain, where a pain sensation is produced (Fig. 1). Nociceptive signals are conveyed by primary afferent fibers from peripheral organs, like the bladder or muscles, to the spinal cord. This is the first relay station involved in the modulation of nociceptive information namely by local inhibitory interneurons that use opioid peptides or aminoacids (γ-amminobutiric acid-GABA- and glycine). Nociceptive information is then transmitted supraspinally, namely to the thalamus, and to several brainstem areas, where additional modulation of the nociceptive signal occurs. The thalamo-cortical pathway ensures that the nociceptive information reaches the somatosensory and prefrontal cortices, where the nociceptive signal is finally perceived as a pain sensation [9, 10]. Some brain areas which directly or indirectly receive nociceptive information from the spinal cord are also involved in descending pain modulation. Both inhibition and facilitation may occur and chronic pain may derive from a reduction of the former and enhancement of the latter [9, 11]. This neurobiological knowledge has been used to design gene therapy studies for chronic pain, namely to choose the somatosensory system areas and neurotransmitters/receptors to be targeted in order to block nociceptive transmission.

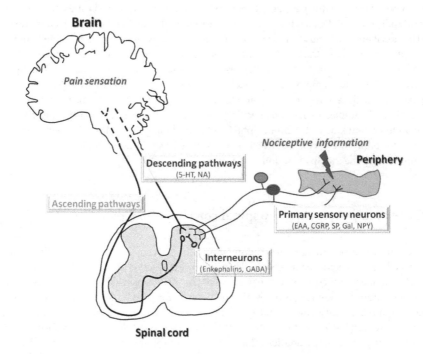

Figure 1. Schematic diagram of pain pathways involved in pain transmission and modulation. **Nociceptive information** is transmitted from the periphery to the spinal dorsal horn by primary sensory neurons. At the spinal level, these neurons transmit nociceptive information to second order neurons ("Ascending pathways") through the release of neurotransmitters like the excitatory amino acids (EAA) glutamate and aspartate, calcitonin gene-related peptide (CGRP), substance P (SP) galanin (Gal) and neuropeptide Y (NPY). In the brain, the nociceptive information is then perceived as a **pain sensation**. The transmission of nociceptive information at the spinal level is modulated by interneurons (mainly inhibitory) through the release of opioid pepides and GABA and also by supraspinal descending neurons ("Descending pathways") through the release of serotonin (5-HT) and noradrenaline (NA). Descending pathways may inhibit or enhance nociceptive transmission from the spinal cord.

Gene therapy is an especially versatile tool for chronic pain management since it is based in a triad of controllable parameters: the vector, the transgene and the promoter. By knowing the neurobiological features of each chronic pain type, namely the neurotransmitters and receptors affected, it is possible to design gene therapy strategies based on the best combination of vectors, transgenes and promoters. As to **vectors**, gene therapy for pain uses mainly "vehicles" which have a "certified" experience in infecting neurons, namely replication-defective forms of viruses. Non-viral vectors have seldom been used in gene therapy studies for pain but their transduction efficiency and specificity are much lower than those of viral vectors. Some of these vectors have the ability to migrate retrogradely (i.e., contrary to the direction of nerve impulse) which is very useful to target neurons that are located in structures of difficult surgical access. A good example is the application of replication-defective forms of Herpes Simplex Virus type 1 (HSV-1) at the periphery (e.g. the skin) to transduce neurons at the spinal ganglia (dorsal root ganglia-DRGs), which are difficult to access due to their bone protection. Regarding the **transgenes** to include in the vectors for gene therapy of pain, it is possible to increase the expression of neurotransmitters and receptors involved in nociceptive inhibition (e.g. opioids), neurotrophic factors or substances with anti-inflammatory properties. Finally, and in what concerns the **promoters**, it is possible to choose those that restrict transgene expression to a cell type, such as a neuron or a glial cell, or even target selective neurochemical neuronal populations. Examples of neuron-specific promoters are synapsin I, calcium/calmodulin-dependent protein kinase II, tubulin alpha I and neuron-specific enolase [12]. Some possibilities of controlling the vectors, transgenes and promoters will be discussed in the next two sections using gene therapy in animal models.

3. Gene therapy targeting the spinal cord in animal pain models

One of the main advantages of experimental gene therapy studies is that they can be performed using several pain models. This is important since each pain type may induce specific changes in neuronal circuits devoted to the transmission and modulation of nociceptive transmission [13]. Studies of gene therapy for pain have used clinically relevant models of inflammatory [14-22] and neuropathic pain [23-34]. In a much lower incidence, models of acute [35-38], post-operative pain [39] and cancer [40] pain have been used in experimental gene therapy studies. The large majority of studies were performed in pain models affecting the limbs or the trunk, in the latter case being of visceral origin [22, 37]. Two studies used gene therapy to block nociceptive transmission coming from the head/ face in pain models that reproduces some types of craniofacial pain, like trigeminal neuralgia [41] or temporomandibular joint disorders [42].

Gene therapy studies for pain in animal models may be divided in studies targeting the spinal cord (Table 1) and studies directed to pain control centres located in the brain (Table 2). Studies directed to the spinal cord mainly aim to manipulate the expression of transgenes in order to block the transmission of nociceptive input at the spinal dorsal horn (Table 1). Most of the spinal cord studies using gene therapy for pain elected HSV-1 as the most suitable vector, due to its natural affinity to the neuron and its ability for retrograde transport [43]. HSV-1 has the additional advantage over other vectors of carrying multiple transgenes or large transgenes and not integrating in the host genome, which reduces the possibility of mutagenic events [44, 45]. After application of replication-defective forms of HSV-1 at the periphery in order to transduce DRG neurons (or trigeminal ganglion neurons), delivery of the transgene product by the spinal branch of transduced neurons at the spinal dorsal horn induced analgesia in several rodent models of pain (Table 1). Gene therapy in animal models of craniofacial pain [41, 42] aimed to release the transgene products at the level of the spinal trigeminal nucleus and this structure is homolog of the spinal cord, which prompted to include these studies in the section devoted to spinal cord studies.

Pain models	Gene product	Inoculation	References
Herpes Simplex type 1			
Acute pain	Pre-proenkephalin	Subcutaneous	[35]
Inflammatory pain	Pre-proenkephalin A	Subcutaneous	[14]
Neuropathic pain	Pre-proenkephalin A	Subcutaneous	[41]
Cutaneous hyperalgesia	Pre-preproenkephalin	Subcutaneous	[36]
Bladder hyperactivity	Pre-preproenkephalin	Bladder wall	[37]
Inflammatory pain	Endomorphin-2	Subcutaneous	[15]
Neuropathic pain	Endomorphin-2	Subcutaneous	[23]
Neuropathic pain	IL-4	Subcutaneous	[24]
Neuropathic pain	sTNFRs	Subcutaneous	[25]
Neuropathic pain	GAD	Subcutaneous	[26, 47]
Chronic pancreatitis	Pre-proenkephalin	Pancreas surface	[22]
Inflammatory pain	$Na_v1.7$ antisense	Subcutaneous	[16]
Incision pain	Pre-proenkephalin	Subcutaneous	[39]
Cancer pain	Pre-proenkephalin	Subcutaneous	[40]
Adenovirus			
Inflammatory pain	GAD	Trigeminal ganglion	[42]
Neuropathic pain	IL-10	Intrathecal	[27]
Inflammatory pain	β-endorphin	Intrathecal	[17]
Neuropathic pain	IL-2	Intrathecal	[28]
Adeno-associated vectors			
Neuropathic pain	IL-10	Intrathecal	[29]
Neuropathic pain	shGCH1	Intrathecal	[30]
Neuropathic pain	Prepro- β-endorphin	Intrathecal	[31]
Inflammatory pain	μ-opioid receptors	DRG	[18]
Lentivirus			
Neuropathic pain	GDNF	Intraspinal	[32]
Neuropathic pain	NFκB Repressor	Intraspinal	[33]

Table 1. Summary of experimental studies using viral vectors for gene transfer to the spinal cord.

As to the transgenes included in the HSV-1 vectors, opioid peptides or their precursors largely prevail due to their well-known ability to block nociceptive transmission at the spinal cord. HSV-1-based delivery of opioids has additional advantages over classic opioids, namely by being deprived of major side-effects and preventing tolerance after repeated administrations of the vector [46]. Furthermore, opioid-based gene therapy can be very powerful in inducing analgesia if combined with administration of very low doses of classical opioids [46]. Besides opioid peptides, other transgenes were included in the HSV-1 vectors constructs. A transgene that increases the levels of the inhibitory neurotransmitter GABA, namely by overexpressing its synthetizing enzyme glutamate decarboxylase (GAD), induced analgesia in neuropathic pain models [26, 47]. HSV-1 based vectors have also been used to deliver transgenes that overexpress anti-inflammatory interleukins [24, 48] or the soluble receptor for tumor necrosis factor-α (TNF-α), which act as an antagonist of TNF-α in order to block its role as a pro-inflammatory mediator [25, 49]. A decrease in the levels of the α subunit of the voltage-gated sodium channel 1.7 (Nav 1.7) was also achieved using HSV-1 constructs but with the transgene inserted in antisense orientation [16].

Other viral vectors, namely adenoviruses, adeno-associated viruses and lentiviruses have been used to target the spinal cord, but unlike HSV-1 vectors which have been administered at the periphery following its natural route of retrograde transport to DRG neurons, these vectors were either directly injected into DRGs or trigeminal ganglion neurons, intrathecally or intraspinally (Table 1). The transgenes included in adenoviruses, adeno-associated viruses are similar to those used in HSV-1 vectors, namely opioids [17, 31], interleukins [27-29] and GAD [42]. Adeno-associated vectors have also carried transgenes that overexpress μ-opioid receptors [18] or block the expression of GTP cyclohydroxilase (GCH1) using small hairpin RNAs [30]. GCH1 is the rate-limiting enzyme of an essential co-factor for nitric oxide synthase (NOS), which modulates nociceptive transmission. Finally, lentiviral vectors have also been used in gene transfer studies directed to the spinal cord. Based on its ability to restrict transduction to the injection site, lentiviral vectors have been administered intraspinally in the dorsal horn to increase the levels of a neurotrophic factor (glial-derived neurotrofic factor, GDNF) [32] or decrease the expression of Nuclear Factor kB (NFκB), which regulates cellular inflammation responses [33]. In the latter study, microdelivery of an HIV pseudotyped lentiviral vector into the spinal dorsal horn led to a preferential transgene expression in glial cells. This shows that, besides the promoter, pseudotyping the vector is a way of directing transgene expression and glia is an important target in pain, inasmuch that chronic pain is associated to the activation of glial cells which produce algogenic mediators that exacerbate pain, namely NFκB. All of these approaches showed considerable analgesic efficacy and reduced side effects.

4. Gene therapy targeting for pain: The challenge of targeting pain control circuits in the brain

Abnormal descending pain modulation from the brain is a common feature of several chronic pain conditions, namely those characterized by widespread pain, like fibromyalgia, which derive from impairments in descending pain inhibition [50]. Studies with gene delivery into the brain (Table 2) are much scarcer than spinal cord deliveries. This is due both to the higher difficulty of surgical approaches to deliver the vectors into the brain and challenges to manipulate the complex brain neuronal circuits involved in pain modulation. The spinal cord constitutes a less invasive delivery route when the aim is to manipulate descending modulatory pathways (Fig. 1). This delivery route was recently explored by injecting intraspinally an adenovirus vector targeting the expression of a potassium channel into noradrenergic pontospinal neurons, which decreased the activity of those pontospinal neurons and induced hyperalgesia [51]. These experiments confirm the pain inhibiting role of the noradrenergic projections to the spinal cord [52].

Pain models	Gene product	Delivery	References
Acute pain	Proenkephalin	Medullary dorsal reticular nucleus (DRt)	[55]
Neuropathic	Tyrosine Hydroxylase antisense	Medullary dorsal reticular nucleus (DRt)	[34]
Inflammatory	Proenkephalin	Medullary ventral reticular nucleus (VLM)	[19]
Inflammatory	Proenkephalin	Medullary dorsal reticular nucleus (DRt)	[20]
Acute pain	GAD	Insular Cortex	[38]
Inflammatory pain	Preproenkephalin	Amygdala	[21]
Acute and Inflammatory pain	NMDA antisense	Medullary nucleus of the solitary tract	[56]
Inflammatory and neuropathic pain model	Potassium channel (hKir$_{2.1}$)	Pontospinal noradrenergic neurons	[51]

Table 2. Summary of animal studies using viral vectors for gene transfer to pain control centers in the brain.

Gene transfer in the brain used almost exclusively HSV-1 vectors to overexpress opioid peptides [19-21, 38] and, in a much more limited extent, GAD [38]. Our research group has a large experience in gene transfer to pain control centres at the medulla oblongata, namely the dorsal reticular nucleus (DRt), the caudal ventrolateral medulla (VLM) and the nucleus of the solitary tract (NTS). These areas were elected based on the extensive neurobiological knowledge of their role in pain modulation [53, 54]. Overexpression of opioid precursors in the DRt and VLM induced analgesia in acute pain tests and models of sustained or chronic inflammatory pain [19, 20, 55]. Brain areas involved in pain control and which are of easier neurosurgical access are the amygdala and the rostral agranular insular cortex. Overexpression of opioid precursors in the central amygdalar nucleus [21] or GAD in the rostral agranular insular cortex induced analgesia in acute pain models [38]. Lentiviral vectors were delivered to the NTS, an area which is crucial in pain and cardiovascular integration, to decrease local expression of N-methyl-D-aspartate (NMDA) receptor, a key receptor for the action of glutamate, and this approach was shown to decrease acute and inflammatory pain [56]. Since glutamate, is the most ubiquitous mediator of excitatory synaptic transmission in the central nervous system and NMDA receptors are also expressed by glial cells, the effects of gene therapy were restricted to NTS neurons by using the rat synapsin promoter.

There is a puzzling difference between gene therapy studies using HSV-1 vectors at the periphery or the brain. Whereas the ability for HSV-1 to migrate retrogradely is the main feature of studies at the periphery, the migration of HSV-1 in the brain is seldom evaluated. This can confound the effects of gene therapy on pain responses since the effect may derive from transduction of neurons that project to the injected area, and not at the targeted area itself. Our research group has pioneer work in studying the dynamics of HSV-1 migration in the brain after injections of the vector in pain control centres of the medulla oblongata, namely the caudal medulla oblongata (VLM) and the dorsal reticular nucleus (DRt). After injections of a HSV-1 vector expressing the lacZ reporter gene, under control of the human cytomegalovirus promoter (hCMV), in pain control centres of the medulla oblongata, migration in VLM and DRt afferents was detected [19, 55] (Fig. 2). However, not all the brain afferents of the VLM and DRt exhibited β-galactosidase (β-gal), the product of *lacZ* expression. For example, the amygdala and the cortex, which are important VLM and DRt afferents [57, 58] did not show neurons expressing β-gal.

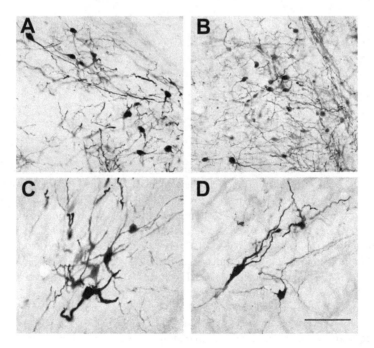

Figure 2. Dynamics of HSV-1 migration in the brain after injection into the DRt. Photomicrographs of β-gal positive neurons in the cerebellum (A), the parabrachial complex (B), the locus *coeruleus* (C) and the VLM (D) at 7 days post-injection Scale bar D: 100 μm (photomicrographs A-C are at the same magnification).

Although it could be argued that this is due to lack of activity of the hCMV promoter in amygdalar and cortical neurons, other studies showed that hCMV is active in those neurons [21, 59]. These results rather point to a selective uptake of HSV-1 vectors injected in the brain parenchyma, probably due to interactions between neuronal receptors and glycoproteins of the HSV-1 envelope. By carefully mapping the brain areas exhibiting retrograde transport after HSV-1 injections in the brain using immunohistochemical detection of the gene reporter and in situ hybridization against the DNA of HSV-1, the problems of affecting brain afferents of the injected area can be circumvented.

The selective migration of HSV-1 in the brain can be a useful feature of the vector. After establishing the dynamics of the migration of HSV-1 in the brain after injection into the DRt (a facilitatory pain control centre of the brain), we used a tissue specific promoter (tyrosine hydroxylase-TH) to direct the expression of the vector to the noradrenergic afferents of the DRt (Fig. 3). Based on the analgesic effects of the administration of α1-adrenorecetor antagonists into the DRt, the TH transgene was inserted in antisense orientation into the vector in order to decrease the levels of noradrenaline in the DRt [34]. A sustained analgesic effect was achieved in a model of neuropathic pain, which reproduces clinically relevant features of neuropathic pain. The fact that the analgesic effects were so long, lasting for 2 months with a single vector injection, and reversed several pain modalities, indicates that targeting pain control centres of the brain needs to be considered both in animal and pre-clinical studies.

5. Gene therapy for chronic pain at the bedside: Human studies

The translational perspectives of the studies summarized in section 2, namely those using replication-defective HSV-1 vectors, favoured the approval of clinical trials for gene therapy for chronic pain. An important reinforcement of the proof-of-concept for the potential utility of HSV-based vector in rodent pain models was provided by equivalent studies performed in primates [36]. These studies were important since the translational perspectives of the rodent results were questioned for several reasons, such as the larger size of dermatomes of humans. The first clinical trial of gene therapy for pain was a safety and dose-escalation Phase I study in ten patients with mild to severe intractable pain due to terminal cancer [60]. The protocol consisted in the administration directly in the pain-reporting area of an HSV-1 replication-defective vector containing the transgene of the precursor of enkephalin [61]. A dose-dependent analgesic effect was demonstrated with a reduction of pain scores lasting for at least 2 weeks and with no adverse effects. These encouraging results prompt to implement a Phase II trial in a larger cancer population and the study includes placebo controls, evaluation of the effects of reinoculation of the vector and assessment of the maximal dose [45, 62].

The progress of the clinical trials for cancer pain opened avenues to test gene therapy to block nociceptive transmission in the spinal cord in other pain conditions, such as painful diabetic neuropathy. This pain type, which is increasing to the pandemic occurrence of diabetes, is difficult to treat with conventional analgesics and only about one third of the patients achieve a 50% pain reduction beyond the placebo effect [63]. A clinical trial has recently been approved

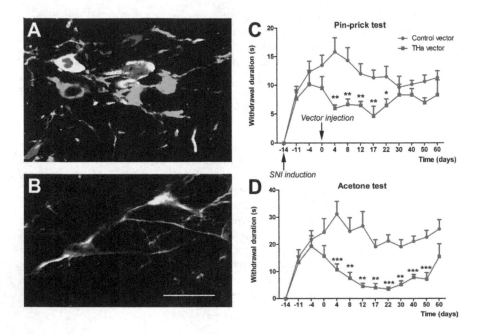

Figure 3. HSV-1 injected at the DRt transduces noradrenergic afferents of the nucleus (**A**, **B**). Photomicrographs representing double-labeled neurons for β-gal and TH (yellowish) in the locus *coeruleus* (**A**) and the A$_5$ noradrenergic cell group (**B**). β-gal positive neurons are shown in red and TH positive neurons are shown in green (**A**). Scale bar in B: 40 μm (A is at the same magnification). The insertion of TH in antisense orientation into HSV-1 (THa vector) induced analgesia in the spared nerve injury (SNI) model of neuropathic pain (**C**, **D**). THa induced a sustained attenuation of mechanical hyperalgesia evaluated by the pin-prick test (**C**) and cold allodynia evaluated by the acetone test (**D**). THa and the control vector were injected at time 0, i.e., 2 weeks after SNI induction. Data are presented as mean ± SEM (n=6 for each group); *P<0.05, **P<0.01, ***P<0.001 THa- *vs.* control- vector.

to use an HSV-1 vector that overexpress GAD to relief painful diabetic neuropathy [45]. Other therapeutic transgenes are being considered for future clinical trials of gene therapy, namely the overexpression of interleukins [45]. The future of gene therapy for chronic pain in humans will depend on the results of the clinical trials that are currently being performed but the promising results obtained so far indicate that gene therapy will add to the armamentarium of available pain treatments.

The application of gene therapy to block nociceptive transmission at supraspinal levels has been proposed by several pain specialists [64]. However, most experimental studies dealing with gene delivery at the brain were directed to pain control areas of the medulla oblongata, which are of difficult neurosurgical approach since they are in close vicinity to areas involved in the control of vital functions, such as cardiovascular and respiratory controls. Moving the focus of the gene delivery studies to areas that are more easy to approach may be useful namely in the context of widespread chronic pain, such as fibromyalgia and complex regional pain syndrome [65]. This can only be considered after a thorough characterization of the pain control circuits in the brain namely in what concerns the functional changes induced by the chronic pain condition in order to select the best brain areas to target to maximise the balance between efficacy and risk.

6. Future challenges

The advances of gene therapy in other diseases of the nervous system rather than pain will be crucial to define the future of gene therapy for chronic pain, namely by the improvements in the delivery systems. Studies which improved the efficacy of non-viral vectors already inspired the construction of a non-viral, non plasmid immunologically defined gene expression (MIDGE) vector that overexpress β-endorphin and induced analgesia after injection into inflamed paws by increasing the concentration of β-endorphin in leukocytes [66]. Since chronic pain requires long-term transgene expression, the duration of the activity of promoters needs to be increased. It could be useful to design constructs that are activated only when pain lasts for longer periods and rises over a certain threshold. This would allow treating chronic pain but still preserve acute pain as an alert signal. An interesting possibility could be to control the activity of the promoter using inducible promoters, which have been used in gene therapy studies other than pain. The activity of these promoters can be induced exogenously, for example, by antibiotics. An ingenious idea was recently applied by using a ligand (glycine) which normally is not expressed in DRG neurons but can be administered to activate HSV-1 vectors to express glycine receptors in animal models of somatic and visceral pain [67]. Besides the vectors and the promoters, an election of effective transgenes for chronic pain will be important to define the future of gene therapy for chronic pain. Transgenes for opioid peptides have been overused in gene therapy studies in animal models but long-term treatments with classic opioids may induce pain, a phenomena known as opioid-induced hyperalgesia [68]. By achieving more sustained and strong transgene expression, it is possible that opioid-induced hyperalgesia could also be induced by gene therapy. New transgenes should be considered in future studies of gene therapy for chronic pain. Based on the role of the vanilloid receptor TRPV-1 (Transient Receptor Potential channel Vanilloid 1) as a pro-nociceptive cationic channel involved in pain signalling, and the clinical relevance of desensitization of TRPV1 receptors [69], this may be an important target molecule in the future. By decreasing the expression of protein kinase C-epsilon (PKC), which phosphorylates TRPV1 receptors, it was possible to induce analgesia in animal models [70]. Even more challenging is the possibility of targeting pain control centres in the brain using gene therapy. These studies will continue for large years to focus on animal pain models in order to determine neurobiological effects of chronic pain installation in pain control centres, using gene therapy as a method to prevent those changes. Finally, the emergent new field in pain research of genetics of pain has recently provided data which may explain the higher susceptibility of some persons to develop chronic pain [71]. Due to its versatility and the possibility of direct gene targeting, gene therapy can be the perfect tool to verify if the holy grail of a personalized pain treatment can be implemented.

Financial support

This work was supported by FCT and COMPTE project PTDC/SAU-NSC/110954/2009.

List of abbreviations

β-gal- β-galactosidase

DRG- Dorsal root ganglion

DRt- Dorsal reticular nucleus

GABA- γ-amminobutiric acid

GAD- glutamate decarboxylase

GDNF- Glial-derived neurotrofic factor

hCMV- Human cytomegalovirus

HSV-1- Herpes Simplex Virus type 1

IASP- International Association for the Study of Pain

IL_2- Interleukin 2

IL_4- Interleukin 4

IL_{10}- Interleukin 10

MIDGE- Non plasmid immunologically defined gene expression

Nav 1.7- Voltage-gated sodium channel 1.7

NFκB- Nuclear Factor kB

NMDA- N-methyl-D-aspartate

NTS- Nucleus of the solitary tract

PKC- Protein kinase C-epsilon

shGCH1- small hairpin RNAs for GTP cyclohydroxilase

sTNFRs- tumor necrosis factor-α

TH- Tyrosine hydroxylase

TRPV-1- Transient Receptor Potential channel Vanilloid 1

VLM- Caudal ventrolateral medulla

Author details

Isaura Tavares[1,2] and Isabel Martins[1,2]

*Address all correspondence to: isatav@med.up.pt

1 Department of Experimental Biology, Faculty of Medicine of Porto, University of Porto, Portugal

2 IBMC - Instituto de Biologia Molecular e Celular, University of Porto, Portugal

References

[1] Merskey, H., et al., Pain terms: a list with definitions and notes on usage. Recommended by the IASP Subcommittee on Taxonomy. Pain, 1979. 6(3): p. 249.

[2] Classification of chronic pain. Descriptions of chronic pain syndromes and definitions of pain terms. Prepared by the International Association for the Study of Pain, Subcommittee on Taxonomy. Pain Suppl, 1986. 3: p. S1-226.

[3] Thienhaus, O. and B.E. Cole, Classification of pain. Weiner RS, 6th ed. 2002: American Academy of Pain Management.

[4] Breivik, H., et al., Survey of chronic pain in Europe: prevalence, impact on daily life, and treatment. Eur J Pain, 2006. 10(4): p. 287-333.

[5] Verhaak, P.F., et al., Prevalence of chronic benign pain disorder among adults: a review of the literature. Pain, 1998. 77(3): p. 231-9.

[6] Gaskin, D.J. and P. Richard, The economic costs of pain in the United States. J Pain, 2012. 13(8): p. 715-24.

[7] Benyamin, R., et al., Opioid complications and side effects. Pain Physician, 2008. 11(2 Suppl): p. S105-20.

[8] Mao, J., M.S. Gold, and M.M. Backonja, Combination drug therapy for chronic pain: a call for more clinical studies. J Pain, 2011. 12(2): p. 157-66.

[9] Tracey, I. and P.W. Mantyh, The cerebral signature for pain perception and its modulation. Neuron, 2007. 55(3): p. 377-91.

[10] Basbaum, A.I., et al., Cellular and molecular mechanisms of pain. Cell, 2009. 139(2): p. 267-84.

[11] Heinricher, M.M., et al., Descending control of nociception: Specificity, recruitment and plasticity. Brain Res Rev, 2009. 60(1): p. 214-25.

[12] Hioki, H., et al., Efficient gene transduction of neurons by lentivirus with enhanced neuron-specific promoters. Gene Ther, 2007. 14(11): p. 872-82.

[13] Porreca, F., M.H. Ossipov, and G.F. Gebhart, Chronic pain and medullary descending facilitation. Trends Neurosci, 2002. 25(6): p. 319-25.

[14] Braz, J., et al., Therapeutic efficacy in experimental polyarthritis of viral-driven enkephalin overproduction in sensory neurons. J Neurosci, 2001. 21(20): p. 7881-8.

[15] Hao, S., et al., Effects of transgene-mediated endomorphin-2 in inflammatory pain. Eur J Pain, 2009. 13(4): p. 380-6.

[16] Yeomans, D.C., et al., Decrease in inflammatory hyperalgesia by herpes vector-mediated knockdown of Nav1.7 sodium channels in primary afferents. Hum Gene Ther, 2005. 16(2): p. 271-7.

[17] Finegold, A.A., A.J. Mannes, and M.J. Iadarola, A paracrine paradigm for in vivo gene therapy in the central nervous system: treatment of chronic pain. Hum Gene Ther, 1999. 10(7): p. 1251-7.

[18] Xu, Y., et al., Adeno-associated viral transfer of opioid receptor gene to primary sensory neurons: a strategy to increase opioid antinociception. Proc Natl Acad Sci U S A, 2003. 100(10): p. 6204-9.

[19] Martins, I., et al., Reversal of inflammatory pain by HSV-1-mediated overexpression of enkephalin in the caudal ventrolateral medulla. Eur J Pain, 2011. 15(10): p. 1008-14.

[20] Pinto, M., et al., Opioids modulate pain facilitation from the dorsal reticular nucleus. Mol Cell Neurosci, 2008. 39(4): p. 508-18.

[21] Kang, W., et al., Herpes virus-mediated preproenkephalin gene transfer to the amygdala is antinociceptive. Brain Res, 1998. 792(1): p. 133-5.

[22] Lu, Y., et al., Treatment of inflamed pancreas with enkephalin encoding HSV-1 recombinant vector reduces inflammatory damage and behavioral sequelae. Mol Ther, 2007. 15(10): p. 1812-9.

[23] Wolfe, D., et al., Engineering an endomorphin-2 gene for use in neuropathic pain therapy. Pain, 2007. 133(1-3): p. 29-38.

[24] Hao, S., et al., HSV-mediated expression of interleukin-4 in dorsal root ganglion neurons reduces neuropathic pain. Mol Pain, 2006. 2: p. 6.

[25] Peng, X.M., et al., Tumor necrosis factor-alpha contributes to below-level neuropathic pain after spinal cord injury. Ann Neurol, 2006. 59(5): p. 843-51.

[26] Hao, S., et al., Gene transfer of glutamic acid decarboxylase reduces neuropathic pain. Ann Neurol, 2005. 57(6): p. 914-8.

[27] Milligan, E.D., et al., Controlling pathological pain by adenovirally driven spinal pro-
      duction of the anti-inflammatory cytokine, interleukin-10. Eur J Neurosci, 2005. 21(8):
      p. 2136-48.

[28] Yao, M.Z., et al., Adenovirus-mediated interleukin-2 gene therapy of nociception.
      Gene Ther, 2003. 10(16): p. 1392-9.

[29] Milligan, E.D., et al., Controlling neuropathic pain by adeno-associated virus driven
      production of the anti-inflammatory cytokine, interleukin-10. Mol Pain, 2005. 1: p. 9.

[30] Kim, S.J., et al., Effective relief of neuropathic pain by adeno-associated virus-mediat-
      ed expression of a small hairpin RNA against GTP cyclohydrolase 1. Mol Pain, 2009.
      5: p. 67.

[31] Storek, B., et al., Sensory neuron targeting by self-complementary AAV8 via lumbar
      puncture for chronic pain. Proc Natl Acad Sci U S A, 2008. 105(3): p. 1055-60.

[32] Pezet, S., et al., Reversal of neurochemical changes and pain-related behavior in a
      model of neuropathic pain using modified lentiviral vectors expressing GDNF. Mol
      Ther, 2006. 13(6): p. 1101-9.

[33] Meunier, A., et al., Lentiviral-mediated targeted NF-kappaB blockade in dorsal spi-
      nal cord glia attenuates sciatic nerve injury-induced neuropathic pain in the rat. Mol
      Ther, 2007. 15(4): p. 687-97.

[34] Martins, I., et al., Reversal of neuropathic pain by HSV-1-mediated decrease of nora-
      drenaline in a pain facilitatory area of the brain. Pain, 2010. 151(1): p. 137-45.

[35] Wilson, S.P., et al., Antihyperalgesic effects of infection with a preproenkephalin-en-
      coding herpes virus. Proc Natl Acad Sci U S A, 1999. 96(6): p. 3211-6.

[36] Yeomans, D.C., et al., Recombinant herpes vector-mediated analgesia in a primate
      model of hyperalgesia. Mol Ther, 2006. 13(3): p. 589-97.

[37] Yokoyama, H., et al., Gene therapy for bladder overactivity and nociception with
      herpes simplex virus vectors expressing preproenkephalin. Hum Gene Ther, 2009.
      20(1): p. 63-71.

[38] Jasmin, L., et al., Analgesia and hyperalgesia from GABA-mediated modulation of
      the cerebral cortex. Nature, 2003. 424(6946): p. 316-20.

[39] Cabanero, D., et al., The pro-nociceptive effects of remifentanil or surgical injury in
      mice are associated with a decrease in delta-opioid receptor mRNA levels: Preven-
      tion of the nociceptive response by on-site delivery of enkephalins. Pain, 2009.
      141(1-2): p. 88-96.

[40] Goss, J.R., et al., Herpes vector-mediated expression of proenkephalin reduces bone
      cancer pain. Ann Neurol, 2002. 52(5): p. 662-5.

[41] Meunier, A., et al., Attenuation of pain-related behavior in a rat model of trigeminal neuropathic pain by viral-driven enkephalin overproduction in trigeminal ganglion neurons. Mol Ther, 2005. 11(4): p. 608-16.

[42] Vit, J.P., et al., Adenovector GAD65 gene delivery into the rat trigeminal ganglion produces orofacial analgesia. Mol Pain, 2009. 5: p. 42.

[43] Glorioso, J.C. and D.J. Fink, Herpes vector-mediated gene transfer in the treatment of chronic pain. Mol Ther, 2009. 17(1): p. 13-8.

[44] Goss, J.R., M.S. Gold, and J.C. Glorioso, HSV vector-mediated modification of primary nociceptor afferents: an approach to inhibit chronic pain. Gene Ther, 2009. 16(4): p. 493-501.

[45] Goins, W.F., J.B. Cohen, and J.C. Glorioso, Gene therapy for the treatment of chronic peripheral nervous system pain. Neurobiol Dis, 2012. 48(2): p. 255-70.

[46] Hao, S., et al., Transgene-mediated enkephalin release enhances the effect of morphine and evades tolerance to produce a sustained antiallodynic effect in neuropathic pain. Pain, 2003. 102(1-2): p. 135-42.

[47] Liu, J., et al., Peripherally delivered glutamic acid decarboxylase gene therapy for spinal cord injury pain. Mol Ther, 2004. 10(1): p. 57-66.

[48] Zhou, Z., et al., HSV-mediated transfer of interleukin-10 reduces inflammatory pain through modulation of membrane tumor necrosis factor alpha in spinal cord microglia. Gene Ther, 2008. 15(3): p. 183-90.

[49] Hao, S., et al., Gene transfer to interfere with TNFalpha signaling in neuropathic pain. Gene Ther, 2007. 14(13): p. 1010-6.

[50] Staud, R., Evidence for shared pain mechanisms in osteoarthritis, low back pain, and fibromyalgia. Curr Rheumatol Rep, 2011. 13(6): p. 513-20.

[51] Howorth, P.W., et al., Retrograde viral vector-mediated inhibition of pontospinal noradrenergic neurons causes hyperalgesia in rats. J Neurosci, 2009. 29(41): p. 12855-64.

[52] Pertovaara, A., Noradrenergic pain modulation. Prog Neurobiol, 2006. 80(2): p. 53-83.

[53] Tavares, I. and D. Lima, The caudal ventrolateral medulla as an important inhibitory modulator of pain transmission in the spinal cord. J Pain, 2002. 3(5): p. 337-46.

[54] Lima, D. and A. Almeida, The medullary dorsal reticular nucleus as a pronociceptive centre of the pain control system. Prog Neurobiol, 2002. 66(2): p. 81-108.

[55] Martins, I., et al., Dynamic of migration of HSV-1 from a medullary pronociceptive centre: antinociception by overexpression of the preproenkephalin transgene. Eur J Neurosci, 2008. 28(10): p. 2075-83.

[56] Marques-Lopes, J., et al., Decrease in the expression of N-methyl-D-aspartate receptors in the nucleus tractus solitarii induces antinociception and increases blood pressure. J Neurosci Res, 2012. 90(2): p. 356-66.

[57] Almeida, A., et al., Brain afferents to the medullary dorsal reticular nucleus: a retrograde and anterograde tracing study in the rat. Eur J Neurosci, 2002. 16(1): p. 81-95.

[58] Cobos, A., et al., Brain afferents to the lateral caudal ventrolateral medulla: a retrograde and anterograde tracing study in the rat. Neuroscience, 2003. 120(2): p. 485-98.

[59] Chiocca, E.A., et al., Transfer and expression of the lacZ gene in rat brain neurons mediated by herpes simplex virus mutants. New Biol, 1990. 2(8): p. 739-46.

[60] Fink, D.J., et al., Gene therapy for pain: results of a phase I clinical trial. Ann Neurol, 2011. 70(2): p. 207-12.

[61] Akil, H., et al., Endogenous opioids: biology and function. Annu Rev Neurosci, 1984. 7: p. 223-55.

[62] Fink, D.J. and D. Wolfe, Gene Therapy for Pain: A Perspective. Pain Manag, 2011. 1(5): p. 379-381.

[63] Turk, D.C., Clinical effectiveness and cost-effectiveness of treatments for patients with chronic pain. Clin J Pain, 2002. 18(6): p. 355-65.

[64] Wu, C.L., et al., Gene therapy for the management of pain: Part I: Methods and strategies. Anesthesiology, 2001. 94(6): p. 1119-32.

[65] Weiss, K. and N.M. Boulis, Herpes Simplex Virus-Based Gene Therapies for Chronic Pain. J Pain Palliat Care Pharmacother, 2012. 26(3): p. 291-3.

[66] Machelska, H., et al., Peripheral non-viral MIDGE vector-driven delivery of beta-endorphin in inflammatory pain. Mol Pain, 2009. 5: p. 72.

[67] Goss, J.R., et al., HSV delivery of a ligand-regulated endogenous ion channel gene to sensory neurons results in pain control following channel activation. Mol Ther, 2011. 19(3): p. 500-6.

[68] Lee, M., et al., A comprehensive review of opioid-induced hyperalgesia. Pain Physician, 2011. 14(2): p. 145-61.

[69] Kissin, I. and A. Szallasi, Therapeutic targeting of TRPV1 by resiniferatoxin, from preclinical studies to clinical trials. Curr Top Med Chem, 2011. 11(17): p. 2159-70.

[70] Srinivasan, R., et al., Protein kinase C epsilon contributes to basal and sensitizing responses of TRPV1 to capsaicin in rat dorsal root ganglion neurons. Eur J Neurosci, 2008. 28(7): p. 1241-54.

[71] Doehring, A., G. Geisslinger, and J. Lotsch, Epigenetics in pain and analgesia: an imminent research field. Eur J Pain, 2011. 15(1): p. 11-6.

Chapter 10

Insulin Trafficking in a Glucose Responsive Engineered Human Liver Cell Line is Regulated by the Interaction of ATP-Sensitive Potassium Channels and Voltage-Gated Calcium Channels

Ann M. Simpson, M. Anne Swan, Guo Jun Liu,
Chang Tao, Bronwyn A O'Brien, Edwin Ch'ng,
Leticia M. Castro, Julia Ting, Zehra Elgundi, Tony An,
Mark Lutherborrow, Fraser Torpy, Donald K. Martin,
Bernard E. Tuch and Graham M. Nicholson

Additional information is available at the end of the chapter

1. Introduction

Type I diabetes is caused by the autoimmune destruction of pancreatic beta (β) cells [1]. Current treatment requires multiple daily injections of insulin to control blood glucose levels. Tight glucose control lowers, but does not eliminate, the onset of diabetic complications, which greatly reduce the quality and longevity of life for patients. Transplantation of pancreatic tissue as a treatment is restricted by the scarcity of donors and the requirement for lifelong immunosuppression to preserve the graft, which carries adverse side-effects. This is of particular concern as Type 1 diabetes predominantly affects children. Lack of glucose control could be overcome by genetically engineering "an artificial β-cell" that is capable of synthesising, storing and secreting insulin in response to metabolic signals. The donor cell type must be readily accessible and capable of being engineered to synthesise, process, store and secrete insulin under physiological conditions.

The cell type of choice for the gene therapy of diabetes is not the β-cell. β-cells are greatly reduced or absent in people with Type I diabetes because of their autoimmune destruction. This fact will actively work against gene therapists trying to derive surrogate β-cells from stem cells. There are innumerable theories describing putative mechanisms for preventing a patient's immune system from re-attacking transplanted β-cells, but the fact that the basic processes of islet cell attack have not been fully elucidated makes the search for relevant genes problematic. Thus, the engineering of non-pancreatic β-cells to synthesise, process, store and secrete insulin has several advantages, the most important of which is the ready availability of donor cells. If non β-cells from a diabetic individual can be engineered to produce insulin, then cellular rejection is less likely to occur since donor and recipient are autologous. In pursuit of this goal, hepatocytes have been shown to be suitable target cells for the generation of artificial β-cells [2-9]. Moreover, liver cells that produce insulin may not be prone to autoimmune attack [10]. The suitability of hepatocytes as a β-cell replacement is attributable, in part, to their inherent glucose responsiveness and their embryonic origin from the same endodermal precursor cells as the β-cell. Most importantly, liver cells express the high capacity glucose transporter, GLUT 2 [11], and the high capacity phosphorylation enzyme, glucokinase [12], which constitute the key elements of the "glucose sensing system" that regulates insulin release from pancreatic β-cells in response to small extracellular nutrient changes.

In pancreatic β-cells, a small increase in plasma glucose concentration stimulates significant insulin secretion. Therefore, glucose is the major modulator of β-cell function and this behaviour must be mimicked in insulin-secreting liver cells. In pancreatic β-cells, K_{ATP} channels, which are composed of four sulphonylurea receptor (SUR) subunits and four inwardly-rectifying potassium channel ($K_{IR}6.2$) subunits [13-18], maintain resting membrane potentials and link plasma glucose concentrations to the insulin secretory machinery. The triggering pathway for insulin release begins with the uptake of glucose via the glucose carrier, GLUT2, and an acceleration of metabolism, such that glucose is used to generate ATP. An increase in the absolute intracellular concentration of ATP, with respect to ADP, stimulates the closure of K_{ATP} channels [19, 20]. Potassium conductance of the plasma membrane decreases, allowing a background current to shift the membrane potential away from the equilibrium potential for K^+, thus depolarising the membrane. Consequently, the pancreatic β-cell is able to translate metabolic signals to electrical signals, the latter regulating insulin secretion. Lack of functional K_{ATP} channels in insulin-secreting NES2Y cells resulted in the unregulated release of insulin, which was restored by expression of both $K_{IR}6.2$ and SUR1 [21].

When depolarisation of the pancreatic β-cell reaches the threshold for activation of L-type ($Ca_V1.3$), and to a lesser extent P/Q ($Ca_V1.2$) and T-type ($Ca_V3.x$) voltage-gated calcium channels, these open allowing Ca^{2+} influx down their electrochemical gradient [22]. The opening of Ca_V channels is intermittent, fluctuating with the membrane potential, therefore generating oscillations in the intracellular (cytosolic) calcium concentration ($[Ca^{2+}]_i$), which, in turn, triggers pulsatile insulin secretion. In β-cells, elevation of $[Ca^{2+}]_i$ occurs via the release of Ca^{2+} from intracellular stores (endoplasmic reticulum, mitochondria and secretory granules) and/or influx of extracellular Ca^{2+} through Ca_V channels [23, 24]. No functional Ca_V channels have been previously described in liver cells, however the presence of an α1-subunit lacking the voltage sensor has been reported in the rat liver cell line H4IIE [25] and an L-type α1-subunit has been detected at low levels in rat liver by RT-PCR [26].

For an insulin-producing liver cell to be of maximum benefit *in vivo* it must be capable of rapid responsive secretion of biologically active insulin. This characteristic demands that artificial β-cells process proinsulin to insulin and store it in granules. Our previous studies have shown that the insertion of genes encoding for insulin and the glucose transporter, GLUT2, into the HEPG2 human hepatoma cell line, resulted in synthesis and storage of (pro)insulin in structures resembling the secretory granules of pancreatic β-cells (HEPG2/ins/g), and the near physiological secretion of (pro)insulin in response to glucose [2, 3]. Similar to pancreatic β-cells, HEPG2ins/g cells responded to glucose via signalling pathways dependent upon K_{ATP} channels [27]. Therefore, expression of both insulin and GLUT2 in HEPG2 liver cells appeared to be sufficient for the generation of functional K_{ATP} channels, unlike the parental cell line that required pharmacological stimulation to activate the K_{ATP} channels [28]. It has previously been shown that stable transfection of the insulin gene into the human liver cell line, Huh7 (which endogenously expresses GLUT2), resulted in synthesis, storage, and regulated release of insulin to the physiological stimulus glucose (Huh7ins cells) [7]. Huh7ins cells are more akin to pancreatic β-cells than HEPG2/ins/g cells. They express a range of β-cell transcription factors [7, 29] and possess storage granules that cleave proinsulin to biologically active diarginyl insulin, due to the expression of the proconvertases PC1 and PC2 [7]. As Huh7ins cells also rapidly secrete insulin in a tightly regulated manner in response to glucose, the Huh7ins cells were able to reverse chemically induced diabetes when transplanted into an animal model [7], which HEPG2ins/g cells [3] failed to achieve [Tuch, unpublished results].

This chapter will detail the use of electrophysiological and biochemical techniques to show that Huh7ins cells respond to a glucose stimulus by closure of K_{ATP} channels and activation of Ca_V channels, which is an analogous mechanism to pancreatic β-cells. Patch-clamp electrophysiology of Huh7ins cells yielded current-voltage (*I-V*) curves that indicated the presence of potassium-selective currents; in contrast, currents recorded from Huh7 cells were non-selective. The presence of functional ATP-sensitive potassium (K_{ATP}) channels and voltage-gated calcium (Ca_V) channels was further validated by measurement of acute insulin secretion by Huh7ins cells in response to pharmacological channel inhibitors and activators and by calcium imaging and patch-clamp electrophysiology experiments. Molecular analyses were used to confirm that the Huh7ins cells express Ca_V and all the subunits of K_{ATP} channels. The secretion of insulin from granules in live Huh7ins cells was revealed by confocal microscopy which allowed visualization of secretion of insulin to a zinquin probe or an insulin-enhanced green fluorescent protein (EGFP) fusion protein (EGFP-ins). The glucose responsive mechanism that we observed in the Huh7ins cells was the same as that reported for the pancreatic β-cell line, MIN6 [30]. Prior to this study, the physiological interaction of K_{ATP} channels and Ca_V channels had never been shown in liver cells engineered to secrete insulin. As the biochemical properties of Huh7ins cells are akin to those of pancreatic β-cells, engineering hepatocytes in this way opens a promising avenue for the ultimate replacement of the endogenous β-cell function that is lost in Type I diabetes, by modifying a patient's own liver cells to become artificial β-cells. This is the first study that clearly delineates the control of insulin trafficking in a functioning artificial β-cell line that was derived from a human liver cell.

2. Understanding the mechanism by which liver-derived artificial beta cells respond to glucose and pharmacological stimulators and inhibitors of insulin secretion:

The mechanisms by which liver-derived artificial β-cells respond to glucose are poorly understood. Indeed, the majority of engineered insulin-secreting liver cells lack a truly regulated pathway of insulin release [31]. As pancreas and liver are derived from the same endodermal origin, the capacity of liver cells to differentiate into cells bearing pancreatic characteristics is well documented. A number of studies have shown that the expression of β-cell transcription factors in liver cells leads to pancreatic transdifferentiation, glucose-regulated insulin secretion and reversal of diabetes [4-7, 9, 32, 33]. Spontaneous pancreatic transdifferentiation and glucose-regulated insulin secretion have also been shown in dedifferentiated liver cells that express β-cell transcription factors such as the HEPG2ins/g and Huh7ins liver cell lines [3, 7, 9], as well as liver cells that have experienced a metabolic insult such as hepatic oval cells cultured in high glucose [34]. Consistent with this, our laboratory has shown spontaneous pancreatic transdifferentiation in hyperglycaemic rat livers and reversal of diabetes following the delivery of the insulin gene using a lentiviral vector [8]. Other recent studies in our laboratory have employed the H4IIE liver cell line, which does not express β-cell transcription factors and lacks a regulated pathway of insulin release [31]. When engineered to express the β-cell transcription factor *Neurod1* and rat insulin (H4IIEins/ND), H4IIE cells underwent pancreatic transdifferentiation and glucose-regulated insulin secretion from secretory granules. However, when *Neurod1* alone was expressed, an array of β-cell transcription factors and pancreatic hormones were expressed, but glucose-regulated insulin-secretion was not observed [9]. The Huh7 parent cell line, from which the insulin-secreting Huh7ins cells were derived, represents an ideal candidate for the engineering of an artificial β-cell. These cells possess several characteristics inherent to β-cells but not intrinsic to primary hepatocytes, such as the expression of β-cell transcription factors *Neurod1* [7], *Pdx1, Nkx2-2, Nkx6-1, Neurog3* and *Pax 6* [29]. Importantly, however, the process of transfection with insulin resulted in the formation of insulin secretory granules and the development of a regulated insulin secretory pathway [7] as was observed in the rodent H4IIEins/ND cells. Results of a mechanistic microarray analysis comparing Huh and Huh7ins cells following insulin transfection indicated that the formation of secretory granules and the development of a regulated secretory pathway was likely related to a protein interaction or posttranslational effect in combination with increased gene expression of secretory granule proteins such as chromgranin A [29]..

2.1. Huh7ins cells possess potassium-selective plasma membrane channels

Huh7 (parental human liver cell line), Huh7ins (parental human liver cell line transfected with human insulin cDNA) [7] were maintained in Dulbecco's Modified Eagle's Medium

(DMEM) supplemented with 10% v/v fetal calf serum (FCS) (Trace Biosciences, Australia) in 5% CO_2 at 37°C. Although of murine origin, MIN6 cells are one of the few β-cell lines that are responsive to glucose in the physiological range, and, accordingly provide an established β-cell-like cell line for comparative purposes [30]. MIN6 cells were grown in DMEM supplemented with 15% v/v FCS (37°C, 5% CO_2). For the Huh7ins cell line, the selective antibiotic G418 (0.55 mg/ml) was added to maintain stable transfectants.

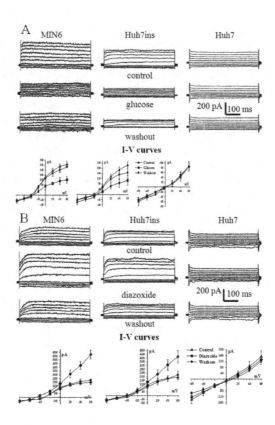

Figure 1. Sensitivity of potassium channels to glucose and diazoxide in Huh7ins cells. The upper three sets of current traces in panels A and B show superimposed families of whole-cell K⁺ currents elicited by 450 ms test pulses from –80 to +80 mV in 10-mV steps. Lower graphs show the I-V relationship of the late current measured at the end of the test pulse and shows the mean ± SEM at each potential. (A) Glucose (20 mM) reversibly inhibited the potassium currents of MIN6 and Huh7ins cells (left and centre columns; n = 4), however glucose did not affect the non-selective currents of Huh7 cells (right column; n = 3). (B) The channel opener diazoxide (100 µM) reversibly increased the potassium currents of MIN6 and Huh7ins cells (left and centre columns; n = 9), but did not effect the non-selective currents of Huh7 cells (right column; n = 3).

To determine if functional K_{ATP} channels were present in Huh7ins or Huh7 cells, K_{ATP} channel currents were recorded using whole-cell patch-clamp electrophysiology, with MIN6 cells being included as the positive control. Whole-cell patch-clamp recordings from potassium channels were made as previously described [27]. Cells grown on coverslips were transferred to a recording chamber and were perfused with a bath solution of the following composition (in mM): 140 Na acetate, 1 $CaCl_2$, 1 $MgCl_2$, 10 HEPES (pH 7.4). Patch pipettes were filled with an internal solution containing (in mM): 136 K acetate, 5 CsF, 5 KCl, 1 EGTA, 10 HEPES (pH 7.3). For inside-out patch-clamp recordings, the patch pipette was filled with (in mM): 135 NaCl, 5 KCl, 5 $CaCl_2$, 2 $MgSO_4$, 5 HEPES or a high K^+ extracellular solution in which KCl replaced NaCl. The bath solution contained (in mM): 107 KCl, 11 EGTA, 2 $MgSO_4$, 1 $CaCl_2$, 11 HEPES (pH 7.2). For Ca_V channel analyses the bath solution contained (in mM): 115 NaCl, 5 KCl, 10 $CaCl_2$, 10 HEPES, 2 D-glucose and 100 µM tetrodotoxin (pH 7.4) and the internal solution contained (in mM): 10 CsCl, 115 Cs aspartate, 2.5 EGTA, 10 HEPES (pH 7.2). Channel currents were amplified and filtered using a MultiClamp amplifier (Molecular Devices, MDS Analytical Technologies, Toronto, Canada) and sampled on-line using a Digidata 1322 (A/D converter) and pClamp 8.2 software program (Molecular Devices).

The electrophysiological properties of the K_{ATP} channel in the Huh7ins cells closely resemble those reported for normal pancreatic β-cells [19]. The outward potassium currents of MIN6 and Huh7ins cells were sensitive to glucose and inhibited by perfusing 20 mM glucose for 5 min, with partial recovery of current amplitude after the washout of glucose for 10 min. In contrast, the non-selective outward and inward currents of Huh7 cells were not altered by the addition of 20 mM glucose (Figure 1A). The outward potassium currents of MIN6 and Huh7ins cells were also reversibly increased by perfusing with the K_{ATP} channel opener, diazoxide, 100 µM (Figure 1B), whereas the non-selective currents of Huh7 cells were unaffected by diazoxide.

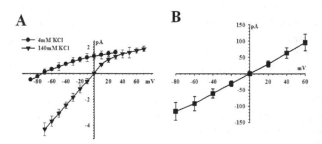

Figure 2. I-V curves of Huh7ins and Huh7 cells. (A) Mean current-voltage relations for inside-out patches of Huh7ins cells exposed to an external K^+ concentration of either 140 mM or 5 mM K^+ (n = 6). (B) Using an internal and external K $^+$ concentration of 5 mM and 140 mM respectively, the reversal potential (E_{rev}) of Huh7 whole-cell currents (n = 6), was approximately 0 mV, indicating a non-selective current. Values represent means ± SEM.

Further support for the presence of functional K_{ATP} channels in Huh7ins cells was obtained by analysis of current-voltage (I-V) relationships of single channel currents, which had similar kinetics to that of pancreatic β-cells. Recordings were made from inside-out patches exposed to 140 mM $[K^+]_i$ and either 140 mM K^+ $[K^+]_o$ or 5 mM K^+ $[K^+]_o$. As would be expected for a K^+-selective channel, the single channel currents recorded with symmetrical $[K^+]$ reversed close to 0 mV, with a mean slope conductance of 48.5 pS (−80 to −10 mV). In comparison, the slope conductance was reduced to 12.4 pS (0 to +60 mV) when the $[K^+]_o$ was reduced to 5 mM, indicating that the channel was K^+-selective (Figure 2A). In contrast the I-V curve for K_{ATP} channels in Huh7 cells indicated that currents from these cells were non-selective as the reversal potential was closer to 0 mV (Figure 2B). As secretory granules require K_{ATP} channels for the appropriate release of insulin [35, 36], it is likely that Huh7ins cells also contained K_{ATP} channels located intracellularly at the secretory granule membrane.

2.2. Secretion of insulin observed in real time in response to glucose and K_{ATP} channel blockers

In order to observe, in real time, the secretion of insulin from granules in response to stimulators and inhibitors of insulin secretion by confocal microscopy, Huh7 and MIN 6 cells were engineered to express insulin fused to EGFP. To accomplish this, human insulin cDNA pC_2 (a gift from Dr. M. Walker, Weizmann Institute, Israel) [7] was cloned into the multicloning site of the pEGFP-N1 vector (Clontech, CA, USA). As there were no intervening stop codons, EGFP/insulin (EGFPins) was expressed as a fusion protein, which allowed visualization and localization of the fusion protein in cells. The construct (20 µg) or vector alone was introduced into Huh7 and MIN6 cells using Lipofectamine 2000 (Invitrogen, Carlsbad, CA), following the instructions of the manufacturer. To obtain stable transfectants, containing the construct (EGFPins) or empty vector (EGFP), G418 antibiotic (0.55 mg/ml) (Gibco Laboratories, Grand Island, NY) was added to the culture medium after 48 h. Media and G418 were changed every 2–3 days. After 3–4 weeks of selection, 25 colonies were chosen and screened for production of insulin by radioimmunoassay (RIA) [7] and EGFP by fluorescence microscopy. Human c-peptide was measured as previously described [8]. Clones were expanded into mass cultures and maintained in G418 selection media (37°C, 5% CO$_2$). Huh7-EGFP (parental human liver cell line expressing EGFP) and Huh7-EGFPins (parental human liver cell line expressing EGFPins) cells were maintained in DMEM supplemented with 10% v/v fetal calf serum (FCS) (Trace Biosciences, Australia) in 5% CO$_2$ at 37°C. MIN6-EGFP (EGFP-expressing MIN6 cells) and MIN6-EGFPins (EGFPins-expressing MIN6 cells) cells were grown in DMEM supplemented with 15% v/v FCS (37°C, 5% CO$_2$). For these transfected cell lines, the selective antibiotic G418 (0.55 mg/ml) was added.

To compare the function of Huh7-EGFPins and Huh7ins cells, chronic insulin secretion, insulin storage, and glucose-responsiveness were assessed. Acute insulin secretion was measured by static stimulation in basal medium consisting of PBS supplemented with (in mM): 1 CaCl$_2$, 20 HEPES, 2 mg/ml BSA, 1.0 D-glucose; pH 7.4, as previously described [7]. Insulin was measured by RIA using human or rodent standards as previously described [7]. To assay insulin content, insulin was extracted from cells using 0.18 N HCl in 70% ethanol for 18 h at 4°C, as previously described [7]. To assess the quantity of human as compared to rodent insulin secreted by MIN6-EGFPins cells, a commercial RIA for human insulin (Linco Research, MO, USA), was used. This has less than 1% and 6% cross-reactivity with rodent insulin and human proinsulin, respectively.

Of the 25 clones of Huh7-EGFPins isolated for analysis, insulin secretion differed 3-fold (0.11 ± 0.2 vs. 0.32 ± 0.2 pmol insulin/10^6 cells/24 h; $n = 6$) and insulin storage varied 2-fold (3.4 ± 1.2 vs. 7.1 ± 0.3 pmol insulin/10^6 cells; $n = 6$). Subsequently, six clones which secreted and stored the highest levels of insulin and exhibited consistently bright EGFP fluorescence, were examined for glucose responsiveness. Whilst all clones were glucose responsive, one clone (clone 16) was most comparable to Huh7ins cells [7] as it secreted equal amounts of insulin over a 24 h period (0.32 ± 0.2 vs. 0.30 ± 0.1 pmol insulin/10^6 cells for Huh7ins cells; $n = 6$). Insulin storage was also comparable between the two cell lines with Huh7-EGFPins (clone 16) and Huh7ins cells storing 7.1 ± 0.3 and 7.0 ± 0.2 pmol/10^6 cells ($n = 6$), respectively. Glucose concentration-response curves for the Huh7-EGFPins (clone 16) and Huh7ins cell lines were also determined and revealed that there was no significant difference to previously published values [7] (data not shown). Levels of human proinsulin (not insulin) were 11.4 ± 1.2% of total insulin ($n = 6$). Human c-peptide levels were 1.0 ± 0.4% of total insulin activity ($n = 6$). Therefore clone 16 was used for all subsequent analyses, and is referred to as Huh7-EGFPins hereafter. As expected, Huh7-EGFP cells did not synthesize, store nor secrete insulin. Examination of the insulin secreted chronically by MIN6-EGFPins cells revealed that 20.5 ± 2.3% ($n = 6$) was of human origin, the remainder being rodent insulin. Of the insulin stored by MIN6-EGFPins cells, 17.9 ± 2.4% ($n = 6$) was human insulin. As expected, all of the insulin stored and secreted by MIN6-EGFP cells was of rodent origin. These data suggest that MIN6 cells handled EGFPins in a similar fashion to native rodent insulin.

In order to perform confocal microscopy, cells were plated on coverslips (Marienfeld superior 22 mm diameter) and grown for 2–4 days. Each coverslip was inserted into a Perspex cell chamber, sealed with silicone grease, and overlaid with 1 ml DMEM containing 5 mM glucose (confocal scanning laser microscope [CSLM] medium). For Zinquin-E (zinquin ester, ethyl[2-methyl-8-p-toluenesulphonamido-6-quinolyloxy]acetate) staining, cells were incubated at 37°C for 30 min with CSLM medium containing 25 µM zinquin E (Luminis Pty Ltd, Australia), as previously described [27]. After incubation, cells were rinsed with CSLM medium before recording confocal images with a Leica TCSNT (Wetzlar, Germany) with an inverted microscope (Leica DMRBE). Cells were imaged with a UV laser, oil 100x (N.A.1.4 UV-corrected Planapo) or oil 63x (N.A.1.32 UV-corrected Planapo). Emissions were collected with a BP490/440 filter. For analyses of stable transfectants expressing EGFP, incubation with a fluorescent probe was not required. These cells were imaged with an Ar/Kr laser and DP488/568 dichroic and emissions were collected with a BP525/550 filter.

CSLM medium or test solutions containing glibenclamide (20 µM), or diazoxide (150 µM) in CSLM medium, or DMEM containing 20 mM glucose, were exchanged at 37°C. Density measurements on images were performed using the public domain NIH Image program [37].

Defined regions of interest (ROI) for individual cells (10–30 cells per experiment) were followed through a time series before, and after, addition of test solutions. All values were normalized by subtracting the initial density, before addition of the test solution, from all the measurements in the series for each individual ROI to give a value of zero density for the

initial time point. Confocal microscopy detected intracellular EGFP-ins or Zinquin-E as
punctuate fluorescence, which was indicative of insulin stored within secretion granules.

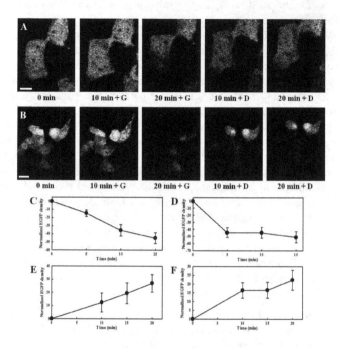

Figure 3. Confocal microscopic visualization of HuH7-EGFPins cells after exposure to glucose and diazoxide. (A) Huh7-
EGFPins and (B) MIN6-EGFPins cells were incubated in DMEM containing 5 mM glucose (CLSM medium), then stimulated with glucose (20 mM, G) and diazoxide (150 μM, D). Images were recorded in CLSM medium at 0, 10 and 20 min
after glucose addition. At 20 min, cells were placed in CLSM medium containing diazoxide and images were recorded
at 10 and 20 min after diazoxide exposure (bars = 10 μm). Normalized EGFP density indicated that (C) Huh7-EGFPins
(n = 60) and (D) MIN6-EGFPins cells (n = 42) showed decreasing EGFP density after addition of glucose, whereas (E)
Huh7-EGFP (n = 19) and (F) MIN6-EGFP cells (n = 12) showed increasing EGFP density after addition of glucose. Values
represent the mean ± SEM.

For statistical analysis of all the confocal measurements described below SPSS version 11.5
(SPSS Inc) was used to determine a one-way analysis of variance after testing for homogene-
ity of variance using the Levene statistic. Huh7-EGFPins and MIN6-EGFPins cells responded in the same way to 20 mM glucose after 10 and 15 min, with loss of fluorescence from the
ROI indicative of insulin secretion (Figure 3A-D). There was no significant difference between the response of Huh7-EGFPins and MIN6-EGFPins cells at 10 min ($p > 0.5$, $n = 60$) and
15 min ($p \geq 0.7$, $n = 42$). The MIN6-EGFPins cells responded more rapidly to the glucose
stimulus than the Huh7ins-EGFP cells, with close to maximum loss of fluorescence achieved
at 5 min, but after 10 min the two cell lines had achieved the same response level (Figure 3C-
D). When diazoxide (150 μM) was added to cells that had been stimulated by 20 mM glucose for 20 min, cytoplasmic fluorescence accumulated, as the release of insulin from

secretory granules was blocked (Figure 3A-B). The response of the control cell lines, Huh7-EGFP and Min6-EGFP to 20 mM glucose was significantly different ($p < 0.00001$) at all time points from that of the engineered cell lines. In the control cell lines fluorescence increased over time (Figure 3E-F) since cells accumulated considerable amounts of EGFP within their cytoplasm and they were unresponsive to 20 mM glucose. Presumably this phenomenon is attributable to an inability of the parental cell lines to direct EGFP to secretory granules, whereas the cells engineered to synthesize insulin responded by releasing insulin from secretory granules so that their fluorescence decreased (Figure 3C-D).

Huh7ins and Min6 cells stained with the zinquin-E probe responded to 20 mM glucose with decreasing fluorescence. There was no significant difference between Huh7ins cells labelled with zinquin-E and Huh7-EGFPins cells in their response to 20 mM glucose after 5 min ($p > 0.8$, $n = 41$) and 15 min ($P > 0.1$, $n = 59$). After incubation with the K_{ATP} channel blocking sulphonylurea, glibenclamide (20 µM), the two cell lines responded as they did in the presence of glucose (i.e. decreasing fluorescence was observed). Conversely, treatment with 150 µM diazoxide, which inhibits glucose-activated β-cell depolarisation by suppressing closure of K_{ATP} channels, caused increased fluorescence, showing that secretion of insulin was blocked in Huh7ins-EGFP cells (Figure 3A) and Huh7ins cells (with zinquin-E probe).

Huh7ins-EGFP and MIN6ins-EGFP cells responded to either glucose or glibenclamide with a decrease in fluorescence (indicative of insulin secretion). The same secretory response to glucose or glibenclamide was seen in MIN6 and Huh7ins cells using the zinquin probe. Through its high affinity for the sulphonylurea subunit of the K_{ATP} channel, glibenclamide renders the K_{ATP} channel inactive and calcium influx through Ca_V channels ensues due to depolarisation of the cell membrane. The release of insulin from intracellular storage granules is the net result of these processes. As this response to glibenclamide was observed for Huh7ins, Huh7-EGFPins, MIN6 and MIN6-EGFPins cells, insulin secretion likely occurred via the classic insulin triggering pathway utilized by pancreatic β-cells. In contrast, the negative controls (Huh7-EGFP and MIN6-EGFP cells) or Huh7 cells in the case of Zinquin-E labelling, were unresponsive to glucose or glibenclamide. The increased fluorescence of the negative control cells MIN6-EGFP and Huh7-EGFP after glucose stimulation showed that there was no trafficking of EGFP to secretory granules. In an earlier publication, Arvan and Halban [38] questioned the specificity of the trans Golgi network sorting process, but the fact that in our cell lines the secretion of EGFP-ins was regulated while EGFP was not, shows that the sorting of EGFP was specific, with only EGFP-insulin being trafficked to secretory granules.

2.3. Huh7ins cells express the K_{ATP} channel subunits, $K_{IR}6.2$, SUR2A and SUR2B, and the α1-subunit of the $Ca_V1.3$ channel

Primers were designed to the cDNA sequences encoding the human K_{ATP} subunits, $K_{IR}6.2$ (F: AGCCCAAGTTCAGCATCTCTCC, R:CCAGAAATAGCATAGTGACAAGTGCC), SUR1 (F: TCAGGGTTGTGAACCGCA, R: GTTTCTGCGAAGCATAGGC), SUR2A (F:

GGCAGGTGGGAAATCATCGTTA, R: TCCCCACCTTCAGTGACAA') and SUR2B (F: GATGCGGTTGTCACTGAA, R: ACTCCTTCACATGTCTGC). Primers were also designed to amplify the α1-subunit of the $Ca_V1.3$ channel of pancreatic β-cells (F: TGGCAGGAGAT-CATGCTGG, R: CTAATCTCTTGCTCGCTACC). RT-PCR analyses were performed using the cDNA synthesised from RNA isolated from Huh7 and Huh7ins cells using TRIzol® Reagent (Invitrogen). Positive controls were HEPG2 cells that express the human $K_{IR}6.2$ and SUR2A subunits [27], or human pancreatic islets.

Immunoblot analyses were performed using protein extracted from Huh7 and Huh7ins cells and human pancreatic islets to detect the human K_{ATP} subunits, SUR1, SUR2A and SUR2B, and the α1-subunit of the $Ca_V1.3$ channel. Detection of the $K_{IR}6.2$ subunit was determined as previously described [27]. For detection of $K_{IR}6.2$, SUR1, SUR2A, SUR2B and the α1-subunit of the $Ca_V1.3$ channel, cell supernatants were suspended in buffer I containing (in mM): 10 Tris, 20 NaH_2PO_4, 1 EDTA, 0.1 PMSF, 10 µg/ml pepstatin, 10 µl/ml leupeptin (pH 7.8), subjected to three freeze-thaw cycles, and then incubated for 20 min at 4°C. The protein concentration of the supernatant was determined using a Micro Bicinchoninic Protein Assay Reagent Kit (PIERCE, Thermo Fisher Scientific, Rockford, Il, USA). Protein samples (15 µg) were electrophoresed in 10% polyacrylamide gels (100 V) and then transferred to nitrocellulose membranes (Millipore Corporation, USA) for immunoblot analyses. Nitrocellulose membranes were blocked in PBS with 5% w/v skim milk overnight at 4°C. Immunoblotting was performed using a 1:1000 dilution of goat anti-human $K_{IR}6.2$, SUR1, SUR2A, SUR2B and the α1-subunit of the $Ca_V1.3$ channel polyclonal IgGs (Santa Cruz Biotech. USA) and detection was achieved using monoclonal (mouse) anti-goat/sheep horseradish peroxidase IgG conjugate (1:800 dilution) (Sigma).

RT-PCR analysis revealed that the Huh7 and Huh7ins cells expressed the human K_{ATP} channel subunit, $K_{IR}6.2$, and the β-cell sulfonylurea receptor subunits, SUR2A and SUR2B (Figure 4A-C), together with the human α1-subunit of the $Ca_V1.3$ channel (Figure 4E). SUR1 was only detected in the Huh7ins liver cell line (Figure 4D). Immunoblot analysis for the presence of $K_{IR}6.2$, SUR1, SUR2A and SUR2B, revealed strong expression in Huh7ins cells and human pancreatic islets, with no detectable expression in Huh7 cells (Figure 4F-I). The presence of protein product for the α1-subunit of the $Ca_V1.3$ channel was confirmed by immunoblot analysis of protein extracted from Huh7ins cells, with only low expression in Huh7 cells (Figure 4J).

Thus, unlike the glucose-responsive insulin-secreting cell line, HEPG2ins/g [26], the Huh7ins cells expressed the SUR1 receptor as do pancreatic β-cells. The functional recording of K_{ATP} activity in Huh7ins cells are supported by the immunoblot blot analyses, which suggests that $K_{IR}6.2$, SUR1, SUR2A and SUR2B are strongly expressed in Huh7ins cells. There was no detectable expression of $K_{IR}6.2$, SUR1, SUR2A and SUR2B in Huh7 cells, which is supported by the absence of K_{ATP} currents in the patch-clamp recordings (Figure 2B). Expression of $K_{IR}6.2$ and SUR1, the two relevant subunits of the pancreatic β-cell K_{ATP} channel, is commonly seen in primary hepatocytes, although dedifferentiated cell lines such as HEPG2 [28] and Huh7 cells appear to have lost expression of SUR1 at the mRNA level. It is apparent that the process of pancreatic transdifferentiation, which has caused the formation of secretory granules, has resulted in expression of $K_{IR}6.2$ protein and SUR1 at the mRNA level and protein expression in Huh7ins cells.

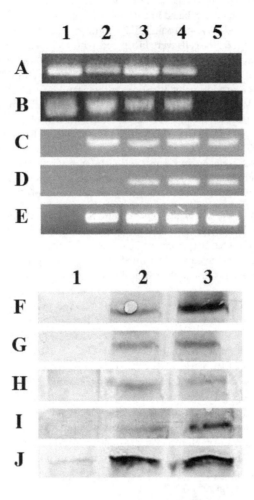

Figure 4. RT-PCR and immunoblot analysis for K_{ATP} and Ca_V channel subunits. RT-PCR analysis of liver cell lines for (A) human $K_{IR}6.2$: HuH7 (lane 1), Huh7ins (lane 2), Huh7-EGFPins (lane 3), HEPG2 (lane 4, positive control), and no cDNA control (lane 5); (B) human SUR2A: Huh7 (lane 1), Huh7ins (lane 2), Huh7-EGFPins (lane 3), HEPG2 (lane 4, positive control), and no cDNA control (lane 5); (C) human SUR2B: no cDNA (lane 1), human pancreas (lane 2, positive control), Huh7 (lane 3), Huh7ins (lane 4), Huh7-EGFPins (lane 5), (D) Human SUR1: no cDNA (lane 1), Huh7 (lane 2), Huh7ins (lane 3), Huh7-EGFPins (lane 4), human pancreas (lane 5, positive control), (E) human α1-subunit of the Ca_V1.3 channel: no cDNA (lane 1), human pancreas (lane 2, positive control), Huh7 (lane 3), Huh7ins (lane 4), Huh7-EGFPins (lane 5). Immunoblot analysis for (F) human $K_{IR}6.2$, (G) human SUR2A, (H) SUR2B, (I) SUR1 and (J) the α1-subunit of the Ca_V1.3 channel in Huh7 (lane 1), Huh7ins (lane 2) and human islet (lane 3).

2.4. Huh7ins cells possess Ca_V channels

The level of intracellular free Ca^{2+} was measured using Fluo4-AM and pluronic F-127 with a Zeiss microscope (Axiovert 200M; Zeiss, Germany). Cells were grown on coverslips until 50–70% confluent and were then incubated in culture medium containing 8 μM Fluo4-AM (Invitrogen, Carlsbad, CA) and 0.1% pluronic F-127 (Invitrogen) at 37°C for 60 min. To remove excess Fluo4-AM and F-127, the cells were incubated with HEPES buffer containing (in mM): 140 NaCl, 5 KCl, 2 $CaCl_2$, 1 $MgCl_2$, 5 D-glucose, 10 HEPES (pH 7.4), for 30 min images were captured. The coverslips were then placed in a chamber containing HEPES buffer. After control images were taken (before addition of glucose or glibenclamide), the cells were exposed to 20 mM glucose or 20 μM glibenclamide until the completion of experiments. For the experiments in the presence of Ca_V channel blocker, the cells were incubated with 10 μM verapamil for 30 min before the addition of glucose or glibenclamide. Fluorescence intensity was observed under a Zeiss microscope and images were captured with a digital camera (Axio-Cam, Zeiss) and the Axiovision program (Zeiss). Images were taken every 20 s and analyzed using ImageJ software [39]. Results were presented as relative fluorescence values (F/F_0), where F_0 represents the fluorescence of controls (before addition of glucose or glibenclamide).

While the expression of Ca_V channels in pancreatic β-cells has been well documented [23, 40], their precise role in hepatocytes is yet to be elucidated. It has been reported that Ca_V1 channels are found in endocrine (pancreatic), cardiac and neural cells [41], but no physiologically-active Ca_V1 channels have been identified in hepatocytes prior to this study. Calcium imaging revealed that an increase in the extracellular glucose concentration from 5 to 20 mM immediately stimulated an elevated level of free $[Ca^{2+}]_i$ in Huh7ins cells, which peaked within 2 min and then gradually recovered to the level observed prior to application of 20 mM glucose (Figure 5A). The F/F_0 value at 2 min after the application of 20 mM glucose in Huh7ins cells was 1.14 ± 0.038 (n = 33, Figure 5B). However, 20 mM glucose did not significantly increase the level of free $[Ca^{2+}]_i$ in Huh7 cells (F/F_0 = 1.02 ± 0.01, n = 19), which was significantly lower than that of Huh7ins cells (Fig 5A-B). To examine if blockade of K_{ATP} channels mimicked the effect of 20 mM glucose, glibenclamide (20 μM) was applied in the bath solution containing 5 mM glucose. Glibenclamide dramatically increased the level of intracellular free Ca^{2+} (F/F_0 = 1.87 ± 0.24, n = 25), which had a similar time course to that observed in the presence of 20 mM glucose, but with a greater peak amplitude. Similar to the effects of 20 mM glucose on Huh7 cells, glibenclamide did not alter calcium flux in Huh7 cells (Figure 5A-B). It should be noted that both 20 mM glucose and 20 μM glibenclamide produced a more delayed increase in the $[Ca^{2+}]_i$ in Huh7 cells in comparison with data recorded in Huh7ins cells (Figure 5A).

Verapamil (10 μM), a phenylalkylamine $Ca_V1.x$ channel blocker, inhibited the increase in $[Ca^{2+}]_i$ in Huh7ins cells produced by 20 mM glucose (1.04 ± 0.02, n = 31) and glibenclamide (0.99 ± 0.02, n = 31; Figure 5A and C). This indicated that the observed glucose-induced block and diazoxide-induced increase in free $[Ca^{2+}]_i$ was mediated by Ca_V channels. To further validate this interpretation, we used the whole-cell patch-clamp technique to measure the effect of increased glucose on membrane currents in Huh7ins and Huh7 cells. The resultant I-V curve indicated that increasing the concentration of glucose from 2 to 20 mM resulted in ac-

Insulin Trafficking in a Glucose Responsive Engineered Human Liver Cell Line is Regulated by
the Interaction of ATP-Sensitive Potassium Channels and Voltage-Gated Calcium Channels

207

tivation of an inwardly-rectifying current in Huh7ins cells (Figure 5D). This current was
blocked by the addition of CsCl thereby lending further support to the premise that it was
mediated via K$^+$ channels. No activation was seen when Huh7 cells were used in these experiments (results not shown). Ca$_V$ channel currents recorded from Huh7ins cells were inhibited by verapamil (10 µM), indicating that Ca$_V$1.x channels were involved in the response
(Figure 5E). This further corroborates the calcium imaging data described above.

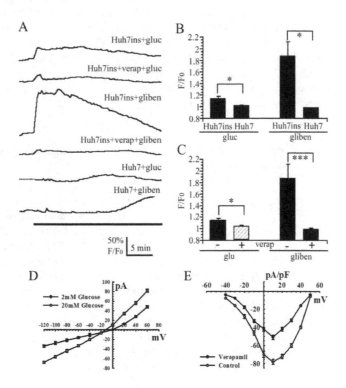

Figure 5. Calcium imaging and patch-clamp electrophysiology of Huh7ins and Huh7 cells. High glucose and blockade
of K$_{ATP}$ channels elevated levels of intracellular free Ca^{2+} in Huh7ins cells. (A) Averaged time courses of relative fluorescence intensity (F/F$_0$) induced by 20 mM glucose (gluc) and 20 µM glibenclamide (gliben) in the presence, and absence, of 10 µM verapamil (verap, Ca$_V$1.x channel blocker) in Huh7ins and Huh7 cells. The black bar at the base of
panel A represents the time of application of glucose or glibenclamide. Each trace represents an average F/F$_0$ value of
the cells investigated. (B) Glucose and glibenclamide increased the level of free [Ca^{2+}], in Huh7ins cells, but not in Huh7
cells. (C) Glucose- and glibenclamide-induced increases in intracellular free Ca^{2+} in Huh7ins cells were significantly inhibited by 10 µM verapamil. The values shown in B and C were taken 2 min after application of glucose or glibenclamide. * $p < 0.05$ and *** $p < 0.001$. (D) Mean I-V relationship in Huh7ins cells under low (2 mM) and high (20 mM)
glucose conditions (n = 4). (E) I-V curves for Ca$_V$ channel currents in Huh7ins cells in the presence of 20 mM glucose
and following the addition of 10 µM verapamil (n = 6). Values are expressed as means ± SEM

The Ca$_V$1.3 α1 subunit (Figure 4J), expressed in pancreatic β-cells [42], was detected in both
Huh7ins cells and the parental Huh7 cells, at both the mRNA and the protein level, suggest-

ing that Huh7ins and Huh7 cells possess $Ca_V1.3$ channels that are similar to those found in pancreatic β-cells. Ca^{2+} imaging and patch-clamp electrophysiology experiments further detected a Ca_V channel current in Huh7ins cells, which was stimulated by glucose and inhibited by verapamil. The expression of functional Ca_V channels in Huh7ins cells may explain, in part, the acute secretion of insulin in response to glucose stimulation. The mechanism of insulin secretion depends upon the activities of ion channels in the plasma membrane, and, more critically, upon the activation of Ca_V channels, caused indirectly by increased glucose metabolism. Influx of Ca^{2+}, through open Ca_V channels, is responsible for the exocytosis of insulin storage granules, emphasising the importance of Ca_V channels in glucose-stimulated insulin secretion [41]. The lack of functional Ca_V channels in Huh7 cells is likely related to the low level of expression of the $Ca_V1.3$ α1-subunit. Once it was determined that Huh7ins cells possessed functional Ca_V channels, static stimulation experiments using the inhibitor verapamil, and the activator BayK8644, established that Ca_V channels in Huh7ins cells function in a similar manner to Ca_V channels in pancreatic β-cells.

2.5. Huh7ins cells appear to be glucose-responsive through the presence of functional K_{ATP} channels and Ca_V channels

To measure insulin secretion, monolayers of cells were incubated with K_{ATP} channel modulators, using concentrations determined from concentration-response curves in the corresponding cell lines. These included the K_{ATP} channel activators tolbutamide (100 µM) or diazoxide (150 µM) and the K_{ATP} channel blocker glibenclamide (20 µM) with or without 20 mM glucose for 1 h. The effects of the Ca_V channel blocker verapamil (10 µM), the Ca_V channel activator Bay K8644 (1 µM), the sarcoplasmic and endoplasmic reticulum family of Ca^{2+}-ATPases (SERCA) blocker ryanodine (20 µM), the SERCA stimulator thapsigargin (1 µM), and the hemi-channel blocker oleic acid (20 µM) were also assessed. Inhibitors and activators were purchased from Sigma, Sydney, Australia. Results were expressed as means ± standard error of the mean (SEM). The statistical analysis of insulin RIA results was by univariate repeated measures analysis of variance using Systat™ version 9. Post-hoc comparisons were made using Tukey's HSD test (Minitab™ version 13, Minitab Inc).

Stimulation with 20 mM glucose resulted in a 3.6- and 5.2-fold increase in insulin secretion by Huh7ins and MIN6 cells, respectively (Figures 6 and 7). Incubation of Huh7-EGFPins cells with the K_{ATP} channel blocker, glibenclamide, significantly increased insulin secretion by Huh7-EGFPins from 0.06 ± 0.01 to 0.26 ± 0.03 pmol/10^6 cells (p< 0.001, n = 6). The K_{ATP} activator, diazoxide, completely inhibited glucose-stimulated insulin release from Huh7-EGFPins (0.05 ± 0.02 pmol/10^6 cells, n = 6) and MIN6-EGFPins cells (data not shown). It was also noted that, diazoxide treatment prevented glucose-induced insulin secretion in Huh7ins and Huh7-EGF-Pins cells. Diazoxide causes sustained opening of K_{ATP} channels causing hyperpolarisation of the cell membrane, thereby preventing the voltage-dependant calcium response and inhibiting insulin exocytosis [43]. Static glucose stimulation experiments demonstrated that the insulin secretory response of Huh7ins and Huh7-EGFPins cells functioned via the channel-dependant pathway of insulin secretion. The responses of Huh7ins and MIN6 cells to diazoxide and glibenclamide treatment were identical to that observed in each of the cell lines in which insulin was fused to EGFP (data not shown). Therefore, fusion of EGFP to insulin did not alter the physiological mechanism of insulin secretion.

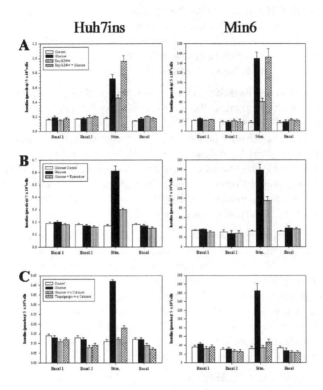

Figure 6. Secretion of insulin from Huh7ins cells and MIN6 cells. Insulin secretion was activated in response to 20 mM glucose alone or (A) 1 μM BayK8644 ± 20 mM glucose. (B) 20 μM ryanodine ± 20 mM glucose; and (C) 1 μM thapsigargin in the absence of extracellular calcium. Cells were incubated in basal medium for two consecutive 1 h periods before being exposed to the stimulus for 1 h, followed by a third period of basal incubation. Cells in the control group were treated throughout with basal medium. Values are expressed as means ± SEM (n = 6).

The application of the $Ca_V1.x$ channel activator, BayK8644 to Huh7ins and MIN6 cells significantly increased insulin secretion above basal levels ($p<0.01$, $n = 6$; Figure 6A). In the presence of 20 mM glucose, BayK8644 further amplified glucose-stimulated insulin secretion in Huh7ins cells ($p<0.05$, $n = 6$, Fig. 6A). Application of the SERCA blocker, ryanodine, which prevents increases in $[Ca^{2+}]_i$, caused a decrease in glucose-stimulated insulin secretion from Huh7ins and MIN6 cells ($p<0.05$, $n = 6$; Figure 6B).

The dihydropyridine, BayK8644, functions as a Ca_V1 channel agonist, which interacts with the α_1 subunit of Ca_V channels to stabilise the channel in the open state, thereby enhancing Ca^{2+} influx to cause the exocytosis of insulin [41]. BayK8644 does not change the membrane potential of resting β-cells [43]. Rather, it acts on the Ca_V channel in the open state, failing to affect basal insulin secretion at non-stimulatory glucose concentrations [43], but exaggerating glucose-stimulated insulin secretion [44, 45]. The addition of BayK8644 increased insulin secretion by both the Huh7ins and MIN6 cells. However, the amount of insulin secreted in the presence of BayK8644 was lower than that released in response to 20 mM glucose alone. Putatively, this concentration of glucose may have stimulated the influx of extracellular Ca^{2+}, the release of $[Ca^{2+}]_i$ from intracellular stores and increased Ca^{2+} via other Ca^{2+}-related pathways to such an extent that the total increase of Ca^{2+} in the cell was higher in the presence of 20 mM glucose as compared to BayK8644 alone.

Consistent with reports that BayK8644 is known to stimulate the opening of Ca_V channels in pancreatic β-cells without altering the membrane potential [44], static stimulation of Huh7ins cells with 1 μM BayK8644 plus 20 mM glucose amplified glucose-stimulated insulin release. However, BayK8644 failed to amplify glucose-stimulated insulin secretion in MIN6 cells. This finding may be attributable to the ability of 20 mM glucose alone to cause the maximum threshold in the activation of insulin release in MIN6 cells, such that the addition of BayK8644 was unable to exert any additional stimulatory effects. Nevertheless, these results demonstrate that the insulin secretory response of the Huh7ins cells is dependent upon the activation of Ca_V channels, as is the case for pancreatic β-cells.

Static stimulation of Huh7ins cells with the highly specific SERCA blocker thapsigargin, which induces the release of Ca^{2+} from intracellular stores resulted in a significant increase (two-fold increase over basal levels), in insulin secretion in the absence of extracellular Ca^{2+} ($p< 0.05$, $n = 6$; Figure 6C). Consistent with results from Tuch $et\ al.$ [7], the response of the Huh7ins cells to glucose was abolished when Ca^{2+} was removed from the basal medium before 20 mM glucose was added ($p> 0.05$ $vs.$ control, $n = 6$; Figure 6C). MIN6 cells showed a similar response; namely, in the absence of extracellular Ca^{2+} the glucose-responsiveness was abolished ($p> 0.05$ $vs.$ control, $n = 6$; Figure 6C), and the presence of 1 μM thapsigargin significantly increased insulin secretion 1.8-fold over basal levels ($P<0.05$, $n = 6$; Figure 6C).

The connexon (hemi-channel blocker), oleic acid, significantly reduced acute insulin secretion by 1.4-fold ($p< 0.05$, $n = 6$; Figure 7A), while verapamil (10 μM) resulted in a significant decrease in insulin secretion to glucose in both cell lines ($p< 0.05$, $n = 6$; Figure 7B). However, the combination of verapamil and ryanodine did not exert an additive effect on insulin secretion, compared to treatment with verapamil alone ($p< 0.05$, $n = 6$; Fig. 7B). Nevertheless, a greater decrease in insulin secretion was observed after the addition of verapamil, ryanodine and oleic acid in both Huh7ins ($p< 0.05$, $n = 6$) and MIN6 cells ($p< 0.05$, $n = 6$; Figure 7C).

SERCA operate to restore diminished intracellular endoplasmic and sarcoplasmic reticulum Ca^{2+} stores, thereby decreasing cytoplasmic Ca^{2+} levels [46-50]. Thapsigargin is a highly selective inhibitor of SERCA. Stimulation of β-cells with glucose causes an initial, thapsigargin-inhibitable, drop in $[Ca^{2+}]_i$ that precedes the increase in $[Ca^{2+}]_i$ due to the pumping of Ca^{2+} into the endoplasmic reticulum [51, 52]. Blocking of SERCA by thapsigargin augments the glucose-induced $[Ca^{2+}]_i$ increase by activating a depolarising store-operated current, which then facilitates the opening of Ca_V channels [51, 53, 54]. Consistent with the results reported by Tuch et al, [7], in the absence of extracellular Ca^{2+}, the glucose responsiveness of both Huh7ins and MIN6 cells in the absence of extracellular Ca^{2+}, was lost, while normal glucose responsiveness was seen when Ca^{2+} was present in the medium. However, thapsigargin, which raises cytosolic Ca^{2+}, stimulated insulin secretion by both Huh7ins and MIN6 cells in the absence of extracellular Ca^{2+}. This finding further supports the role of intracellular Ca^{2+} storage in insulin secretion in both pancreatic β-cells and in the insulin-secreting liver cell line, Huh7ins.

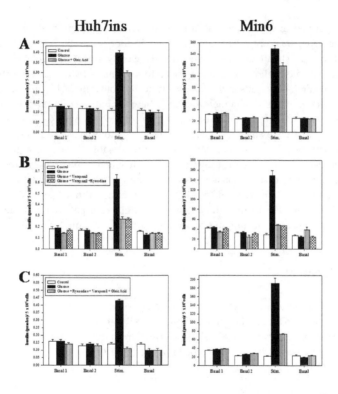

Figure 7. Secretion of insulin from Huh7ins cells and MIN6 cells. Insulin secretion was activated in response to 20 mM glucose alone or in the presence of (A) 20 μM oleic acid; (B) 10 μM verapamil ± 10 μM ryanodine and (C) 10 μM verapamil, 20 μM ryanodine and 20 μM oleic acid. Cells were incubated in basal medium for two consecutive 1 h periods before being exposed to the stimulus for 1 h, followed by a third period of basal incubation. Cells in the control group were treated throughout with basal medium. Values are expressed as means ± SEM (n = 6).

The presence of 20 μM ryanodine, which blocks Ca_V channels at concentrations ≥ 10 μM [55] and prevents the release of Ca^{2+} from the endoplasmic reticulum, reduced the glucose-responsiveness of both Huh7ins cells and MIN6 cells, although to a lesser extent than was observed in the presence of 10 μM verapamil. This finding is consistent with previous reports that intracellular Ca^{2+} stores (and therefore SERCA) contribute to the intracellular Ca^{2+} response during insulin secretion. The application of verapamil to Huh7ins cells caused a complete abrogation of glucose-responsiveness upon extracellular Ca^{2+} levels has been previously reported for pancreatic β-cells [40, 43, 56]. As expected the addition of oleic acid to Huh7ins and MIN6 cells resulted in reduced glucose responsiveness, due to the blockage of hemi-channels, similar to what has been reported in pancreatic β-cells [57].

3. Conclusion

The results described in this chapter indicate that insulin secretion in engineered hepatocytes (Huh7ins cells) was controlled, as precisely as in the pancreatic β-cell, by a fully functional K_{ATP} and Ca_V channel system. The results clearly document that Huh7ins cells respond to glucose via insulin secretion from secretory granules by the same mechanism observed in pancreatic β-cells. This is the first study to demonstrate a clear physiological and biochemical interaction of K_{ATP} channels and Ca_V channels in liver cells, and as such reveals that hepatocytes are ideal candidates for the engineering of artificial β-cells. Testament to this, we have successfully engineered a liver cell line to synthesize, store and secrete insulin. Regardless of whether this hepatoma cell line will be a viable β-cell alternative for transplantation into patients, the present study provides valuable information with regards to the future engineering of glucose-responsive insulin-secreting liver cells. Elucidation of the minimal molecular modifications required for the creation of an artificial β-cell from a hepatocyte may one day provide therapeutic avenues to engineer a patient's own liver cells to synthesize, store and secrete insulin in response to metabolic stimuli.

Acknowledgements

This work was supported by grants from Diabetes Australia Research Trust, Rebecca L. Cooper Medical Research Foundation and the University of Technology Sydney. We would like to thank Wayne Hawthorne and Philip O'Connell from the Westmead Millennium Institute for human pancreatic islets and Richard Limburg for IT support.

Author details

Ann M. Simpson[1*], M. Anne Swan[2], Guo Jun Liu[3], Chang Tao[1], Bronwyn A O'Brien[1], Edwin Ch'ng[1], Leticia M. Castro[1], Julia Ting[1], Zehra Elgundi[1], Tony An[2], Mark Lutherborrow[4], Fraser Torpy[5], Donald K. Martin[1], Bernard E. Tuch[6] and Graham M. Nicholson[1]

*Address all correspondence to: Ann.Simpson@uts.edu.au

1 School of Medical & Molecular Biosciences, University of Technology Sydney, Sydney, Australia

2 School of Medical Sciences (Anatomy & Histology) and Bosch Institute, University of Sydney, Australia

3 Brain and Mind Research Institute, Faculty of Health Sciences, University of Sydney and Life Sciences, Australian Nuclear Science and Technology Organization, Sydney, Australia

4 Australian Foundation for Diabetes Research & Diabetes Transplant Unit, Sydney, Australia

5 School of the Environment, University of Technology Sydney, Sydney, Australia

6 Australian Foundation for Diabetes Research & Diabetes Transplant Unit, Prince of Wales Hospital, and CSIRO, Division of Materials Science and Engineering, Sydney, Australia

References

[1] Eisenbarth, G. S. (1986). Type I diabetes mellitus: a chronic autoimmune disease. *N Engl J Med*, 4-1360.

[2] Simpson, A. M., Tuch, B. E., Swan, Tu. J., & Marshall, G. M. (1995). Functional expression of the human insulin gene in a human hepatoma cell line (HEP G2). *Gene Therapy*, 2-231.

[3] Simpson, A. M., Marshall, G. M., Tuch, B. E., Maxwell, L., Swan, MA, Tu, J., Beynon, S., Szymanska, B., & Camacho, M. (1997). Gene therapy of diabetes: glucose-stimulated insulin secretion in a human hepatoma cell line. *Gene Therapy*, 4-1202.

[4] Ber, I., Shternhall, K., Perl, S., Ohanuna, Z., Goldberg, I., Barshack, I., Benvenisti-Zarum, L., Meivar-Levy, I., & Ferber, S. (2003). Functional, persistent, and extended liver to pancreas transdifferentiation. *J Biol Chem*, 278-31950.

[5] Ferber, S., Halkin, A., Cohen, H., Ber, I., Einav, Y., Goldberg, I., Barshack, I., Seijffers, R., Kopolovic, J., Kaiser, N., & Karasik, A. (2000). Pancreatic and duodenal homeobox gene 1 induces expression of insulin genes in liver and ameliorates streptozotocin-induced hyperglycaemia. *Nature Med*, 6-568.

[6] Kojima, H., Fujimiya, M., Matsumara, K., Yunan, P., Imaeda, H., Maeda, M., & Chan, L. (2003). NeuroD-betacellulin gene therapy induces islet neogenesis in the liver and reverses diabetes in mice. *Nature Med*, 9-596.

[7] Tuch, B. E., Szymanska, B., Yao, M., Tabiin, M., Gross, D., Holman, S., Swan, MA, Humphrey, R., Marshall, G. M., & Simpson, A. M. (2003). Function of a genetically modified human liver cell line that stores, processes and secretes insulin. *Gene Therapy*, 10-490.

[8]   Ren, B. H., O'Brien, B. A., Swan, M. A., Kiona, M. E., Nassif, N., Wei, M. Q., & Simpson, A. M. (2007). Long-term correction of diabetes in rats following lentiviral hepatic insulin gene therapy. *Diabetologia*, 50, 1910-1920.

[9]   Simpson, A. M., Tao, C., Swan, M. A., Ren, B., & O'Brien, B. A. (2008). Glucose regulated production of human insulin in H4IIE rat liver cells. *Diabetes*, 56(1), A120.

[10] Tabiin, M. T., Tuch, B. E., Bai, L., Han-G, X., & Simpson, A. M. (2001). Susceptibility of insulin-secreting hepatocytes to the toxicity of pro-inflammatory cytokines. *J Autoimmunity*, 17-229.

[11] Permutt, MA, Koranyi, L., Keller, K., Lacy, P. E., & Scharp, D. W. (1989). Cloning and functional expression of a human pancreatic islet glucose-transporter cDNA. *Proc Natl Acad Sci USA*, 86(22), 8688-8692.

[12] Weinhouse, S. (1976). *In: Current topics in Cellular regulation. BL Horecker & ER Stadtman., editors. Academic Press.*

[13] Aguilar-Bryan, L., Nichols, C. G., Wechsler, S. W., Clement, J. P., Boyd, A. E., González, G., Herrera-Sosa, H., Nguy, K., Bryan, J., & Nelson, D. A. (1995). Cloning of the beta cell high-affinity sulfonylurea receptor: a regulator of insulin secretion. *Science*, 268-423.

[14] Inagaki, N., Gonoi, T., Clement, J. P., Namba, N., Inazawa, J., Gonzalez, G., Aguilar-Bryan, L., Seino, S., & Bryan, J. (1995). Reconstitution of IK_{ATP}: an inward rectifier subunit plus the sulfonylurea receptor. *Science*, 270-1166.

[15] Inagaki, N., Gonoi, T., & Seino, S. (1997). Subunit stoichiometry of the pancreatic beta-cell ATP-sensitive K^+ channel. *FEBS Lett*, 409, 232-236.

[16] Clement, J. P., Kunjilwar, K., Gonzalez, G., Schwanstecher, M., Panten, U., Aguilar-Bryan, L., & Bryan, J. (1997). Association and stoichiometry of K_{ATP} channel subunits. *Neuron*, 18, 827-838.

[17] Shyng, S., & Nichols, C. G. (1997). Octameric stoichiometry of the K_{ATP} channel complex. *J Gen Physiol*, 110, 655-664.

[18] Aguilar-Bryan, L., Clement, J. P., Gonzalez, G., Kunjilwar, K., Babenko, A., & Bryan, J. (1998). Toward understanding the assembly and structure of K_{ATP} channels. *Physiol Rev*, 78-227.

[19] Ashcroft, F. M., & Rorsman, P. (1989). Electrophysiology of the pancreatic beta-cell. *Prog Biophys Mol Biol*, 54-87.

[20] Lang, J. (1999). Molecular mechanisms and regulation of insulin exocytosis as a paradigm of endocrine secretion. *Eur J Biochem*, 259-3.

[21] Macfarlane, W. M., O'Brien, R. E., Barnes, P. D., Shepherd, R. M., Cosgrove, K. E., Lindley, K. J., Aynsley-Green, A., James, R. F., Docherty, K., & Dunne, MJ. (2000). Sulfonylurea receptor 1 and Kir6.2 expression in the novel human insulin-secreting cell line NES2Y. *Diabetes*, 49-953.

[22] Braun, M., Ramracheya, R., Zhang, Q., Karanauskaite, J., Partridge, C., Johnson, P. R., & Rorsman, P. (2008). Voltage-gated ion channels in human pancreatic β-cells: Electrophysiological characterization and role in insulin secretion. *Diabetes*, 57-1618.

[23] Wollheim, C. B., & Sharp, G. W. (1981). Regulation of insulin release by calcium. *Physiol Rev*, 61-914.

[24] Gilon, P., & Henquin, J. C. (2001). Mechanisms and physiological significance of the cholinergic control of pancreatic beta-cell function. *Endocr Rev*, 22-565.

[25] Bereton, H. M., Harland, M. L., Froscio, M., Petronijevic, T., & Barrit, G. J. (1997). Novel variants of voltage-operated calcium channel alpha 1-subunit transcripts in a rat liver-derived cell line: deletion in the IVS4 voltage sensing region. *Cell Calcium*, 22, 39-52.

[26] Snutch, T. P., Tomlinson, W. J., Leonard, J. P., & Gilbert, M. M. (1991). Distinct calcium channels are generated by alternative splicing and are differentially expressed in the mammalian CNS. *Neuron*, 7, 45-57.

[27] Liu, G. J., Simpson, A. M., Swan, Tao. C., Tuch, B. E., Crawford, R. M., Jovanovic, A., & Martin, D. K. (2003). ATP-sensitive potassium channels induced in liver cells after transfection with insulin cDNA and the GLUT 2 transporter regulate glucose-stimulated insulin secretion. *FASEB J*, 17-1682.

[28] Malhi, H., Irani, A. N., Rajvanshi, P., Suadicani, S. O., Spray, D. C., Mc Donald, T. V., & Gupta, S. (2000). K_{ATP} channels regulate mitogenically induced proliferation in primary rat hepatocytes and human liver cell lines. *J Biol Chem*, 275-26050.

[29] Lutherborrow, M. A., Appavoo, M., Simpson, A. M., & Tuch, B. E. (2009). Gene expression profiling of Huh7ins lack of a granulogenic function for chromagranin A. *Islets*, 1, 60-70.

[30] Miyazaki-I, J., Araki, K., Yamato, E., Ikegami, H., Asano, T., Shibasaki, Y., Oka, Y., & Yamamura, K. (1990). Establishment of a pancreatic beta cell line that retains glucose-inducible insulin secretion: Special reference to expression of glucose transporter. *Endocrinology*, 127-126.

[31] Sapir, T., Shternhall, K., Meivar-Levy, I., Blumenfeld, I., Cohen, H., Skutelsky, E., Eventov-Friedman, S., Barshack, I., Goldberg, I., Pri-Chen, S., Ben-Dor, L., Polak-Charcon, S., Karasik, A., Shimon, I., Mor, E., & Ferber, S. (2005). Cell-replacement therapy for diabetes: generating functional insulin-producing tissue from adult human liver cells. *Proc Natl Acad Sci USA*, 102-7964.

[32] Fodor, A., Harel, C., Fodor, L., Armoni, M., Salmon, P., Trono, D., & Karnielli, E. (2007). Adult rat liver cells transdifferentiated with lentiviral IPF1 vectors reverse diabetes in mice: an ex vivo gene therapy approach. *Diabetologia*, 50-121.

[33] Vollenweider, F., Irminger, J. C., Gross, D. J., Villa-Komaroff, L., & Halban, P. A. (1992). Processing of proinsulin by transfected hepatoma (FAO) cells. *J Biol Chem*, 267-14629.

[34] Yang, L., Li, S., Hatch, H., Ahrens, K., Cornelius, J. G., Petersen, B. E., & Peck, A. B. (2002). In vitro trans-differentiation of adult hepatic stem cells into pancreatic endocrine hormone-producing cells. *Proc Natl Acad Sci USA*, 99-8078.

[35] Nguyen, T., Chin, W. C., & Verdugo, P. (1998). Role of Ca^{2+}/K^+ ion exchange in intracellular storage and release of Ca^{2+}. *Nature*, 395-908.

[36] Quesada, I., Chin, W. C., Steed, J., Campos-Bedolla, P., & Verdugo, P. (2001). Mouse mast cell secretory granules can function as intracellular ionic oscillators. *Biophys J*, 80, 2133-2139.

[37] National Institutes of Health. (2008). NIH Image. http://rsb.info.hih.gov/nih-image/ Accessed 1 July,).

[38] Arvan, P., & Halban, P. A. (2004). Sorting ourselves out: seeking consensus on trafficking in the beta-cell. *Traffic* , 5, 53-61.

[39] National Institutes of Health. (2009). Image J. http://rsb.info.nih.gov/ij/Accessed 20 September).

[40] Yoon, N., Nataliya, S., Jeong-J, M., Lee, T., Lee-S, M., Kim-L, H., Chin, H., Suh-G, P., Kim, S., & Shin-S, H. (2003). Requirement for the L-type Ca^{2+} channel α_{1D} subunit in postnatal pancreatic β-cell generation. *J Clin Inves*, 108, 1015-1022.

[41] Catterall, W. A., & Striessnig, J. (1992). Receptor sites for Ca^{2+} channel antagonists. Trends Pharm Sci; , 13-256.

[42] Henquin, J. C. (2000). Triggering and amplifying pathways of regulation of insulin secretion by glucose. *Diabetes*, 49, 1751-1760.

[43] Ammälä, C., Moorhouse, A., & Ashcroft, F. M. (1996). The sulphonylurea receptor confers diazoxide sensitivity on the inwardly rectifying K^+ channel Kir6.1 expressed in human embryonic kidney cells. *J Physiol*, 494, 709-714.

[44] Larsson-Nyren, G., & Sehlin, J. (1996). Comparison of the effects of perchlorate and Bay K 8644 on the dynamics of cytoplasmic Ca^{2+} concentration and insulin secretion in mouse β-cells. *Biochem J*, 314-167.

[45] Malaisse-Lagae, F., Matthias, P. C. F., & Malaisse, W. J. (1984). Gating and blocking of calcium channels by dihydropyridines in the pancreatic β-cell. *Biochem Biophys Res Comm*, 123-1062.

[46] Lytton, J., Westlin, M., & Hanley, M. R. (1991). Thapsigargin inhibits the sarcoplasmic or endoplasmic reticulum Ca-ATPase family of calcium pumps. *J Biol Chem*, 266-17067.

[47] Kirby, M. S., Sagara, Y., Gaa, S., Inesi, G., Lederer, W. J., & Rogers, T. B. (1992). Thapsigargin inhibits contraction and Ca2+ transient in cardiac cells by specific inhibition of the sarcoplasmic reticulum Ca2+ pump. *J Biol Chem*, 267, 12545-12551.

[48] Gericke, M., Droogmans, G., & Nilius, B. (1993). Thapsigargin discharges intracellular calcium stores and induces transmembrane currents in human endothelial cells. *Pflügers Arch*, 422-552.

[49] Parekh, A. B., Terlau, H., & Stühmer, W. (1993). Depletion of InsP$_3$ stores activates a Ca^{2+} and K$^+$ current by means of a phosphatase and a diffusible messenger. *Nature*, 364-814.

[50] Randriamampita, C., & Tsien, R. Y. (1993). Emptying of intracellular Ca^{2+} stores releases a novel small messenger that stimulates Ca^{2+} influx. *Nature*, 364-809.

[51] Roe, M. W., Mertz, R. J., Lancaster, M. E., Worley, J. F. 3rd, & Dukes, I. D. (1994). Thapsigargin inhibits the glucose-induced decrease of intracellular Ca2+ in mouse islets of Langerhans. *Am J Physiol*, 266, E 852-862.

[52] Miura, Y., Henquin, J. C., & Gilon, P. (1997). Emptying of intracellular Ca^{2+} stores stimulates Ca^{2+} entry in mouse pancreatic beta-cells by both direct and indirect mechanisms. *J Physiol*, 503-387.

[53] Worley, J. F., Mc Intyre, M. S., Spencer, B., & Dukes, I. D. (1994a). Depletion of intracellular Ca2+ stores activates a maitotoxin-sensitive nonselective cationic current in beta-cells. *J Biol Chem*, 269, 32055-32058.

[54] Worley, J. F., Mc Intyre, M. S., Spencer, B., Mertz, R. J., Roe, M. W., & Dukes, I. D. (1994b). Endoplasmic reticulum calcium store regulates membrane potential in mouse islet beta-cells. *J Biol Chem*, 269, 14359-14362.

[55] Meissner, G. (1986). Ryanodine activation of the Ca^{2+} release channel of sarcoplasmic reticulum. *J Biol Chem*, 261-6300.

[56] Nevins, A. K., & Thurmond, D. C. (2003). Glucose regulates the cortical actin network through modulation of Cdc42 cycling to stimulate insulin secretion. *Am J Physiol Cell Physiol*, 285, C698-710.

[57] Meda, P., Bosco, D., Chanson, M., Giordano, E., Vallar, L., Wollheim, C., & Orci, L. (1990). Rapid and reversible secretion changes during uncoupling of rat insulin-producing cells. *J Clin Invest*, 86-759.

Chapter 11

Clinical and Translational Challenges in Gene Therapy of Cardiovascular Diseases

Divya Pankajakshan and Devendra K. Agrawal

Additional information is available at the end of the chapter

1. Introduction

Cardiovascular (CV) disease is the most prevalent life-threatening clinical problem and is a major cause of disability and economic burden worldwide [1]. Despite extensive pharmacotherapies, there remain many vascular conditions for which pharmacological interventions are either non-existent or largely ineffective. CV gene therapy offers the benefit of sustained and/or controlled expression of desired proteins in cell types, which makes it more beneficial in providing durable clinical benefits [2]. The therapeutic gene works by either over-expressing therapeutically beneficial proteins, replacing a deficient gene or its expression proteins, or silencing a particular gene whose expression is not beneficial in the clinical scenario [3]. In addition, success of gene therapy also depends on the choice of the vector and the delivery approach. Blood vessels are among the most feasible targets for gene therapy because of ease of access using a catheter or by systemic delivery. The new genetic material should enter the cells in the vasculature overcoming the anatomical, cellular and physiological barriers and induce the expression of the transfected gene in the target tissue. The target cells in the arteries are endothelial cells (EC), smooth muscle cells (SMC) and fibroblasts, which constitute the intimal, medial and adventitial layers, respectively [4]. In the case of atherosclerotic lesions, macrophages also become a target cell. For the treatment of cardiovascular diseases, gene therapy strategies have been designed to enhance re-endothelialization and EC function to reduce thrombosis, inhibit SMC proliferation and migration to prevent neointimal hyperplasia, and to improve therapeutic neo-vascularization to counteract ischemia.

Viral and non-viral vector systems have been evaluated for gene transfer to the vasculature. Lipoplexes, polyplexes and lipopolyplexes as well as naked DNA have been used as non-viral vectors for gene delivery to vascular tissues. Retroviruses, lentiviruses, adenoviruses and adeno-associated viruses have been tested as viral vectors. Both systems have their own advantages and disadvantages that determine its use for a particular subset of CV diseases. Another challenge is the development of delivery approaches that are clinically viable and are capable of achieving consistent therapy for diseased arterial tissues. The efficiency of localization, restriction of systemic distribution and adequacy of permeation into the target tissue are required for the optimal delivery of the vector. It is also dependent on the requirements of a given patho-physiological situation. Systemic, intravascular and perivascular approaches are used for gene delivery to the vasculature.

In this chapter, our goal is to summarize the current understanding of gene therapy strategies used to treat CV diseases, specifically the therapies targeting thrombosis, atherogenesis, SMC proliferation and migration, modification of extracellular matrix (ECM) and regeneration of the endothelial cell layer. We will discuss various vectors and delivery approaches used in the CV gene therapy and describe, in detail, the challenges associated with each approach.

2. Vectors in vascular gene therapy

The ideal vector for clinical application would target the specific cell, offer the capacity to transfer large DNA sequences, result in therapeutic levels of transgene expression that are not attenuated by the host immune response, express transgene for a duration required to alleviate the clinical problem, pose no risk of toxicity either acutely (as a result of immunogenicity or unregulated transgene expression) or in the long-term (such as oncogenesis), and be cost-effective and easy to produce in therapeutically applicable quantity [5]. Currently, no available vector fulfils all these criteria; therefore, a perfect vector for vascular gene therapy does not exist. Nonetheless, viral and non-viral vector systems have been evaluated for gene transfer to the vasculature.

2.1. Viral vectors

Retroviruses, adenoviruses (Ad) and adeno-associated viruses (AAV) are used as viral vectors in vascular gene transfer. Recombinant retroviruses are RNA viruses that are capable of integrating transgene into the target genome. Disadvantages of this vector include instability, the requirement of cell division for gene transfer and the inability to attain high titers. Since the majority of vascular cells are not undergoing mitosis at the time of exposure to the viral vector, the efficiency of gene delivery to vascular cells by such vectors may be as low as 1% to 2% [6]. Attempts have been made to increase the transduction efficiency in endothelial cell using multiple viral exposures [7] or increasing viral titers by ultracentrifugation [8]. Murine leukemia retroviral vectors (MuLV) pseudotyped with the vesicular stomatitis virus G glycoprotein (VSV-G) have the capacity to transfect human ECs and SMCs *in vitro* with significant improvement in stability and transduction efficiency [9]. Unlike other retroviruses, lentiviruses are able to transduce non-dividing cells, which is an attractive characteristic for CV gene therapy. These vectors demonstrate significantly broadened tropism and high stability and have been used to demonstrate efficient transgene delivery *in vitro* into SMCs and ECs from human saphenous vein [10], human coronary artery SMCs and ECs [11], and cardiomyocytes [12].

Ad vectors are the most commonly used viral vectors in the CV system. They transfect non-dividing cells efficiently [Figure 1], but sustained gene expression is limited to approximately 2 weeks because the gene is kept episomal [2]. The administration of the Ad vectors is almost invariably associated with the development of systemic neutralizing antibodies directed against the vector [13]. Therefore, lowering the immunogenicity of the Ad virus is desirable and can be achieved by deleting genes that encode viral proteins [14]. Another method of reducing the inflammatory reaction to gene transfer by Ad vectors is to preserve the E3 region, which is supposed to modulate the host immune response *in vivo* [15]. When systemically administered, Ad5 poorly transduced ECs but could effectively transduce medial SMCs during endothelial denudation [5]. Efficient myocardial transduction was observed following local delivery of Ad5 vectors in porcine heart, where almost 80% of cardiomyocytes were transduced [16].

AAV vectors have emerged as versatile vehicles for gene delivery due to their efficient infection of dividing and non-dividing cells in the presence of helper virus, sustained maintenance of viral genome leading to long-term expression of the transgene, and a strong clinical safety profile [17]. AAV is non-pathogenic since it cannot replicate without the assistance of a helper virus. Recombinant AAV (rAAV) vectors have almost the entire viral genome removed, thereby yielding a delivery vehicle with enhanced safety and reduced immunogenicity [18]. The AAV *Rep* and *Cap* genes, which are required for viral replication and packaging, are supplied by a helper plasmid during the production process. Wild type AAV preferentially integrates to a specific locus of human chromosome 19. The rAAV has mechanisms for sustained episomal maintenance or semi-randomly integrates at a low rate [19]. Problems with AAV vectors include limited tissue tropism for serotypes that bind heparan sulphate, challenges with preexisting immunity due to prior exposure, and also substantially delayed onset of transgene expression compared to other vectors.

2.2. Non-viral vectors

Even though the transfection efficiency of non-viral vectors are lower than that of their viral counterparts, they are associated with many advantages such as low immunogenic response, the capacity to carry large inserts of DNA (52Kb), the possibility of selective modification using ligand and large scale manufacture [20]. Ideal non-viral vectors should be degradable into low molecular weight components in response to biological stimuli for lower toxicity and effective systemic clearance. They should also be efficient in overcoming extracellular and intracellular barriers and tissue/cell-targeted for specific accumulations [21]. In this group of vectors, naked DNA, cationic liposomes and cationic polymers have been used for vascular gene transfer.

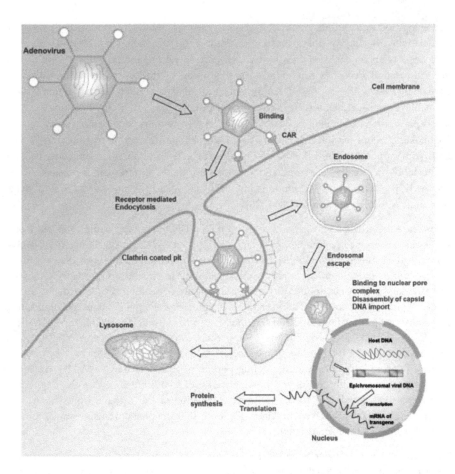

Figure 1. Transduction using adenoviral vectors. Recombinant adenovirus enters cells via CAR-mediated binding allowing internalization via receptor-mediated endocytosis through clathrin-coated vesicles. Inside the cytoplasm, the endocytosed adenoviral vector escapes from the endosomes, disassembles the capsid and the viral DNA enter into the nucleus through the nuclear envelope pore complex. The viral DNA is not incorporated into the host cell genome, but rather assumes an epichromosomal location, where it can still use the transcriptional and translational machinery of the host cell to synthesize recombinant protein. [CAR; Coxsackievirus and adenovirus receptor]

Gene transfer with naked DNA is attractive because of its simplicity and lack of toxicity [22]. However, the efficiency of gene transfer with naked DNA is low due to its negative charge conferred by the phosphate groups, making cellular uptake difficult by the negatively charged cell surface, rapid degradation by nucleases in the serum and clearance by the mononuclear phagocyte system in the systemic circulation. However, site-specific arterial gene transfer of vascular endothelial growth factor (VEGF)-165 could yield efficient gene transfection resulting in accelerated re-endothelialization, inhibition of neointimal thickening, reduced thrombogenicity, and restoration of endothelium-dependent vasomotor reactivity after injury due to balloon angioplasty in a rabbit model [23]. Physical approaches have been explored for plasmid gene transfer into vascular cells *in vitro* and *in vivo*. Ultrasound exposure can induce transient pore formation in the cell membrane, thereby increasing the plasmid DNA uptake. Indeed, microbubble-enhanced ultrasound can achieve transgene expression levels *in vitro* at approximately 300-fold than that of naked plasmid DNA alone in porcine VSMCs [24]. The non-invasive nature of this technique makes it more feasible for clinical use. Local administration of plasmid DNA, coupled with application of brief electric pulses to cells or tissues to increase cellular permeability-- also called electroporation--yields high levels of transgene expression in the arteries [25]. However this technique is limited by its invasive nature and tissue damage associated with high voltages applied [26].

To increase the efficiency of gene transfer by naked DNA, they are complexed with cationic lipids (liposomes or lipoplexes) or polymers (polyplexes). The resulting net positive charge of the cationic lipid/polymer DNA complexes facilitates fusion with the negatively charged cell membrane and also reduces susceptibility to circulating nucleases. Transfection efficiency of cationic lipoplexes varies dramatically depending on the structure of the cationic lipids (the overall geometric shape, the number of charged groups per molecules, the nature of lipid anchors, and linker bonds), the charge ratio used to form DNA–lipid complexes, and the properties of the co-lipid [22]. Although transfection efficiencies of liposomes are generally seen lower in vascular cells [22], the LID vector system, consisting of a liposome (L), an integrin targeting peptide (I), and plasmid DNA (D), transfects primary porcine vascular SMCs and porcine aortic ECs with efficiency levels of 40% and 35%, respectively, under *in vitro* conditions [27]. Some of the cationic lipids have been found to negatively affect cell function. Cationic lipid-mediated transfection of bovine aortic ECs inhibits their attachment [28].

The DNA packaging efficiency and *in vivo* stability are higher for cationic polymers compared to cationic lipids. Furthermore, these complexes can be surface-modified with antibodies or other targeting ligands to deliver nucleic acids to specific cells [29]. Several cationic polymers have been evaluated for their ability to form complexes with DNA, the most significant being poly-lysine (PLL) and polyethylene-imine (PEI) [30]. PEI affects EC function [31]; however, when conjugated with fractured polyamidoamine (PAMAM) dendrimers, less toxic effects were observed on vascular cells in addition to the enhanced transfection efficiencies [32]. Brito *et al.* [33] developed lipo-polyplex nanovector systems that can transfect EC and SMCs with reasonably high efficiency. They used a combination of a cationic biodegradable polymer, poly(beta-amino ester) (PBAE), and a cationic phospholipid, 1,2-dioleoyl-3-trimethylammonium propane (DOTAP) and obtained 20% and 33% transfection efficiencies *in vitro* in SMC and ECs, respectively. Molecular tuning of non-viral vectors via stimuli responsive degradation is another novel approach that can be adopted in vascular gene transfer [21]. Schematic representation of non-viral gene delivery is given in Figure 2.

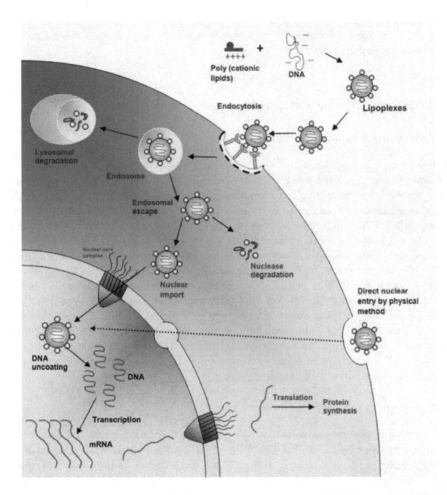

Figure 2. Non-viral gene delivery using lipoplexes: DNA is complexed with cationic liposomes and is internalized through receptor mediated endocytosis. After their internalization large amounts of complexes are degraded in the endolysosomal compartments. Only a small fraction enters into the nucleus and elicits desired gene expression.

2.3. Stem cells

One of the recent approaches is to use stem cells as gene delivery vehicles. Stem cell-based gene therapy approaches are currently being employed in recent studies as an alternative strategy to promote myocardial angiogenesis and regeneration. Indeed, the injection of genetically modified bone marrow-derived mesenchymal stem cells to express angiopoietin-1 improved arteriogenesis and increased collateral blood flow in porcine model of chronic myocardial ischemia [34]. Nanofiber-expanded hematopoietic stem cells over-expressing

VEGF and platelet-derived growth factor (PDGF) had a favorable impact on the improvement of rat myocardial function accompanied by upregulation of tissue connexin 43 and pro-angiogenic molecules after infarction [35].

3. Major targets in vascular gene therapy

3.1. Promotion of re-endothelialization

EC loss because of vascular injury is a major contributing factor to the local activation of patho-physiological events leading to the development of neo-intimal hyperplasia [36]. Previous reports have shown that transplantation of autologous endothelial progenitor cells (EPCs) onto balloon-injured carotid artery leads to rapid re-endothelialization of the denuded vessels [37]. EPCs can be genetically manipulated *ex vivo*, expanded, and reintroduced *in vivo*, where at least a proportion will contribute to a long-lasting pool that can provide therapeutically relevant levels of transgene expression. Chemokine receptor, CXCR4, is a key molecule in regulating EPC homing [38]. Chen *et al.* [38] reported that CXCR4 gene transfer to EPCs contributes to their enhanced *in vivo* re-endothelialization capacity. In another study, Ohno and colleagues over-expressed C-type natriuretic peptide by gene transfer in rabbit jugular vein grafts and observed accelerated re-endothelialization [39]. EPCs over-expressing endothelial nitric oxide synthase (eNOS) further enhance the vasculo-protective properties of these cells [40]. Local intravascular and extra-vascular expression of VEGF, using plasmid DNA, accelerated re-endothelialization and decreased intimal thickening after arterial injury in rabbit models [23, 41].

3.2. Promotion of endothelial cell function

Antithrombotic and anticoagulation therapy generally involves the systemic administration of agents that target a small region of the vasculature. Localized and controlled delivery of specific genes could allow sustained antithrombotic or anticoagulant treatment when prolonged systemic administration is undesirable. Antithrombotic gene therapy strategies could include inhibition of coagulation factors, over-expression of anticoagulant factors, or modulation of EC biology to make thrombus formation or propagation unfavorable [42]. Ad gene transfer of thrombomodulin decreased arterial thrombosis to 28% compared to 86% in control rabbit model [43]. Hemagglutinating virus of Japan (HVJ)-liposome-mediated gene transfer of tissue factor pathway inhibitor (TFPI), a primary inhibitor of TF-induced coagulation, significantly reduced/inhibited thrombosis after angioplasty in atherosclerotic arteries without any significant adverse effects [44]. Ad gene transfer of many mediators, including hirudin to inhibit thrombin [45], tissue plasminogen activator (tPA) to enhance fibrinolysis [43], cyclo-oxygenase to augment prostacyclin synthesis [46], prevents arterial thrombosis and promotes local thromboresistance. Vascular gene delivery of anticoagulants by local infusion of retrovirally-transduced EPCs with tPA and hirudin genes has also been attempted [37].

3.3. Inhibition of atherogenesis

The extensive cross-talk between the immune system and vasculature leading to the infiltration of immune cells into the vascular wall is a major step in atherogenesis. In this process, reactive oxygen species play a crucial role, by inducing the oxidation of low-density lipoprotein (LDL) and the formation of foam cells, and by activating a number of redox-sensitive transcriptional factors, such as nuclear factor kappa B (NFκB), Nuclear factor E2-related factor-2 (Nrf2) [47], or activating protein 1 (AP1) that regulate the expression of multiple pro-and anti-inflammatory genes involved in atherogenesis [48]. Delivery of genes encoding antioxidant defense enzymes, like extracellular superoxide dismutase [49, 50], catalase [51], glutathione peroxidase [51] or heme oxygenase-1 [52], suppresses atherogenesis in animal models.

Apolipoprotein E (ApoE), a blood circulating protein with pleiotropic atheroprotective properties, has emerged as a strong candidate for treating hypercholesterolemia and CV disease. The gene transfer of ApoE Ad vectors produced substantial amounts of plasma ApoE following intravenous injection into ApoE-/- mice, which lowered plasma cholesterol, and after 1 month, slowed aortic atherogenesis [53]. Hepatic expression of human ApoE3 using a second-generation recombinant Ad vector directly induced regression of pre-existing atherosclerotic lesions without reducing plasma cholesterol or altering lipoprotein distribution [54]. High concentrations of atherogenic apolipoprotein (apo) B100 could also be lowered by hepatic gene transfer with the catalytic subunit of apoB mRNA editing enzyme [55].

3.4. Inhibition of SMC proliferation and migration

SMC migration and proliferation as well as deposition and turnover of ECM proteins contribute to the process of Intimal hyperplasia. Several different approaches were introduced to inhibit SMC proliferation during restenosis. Most of the approaches targeted inhibition of cell cycle, where cell cycle inhibitor genes are over-expressed. Non-phosphorylated retinoblastoma gene (Rb) [56]; p21 [57, 58]; p27-p16 fusion gene [59, 60] ; cyclin-dependent kinase inhibitor p57Kip2 [61]; and the growth-arrest homeobox gene gax [62] are few of the genes over-expressed to inhibit cell proliferation and neo-intimal formation. Genes that have a beneficial influence on various aspects of vessel wall physiology also inhibit SMC proliferation. Nitric oxide generation by endothelial nitric oxide synthase inhibits SMC proliferation *in vitro* and modulates vascular tone locally *in vivo* [63].

Another approach was to inhibit growth factor signaling by the introduction of nucleic acid constructs that interfere with mRNA stability, such as antisense oligonucleotides, hammer head ribozymes and siRNA [64]. Gene transfer of a truncated form of fibroblast growth factor (FGF) receptor using Ad vector suppressed SMC proliferation *in vitro* [65]. Hammerhead ribozymes directed against PDGF-A chain [66] and transforming growth factor-β [67] inhibited SMC proliferation and neointima formation in rat carotid artery after balloon injury.

The regulation of a target gene can influence the level of transcription, either by decoy oligonucleotides, which are either short double-stranded oligonucleotides or dumb-bell shaped circular oligonucleotides that represent transcription factor binding sites, and thus compete for binding of a specific transcription factor that is relevant for the respective gene [64]. Administration of AP-1 decoy ODNs *in vivo* using HVJ-liposome method virtually abolished neointimal formation after balloon injury to the rat carotid artery [68]. Transfection of vein grafts with a decoy antisense oligonucleotide to block transcription factor E2F imparted long-term resistance to neointimal hyperplasia and atherosclerosis in rabbits on a cholesterol diet [69]. Another approach was to drive SMC into apoptosis during the process of proliferation and migration. Transduction of rabbit iliac arteries with recombinant Ad vectors for Fas ligand (L) reduced neointima formation, which occurred through the killing of Fas expressing neighboring SMC by FasL-transduced cells [70].

The regulation of SMC migration is mediated partly through the action of matrix metalloproteinases (MMPs) and their endogenous inhibitors, tissue inhibitors of matrix metalloproteinases (TIMPs) [71]. AAV-mediated TIMP1 transduction in SMCs of injured rat carotid arteries significantly reduced the ratio of intima to media (52.4%) after two months of treatment [72]. Overexpression of TIMP-2 [73], TIMP-3 [74] and TIMP-4 [75] has also been demonstrated to inhibit SMC migration and neo-intimal proliferation in human vein grafts and porcine vascular injury models. Gurjar *et al.* [76] demonstrated that eNOS gene transfer inhibits SMC migration and MMP-2 and MMP-9 activities in SMCs *in vitro*. A combination approach of TIMP-1 and plasminogen activator system inhibited vein graft thickening in hypercholesterolemic mice, when plasmids encoding TIMP-1-ATF (amino terminal fragment of urokinase) were incorporated to the vein graft by intravascular electroporation [77].

3.5. Enhancement of therapeutic angiogenesis

Ischemic diseases, including acute myocardial infarction and chronic cardiac ischemia, are characterized by an impaired supply of blood resulting from narrowed or blocked arteries that starve tissues of needed nutrients and oxygen [78]. Delivery of genes encoding angiogenic factors or the whole protein has been shown to induce angiogenesis in numerous animal models with the expression of a functioning product [79]. The successful application of recombinant protein and gene transfer for the treatment of myocardial ischemia was reported by Losordo and colleagues [80] by direct intra-myocardial gene transfer of naked plasmid DNA encoding VEGF-165 in porcine model. These results were confirmed in phase 1 assessment of direct intra-myocardial administration of Ad vector expressing VEGF-121 cDNA in patients with severe coronary artery disease [81]. Ad-mediated FGF-4 gene transfer improved cardiac contractile function and regional blood flow in the ischemic region during stress in pig model [82]. Placebo-controlled trials in humans with chronic stable angina indicate that Ad5FGF-4 increased treadmill exercise duration and improved stress-related ischemia [82]. In another study, following coronary artery occlusion, rabbits treated with Ad vector containing acidic FGF showed a 50% reduction in the risk region for myocardial infarction [83].

4. Challenges in gene therapy

4.1. Cellular and extracellular barriers in gene delivery

Viruses have highly evolved mechanisms for obtaining optimized receptor-mediated internalization, efficient cytosolic release, directed and fast intracellular transport towards compartments and readily disassemble. In contrast, non-viral vectors must overcome multiple extracellular and intracellular barriers [21]. These barriers include binding to the cell surface, traversing the plasma membrane, escaping lysosomal degradation, and overcoming the nuclear envelope. To overcome the delivery barriers in non-viral gene transfer, various strategies have been employed to enhance the circulation time, improve intracellular delivery, and enhance endosomal escape and nuclear import. Lipoplexes have shown rapid hepatic clearance during systemic administration. Modification of lipoplexes with hydrophilic molecules like polyethylene glycol (PEG) and polyethyleneimine (PEI) causes steric hinderance between opsonins and the delivery vectors, increasing their circulation time in the blood. PEGylation of PLL decreases interparticle aggregation, resulting in high transfection efficiency in the presence of serum [29]. One study has demonstrated that when artery wall binding peptide (AWBP), a core peptide of apo B100 -- a major protein component of LDL -- was conjugated to PLL with PEG as the linker, the PLL-PEG-AWBP protected the plasmid DNA from nucleases for more than 120 min in circulation and also showed 100 times higher transfection efficiency when compared to PLL and PLL-g-PEG in bovine aortic ECs and SMCs [84]. In an innovative approach, micellar nanovectors made of PEG-block-polycation, carrying ethylenediamine units in the side chain [PEG-PAsp(DET)], complexed with plasmid DNA to form polyplex micelle effectively transfected vascular smooth muscle cells in vascular lesions without any vessel occlusion by thrombus [85] in rabbit carotid arteries. However, PEI-mediated gene delivery can affect EC function and viability [31].

The size and charge of the lipoplex/polyplex play an important role in their intracellular delivery. Lipoplexes and polyplexes are generally formulated into particles with net positive charges to trigger endocytosis by non-specific electrostatic interaction between the positively charged complexes and negatively charged cell surface [29]. Since drug carriers with a smaller particle size have resulted in higher arterial uptake compared to carriers with larger size, the size of the complexes was expected to be a dominating factor in the arterial wall lesions because of the rapid blood flow which could wash out most of the drugs or therapeutic chemical agents from the arterial wall lesions within 20–30 min. Song *et al.* [86] reported a potentially useful particle size of 70~160 nm for local intraluminal therapy of restenosis.

By taking advantage of high expression levels of receptors or antigens in diseased conditions, gene complexes can be targeted using specific ligands, such as antibodies, peptides and proteins. Cyclic RGD (cRGD) peptide recognizes $\alpha(v)\beta(3)$ and $\alpha(v)\beta(5)$ integrins, which are abundantly expressed in vascular lesions. When cRGD was conjugated to PEG-PAsp(DET) to form polyplex micelles through complexing with plasmid DNA, the micelles achieved significantly more efficient gene expression and cellular uptake as compared to PEG-PAsp(DET) micelles in ECs and SMCs [87]. PAMAM dendrimers with E/P-selectin antibody was used for gene targeting to activated vascular ECs [88]. The lectin-like oxidized LDL receptor (LOX-1) is expressed selectively at low levels on ECs but is strongly upregulated in dysfunctional ECs associated with hypertension and atherogenesis. White and colleagues [89] confirmed the selectivity to LOX-1 for peptides LSIPPKA, FQTPPQL, and LTPATAI, which could be potential targets to dysfunctional ECs expressing LOX-1 receptor. Another approach to increase intracellular delivery is to use cell penetrating peptides (CPPs). CPPs consist of short peptide sequences that are able to translocate large molecules into the cells and increase the transfection efficiency [90].

Following internalization of lipoplexes and polyplexes via endocytosis, endosomal entrapment and subsequent lysosomal degradation are the major hurdles that limit transfection efficiency [29]. Lipoplexes are modified with dioleoylphosphatidylethanolamine (DOPE) or other helper lipids due to its fusogenic functionality and its ability to destabilize endosomal membranes. Small PLLs with cationic lipid DOCSPER [1,3-dioleoyloxy-2-(N(5)-carbamoyl-spermine)-propane] enhanced gene transfer in primary porcine SMCs *in vitro* and *in vivo* in porcine femoral arteries [91]. Polyplexes, PEI and PAMAM are cationic polymers of high efficiency partly because of their ability to burst the endosomal membrane due to 'proton sponge effect'.

A promising new delivery strategy is to use synthetic peptide carriers containing a nuclear localization signal to facilitate nuclear uptake of plasmid DNA. Nuclear import of plasmid DNA is more challenging for transfecting non-dividing cells. Strategies to increase the nuclear import of genes involve tagging the nuclear localization sequence (NLS) with DNA vectors. NLS is a major player that shuttles protein-plasmid complexes through the nuclear pore by interaction with importins and transportin [92, 93]. Incorporation of DNA nuclear targeting sequence SV40 into expression plasmids results in 10-40 fold increases in vascular gene expression in rat mesenteric arteries [94], confirming the function of DNA nuclear targeting sequences *in vivo*.

4.2. Challenges associated with the vectors

4.2.1. Insertional mutagenesis

Insertional mutagenesis is a major concern in gene therapy involving viral vectors. These vectors integrate randomly or quasi-randomly into the host cell's genome, to stably transfect the target cell. The variable site and frequency of integration of the transgene can induce mutagenesis in the host genome, resulting in devastating consequences for the cell and for the organism. [95, 96]. Another disadvantage of the random integration of a transgene is the unpredictability of its stability and its expression. The genomic locus in which the vector integrates can have profound effects on the level of transgene expression, as it can completely silence the transgene, or it can increase or decrease its expression. These effects could not be avoided by sophisticated vector design or inclusion of the gene's own promoter and/or enhancer region in the transgenic vector construct, as the surrounding chromatin can override the activity of the original regulatory regions. Gene targeting by homologous recombination, however, lacks many of these shortcomings [96]. In this process, the transgene recombines with its natural locus in the host genome, thereby ensuring correct transcription. Also, after homologous recombination, the targeted modification of the chromosomal locus is stable, whereas randomly integrated sequences might be lost over time. In their seminal paper, Russel and Hirata [97] reported that DNA vectors based on the AAV could target homologous chromosomal DNA sequences and allow high-fidelity, non-mutagenic gene repair in a host cell. Although the laborious vector design and low transfection efficiencies of AAV vectors compared to the other viral vectors still remains a concern, statistical information neatly outlines the advantage of rAAV gene replacement system over standard viral vectors, which induce strong immune response.

4.2.2. Tissue-specific targeting

The promiscuous tropism of vectors resulting in high-level transgene expression in multiple tissues is another major challenge in vascular gene therapy. After systemic application, most viral vectors are trapped by the liver, hampering delivery to target CV tissues. Approaches to restrict gene delivery to desired cell types *in vivo* relied mostly on cell surface targeting or cell-specific promoters.

The *cis*-acting regulatory elements of the SM (smooth muscle)22α [98-100], telokin [101], smooth muscle myosin heavy chain [102], smooth muscle α- [100] and γ-actin [103], and desmin [104] genes have been shown to direct reporter gene expression to smooth muscle tissues in transgenic mice. In our studies, specific gene transfer to the SMC layer was achieved in swine coronary and peripheral arteries using SM22α promoter in AAV [17]. Although the efficiency of transduction was low when compared to a similar study using AAV vectors with cytomegalovirus (CMV) promoter [105], the use of SM22α promoter caused specific transduction of SMCs *in vivo*. An interesting approach to enhance the transduction efficiency of SM22α -containing plasmid was to incorporate chimeric transcriptional cassettes containing a SM-myosin heavy chain enhancer element combined with the SM22α promoter [106]. The transfection levels obtained using these chimeric constructs in Ad vector were similar to that with CMV promoter when tested in rat carotid arteries. Certain DNA nuclear targeting sequences can be used to restrict DNA nuclear import to specific cell types. Young *et al.* [107] improved the efficiency of transduction in SMCs of rat vasculature using a SMC-specific DNA nuclear targeting sequence.

EC specific gene expression was obtained when promoters of *fms*-like tyrosine kinase-1 (FLT-1) [108], intercellular adhesion molecule (ICAM) -2 [109], angiopoietin-2 [110], eNOS [111], vascular cell adhesion molecule-1 (VCAM-1) [112], von Willebrand factor [113], tyrosine kinase with immunoglobulin and epidermal growth factor homology domains (Tie) [114], kinase-like domain receptor [115] were used in transgenic mouse models. Other EC-specific promoters include the oxidized LDL receptor LOX-1 [116] and ICAM-1 [117], which exhibit upregulation upon cytokine stimulation, a possible advantage depending on the application in inflammatory conditions [118]. With the possible exception of the mouse Tie-2 and human ICAM-2 genes, most of EC–specific promoters tested to-date have been shown to direct expression in distinct and restricted sites of the vascular tree [119]. A combination approach of the Tie2 promoter and enhancer (Tshort) by Minami and collegues [119] direct-ed widespread EC expression *in vivo.*

Another challenge was in generating an EC-specific promoter with comparable efficiency as the CMV promoter. White *et al.* [120] examined several novel Ad expression cassettes for EC-specific gene transfer with CMV, Tshort, ICAM-2, ICAM-1, FLT-1 promoters, respective-ly and found that LOX-1 promoter elements significantly increased reporter gene expression in carotid arteries compared to other promoters. The efficacy of these novel expression cas-settes in large animal models have yet to be established.

An increasingly important area to in-tissue specific targeting is to engineer viral vectors Ads and AAVs with altered cell tropisms to narrow or broaden its efficiency in tissues refractory to infection [19, 121]. Non-genetic approaches typically utilize bispecific antibodies that both neutralize wild-type virus tropism and provide a new cell binding capacity [122]. For genet-ic targeting strategies, the virus capsid are engineered to express foreign ligands that target selected receptors in the absence or presence of additional modification to ablate the natural tropism of the virus [122, 123]. Ad homing to target endothelial cells at specific sites of the body can be achieved by deleting the ability of the virus to interact with its natural receptor, Coxsackievirus and adenovirus receptor (CAR), and a simultaneous addition of a ligand that directs the virus to the angiotensin converting enzyme on the ECs. Retargeting of AAV-2 with novel peptides could increase both transduction efficiency and selectivity [124] in vascular ECs [125] and SMCs [126] *in vitro.*

4.3. Challenges associated with the mode and route of gene delivery

4.3.1. Systemic gene delivery

The vascular system represents an ideal route of substance transport for reaching a specific site for therapeutic intervention. However, in the case of non-viral vectors, which are cation-ic polymers in most cases, it has been found that electrostatic interactions between the sulphated glycosaminoglycans in the serum as well as those expressed on the cell surface cause premature release of plasmid DNA leading to its inactivation and extracellular degra-dation by serum DNAses [21]. Also, after systemic vascular application, non-specific distri-bution of plasmid DNA throughout the vasculature would result in undesired side effects because of accumulation at non-specific sites. Intravenous administration of cationic poly-mers resulted in their localization to liver, lung, kidney, and spleen in pigs and rabbits [127-129]. Other barriers to systemic delivery include rapid clearance of the lipoplexes by the reticulo-endothelial system and target specificity.

Most Ad vectors are trapped by the liver, hampering delivery to target CV tissues after sys-temic application. Systemic tail vein injection of Ad vector in mice resulted in virus DNA deposition liver, lung, kidney and testis [130]. Furthermore, the use of a heterologous viral promoter CMV in the majority of vascular gene transfers causes systemic organ toxicity re-sulting from unrestricted transgene expression [131]. Retargeting of vectors and use of tissue specific promoters offers an enhanced safety profile by reducing ectopic expression in vital organs including the liver and lungs.

4.3.2. Endovascular gene delivery

Endovascular catheter-based gene delivery allows localization of vectors to the vessel wall and has the advantage that smaller quantities of viral vectors can be used when compared to those used in systemic delivery. The localized delivery minimizes widespread bio-distribution of vectors and simultaneously increases the local vector concentration. Several catheters are used for vascular gene delivery [132], and the efficiency of gene transfer depends on multiple physical parameters during the delivery process, including balloon pressure, vessel wall exposure time, concentration, and injection force [133]. Diffusive balloon catheters that include double balloon, channel, microporous and hydrogel balloons, facilitate passive diffusion of the vector to reach only the innermost layers of the artery (intima and inner media) [134]. Although this system has the advantage of causing relatively minor damage to the vessel media and intima, the major drawbacks include tissue ischemia caused due to blood flow blockage following balloon inflation and relatively low gene transfection rates owing to the short exposure time to the vessel wall. The pressure-driven balloon catheters [135], like the circumferential needle injection balloon catheter and the porous balloon catheter, are thought to efficiently delivery vectors to the deeper medial and adventitial layers of the artery compared to passive diffusion catheters, but they increase the risk of vascular injury. Damage to the endothelial lining promotes SMC proliferation and may lead to restenosis. The localized vascular injury can also cause increased inflammatory response. Iontophoretic catheters, a mechanically assisted injection catheter, enhance the vector penetration across the EC lining by generating an electrical current gradient to drive charged or hydrophilic molecules as deep as the adventitial layer of the artery wall, but depends on the charge, size, and concentration of the delivered compound [136]. Despite the theoretical aspects, in most cases of catheter-based gene transfer the vector is not distributed to the target vessels but to the region of tissue surrounding the target vessel or into the systemic circulation.

Gene eluting stents are attractive alternatives for localized gene delivery as they provide a platform for prolonged gene elution and efficient transduction of opposed arterial walls, especially in the treatment of in stent restenosis [132]. Local delivery of naked plasmid DNA encoding for human VEGF-2 via gene-eluting stent could decrease neointima formation while accelerating re-endothelialization in rabbit model [137]. Stents coated with lipoplexes containing eNOS plasmid accelerated re-endothelialization in hypercholesterolemic rabbits [138]. The same research group also demonstrated successful Ad and AAV delivery to the vessel wall by gene eluting stents with no systemic dissemination of the viral vectors [139]. Stents are often coated with synthetic or naturally occurring biopolymers for prolonged release of the gene to the vessel wall [140]. Recently, fully biodegradable stents have shown great promise in the treatment of peripheral arterial disease [141]. A combination approach of therapeutic gene delivery and fully biodegradable stents would be a novel approach to gene therapy.

4.3.3. Perivascular gene delivery

In endovascular approach, most catheters require prolonged total vascular occlusion for efficient gene delivery to the vasculature increasing the risk of ischemia. Delivery of genes directly into the adventitia bypassing intima and media may facilitate relatively rapid and efficient delivery compared to endovascular approaches [132]. The advantages of perivascular gene transfer are that the blood flow and endothelium are not disrupted and the placement of vector particles within tissues will result in enhanced local transduction efficiency compared to that achievable by endoluminal delivery [142]. Moreover, the local gene delivery through this 'outside in' approach has received increased attention due to important findings on the capacity of adventitia to influence neointima formation and vascular remodeling [143]. Localized adventitial delivery of a replication-deficient Ad construct containing a fibroblast-active promoter with the gp19ds portion of NADPH inhibitor was effective in reducing overall vascular superoxide anion O_2^- and neointima formation after angioplasty in rat common carotid artery [144]. Shneider *et al.* [145] showed that the infusion of Ad vectors into the carotid artery adventitia achieved recombinant gene expression at a level equivalent to that achieved by means of intraluminal vector infusion. Further, perivascular approach has been reported to minimize the pro-inflammatory effects of Ad vectors [145]. Adventitial gene delivery are also reported to be performed with silastic or biodegradable collars [146] which act as reservoirs of the vector.

The endovascular access is comparatively difficult in the case of coronary arteries, and the numerous side branches will also permit the run-off of the infused volume. An alternative delivery approach for coronary arteries is the expression of diffusible gene products into the pericardial space surrounding the heart and coronary arteries [147]. Transvascular needle injections of Ad vectors to the adventitia and perivascular tissue of coronary arteries have also been reported [148].

4.4. Immunological barriers to gene transfer

The immune system has evolved to eliminate foreign material and therefore, constrains the successful use of gene-replacement therapy based on viral vectors. There are several reports that suggest innate and adaptive immune responses to gene transfer [149, 150]. The vector dose, the route of administration, the nature of the transgene, and host-related factors responsible for inter-individual variability influence the immune response [151]. The early responses involve mechanisms that include the detection of pathogen-associated molecular patterns (PAMPs) present on the viral structural proteins containing the transgene by pattern recognition receptors (PRRs) on cells of the innate immune system (i.e., macrophages and dendritic cells) and the subsequent elaboration of pro-inflammatory cytokines that can up-regulate later adaptive immune responses [152]. The most studied family of PRRs are the toll-like receptors (TLRs), of which TLR2, TLR3, TLR4, TLR7, TLR8 and TLR9 have been implicated in initiating inflammatory responses to viruses [153]. The adaptive responses can include: the generation of antibodies to the transgene delivery vehicle compromising vector administration, or the generation of antibodies to the transgene product which nullifies transgene expression, or cytotoxicity to vector and/or transgene product which leads to the loss of transduced cells. It also results in a CD8[+] memory T cell response that thwarts further efforts to use the same vector or transgene.

Ad vector particles can elicit strong innate and adaptive immune responses. The interplay of both systems activates CD4+ and CD8+ T cells and B cells as well as facilitates the induction of transgene-specific immune responses. The innate immune responses after systemic administration of Ad vectors are due to several processes: complement system activation, anaphylotoxin release, macrophage activation, release of cytokines and chemokines, including Interleukin (IL)-1, IL-6, tumor necrosis factor (TNF)-α, macrophage inhibitory protein-2, and RANTES (regulated and normal T cell expressed and secreted); EC activation, generalized transcriptome dysregulation in multiple tissues, activation of macrophages and dendritic cells, mobilization of granulocyte and mast cells, and thrombocytopenia [154]. These responses are due to activation of multiple PRRs including RIG-I-like receptors and Toll-like receptors: TLR-2, TLR-4 and TLR-9 [155]. *In vivo* administration of higher doses of Ad vectors can result in one or all of these innate responses or may even lead to mortality in small animal models [156]. Ad infection of ECs is followed by expression of adhesion molecules such as ICAM-1 and VCAM-1 leading to increased leukocyte infiltration within transduced tissues [157]. Kupffer cells, the resident macrophages of the liver, rapidly scavenge and eliminate Ad5-based vectors from the circulation in mice [158], and this interaction contributes to the induction of pro-inflammatory cytokines and chemokines [159]. It has been reported that increasing the dose of Ad vector would probably fail to increase transgene expression, as the CAR adenoviral receptors would become saturated; in addition, the higher dose would induce a stronger inflammatory response responsible for increased elimination of the infected cells expressing the transgene [151].

Ad-based gene transfers can be hindered due to adaptive immune responses to the virus or the transgene it encodes. Ad viruses can induce a cytotoxic T-cell response as well as infiltration by CD4+ and CD8+ T cells. The mechanism involves internalization and priming by dendritic cells of capsid antigens associated with Class II Major histocompatibility complex (MHC) antigens, presentation of these antigens to CD4+ T cells, which become activated, and in turn CD8+ T cell activation by these CD4+ T cells [151]. These adaptive immune responses can limit the duration of transgene expression, and/or limit the ability to re-administer the vector.

Development of new large capacity or gutless (devoid of all viral genes) vectors [160] or modification of capsid sequences [161] are a few of the various strategies devised to reduce the immunogenicity of the Ad viral vectors. Adaptive immunity against these vectors has been substantially reduced through the development of helper-dependent Ad vectors that contain no Ad genes. However, these gutless Ad vectors can efficiently transduce antigen presenting cells (APCs) [162], which readily triggered innate immune responses and further augmented the induction of adaptive immune responses to the transgene product. This problem led to the introduction of tissue-specific promoters in gutless Ad vectors to restrict transgene expression in target cells but not in APCs [162]. Genome modification, capsid modification by Ad capsid-display of immuno-evasive proteins, chimeric Ad vectors and Ad vectors derived from alternative Ad serotypes are few techniques adopted for eluding Ad vector immunity [161]. The tropism modification strategies for targeted gene delivery using Ad vectors have been extensively reviewed [163]. Another method to decrease the immune response is to modify the route of delivery of the vector. In the adventitial delivery of Ad vectors to rabbit carotid arteries, recombinant gene expression was achieved at a level equivalent to that achieved by intraluminal vector infusion. Despite the generation of a systemic immune response, adventitial infusion had no detectable pathologic effects on the vascular intima or media [145]

Pre-existing immunity due to neutralizing antibodies against endemic Ad serotypes in human populations can contribute to pre-existing Ad specific adaptive immune responses [154]. These cellular responses may be more challenging than humoral immune responses, as these cellular adaptive immune responses to Ads have been shown to recognize multiple diverse, cross-clade Ad serotypes subsequent to exposure to only a single Ad serotype [154]. Arterial gene transfer with type 5 Ad vectors did not cause significant levels of gene expression in the majority of humans. Both immune-suppression and further engineering of the vector genome to decrease expression of viral genes show promise in circumventing barriers to Ad-mediated arterial gene transfer [164].

The innate immune response to the AAV capsid has received limited attention due to the minimal responses that AAV2 elicits [162]. According to recent reports by Herzog and others [165], innate immune system also plays important roles in activation of immunity by AAV mediated gene transfer, both in inducing the initial response to the vector and in promoting a deleterious adaptive immune responses. The initial innate immune responses were mediated by the TLR9-MyD88 pathway via a traditional NF-κB pathway to induce type 1 interferon production. Subsequently, alternative NF-κB pathway is triggered, prompting adaptive immune responses [166]. *In vivo*, intravenous injection of AAV-lacZ rapidly induces the expression of messenger RNAs (mRNAs) for the cytokines TNF-α, RANTES, interferon-γ-induced protein 10, macrophage inflammatory protein(MIP)-1β, monocyte chemotactic protein-1, and MIP-2. However, this effect lasts only 6 h, compared to more than 24 h with Ad infection [151]. The adaptive cell-mediated response is far weaker with AAV vectors than with adenoviral vectors probably due to the inability of AAVs to efficiently infect APC, including dendritic cells and macrophages. AAV vectors may be capable of infecting immature dendritic cells, but only when large doses of vector are used. In addition, even though a modest amount of dendritic cells are present at sites of AAV infection *in vivo*, they usually fail to induce a T-cell response of sufficient magnitude to eliminate the infected cells and, therefore, to decrease the duration of transgene expression [151].

Cytotoxic T-cell responses to AAV capsid antigen especially in patients with pre-existing neutralizing antibodies against AAV remain a major road block to achieve persistent therapeutic correction for clinical application. Natural, asymptomatic AAV infection in humans is common, and it estimates that up to 80% of humans possess neutralizing antibodies to some AAV serotypes, especially AAV-2 [167]. Recently, multiple serotypes of AAV in addition to AAV2 have been developed; these serotypes carry different capsid proteins and exhibit different tropism towards different organs [18]. However, changing serotypes may only lead to partial success due to the strong conservation of immune-dominant capsid epitopes in AAVs. In patients with high titers of neutralizing antibodies to gene therapy vectors such as AAV and Ad vectors, IgGs can be removed from blood by plasmapheresis, double filtration plasmapheresis and immune-absorbant plasmapheresis before gene transfer procedure to increase transduction rates of target tissues [168].

Plasmids alone or in combination with naked bacterial DNA can stimulate innate immune responses [152]. Plasmids, composed chiefly of bacterial DNA, contain far greater amounts of unmethylated CpG motifs than do the DNA in eukaryotic cells. DNA devoid of CpG motifs does not induce proinflammatory cytokine synthesis by macrophages *in vitro*. TLR 9 recognizes the unmethylated CpG motifs in immunostimulatory sequences of bacterial DNA which activate the cells responsible for innate immune responses (for example macrophages) after penetration of bacteria into the body [169]. Indeed, elimination or methylation of these sequences could be a method for suppressing the inflammatory response induced by unmethylated CpG sequences in plasmids [168].

5. Conclusion

An enormous amount of research has been done in the past few decades on the choice of the therapeutic gene, vectors and delivery approaches for effective vascular gene transfer. The low efficiency of gene transfer to vascular tissues still remains a major drawback.. Of the several approaches used so far, Ad-mediated gene transfer has been found to be the most efficient when compared to other methods. However, gene transfer using viral vectors has often caused ectopic expression and also an increased immunological response. The use of tropism modified vectors and plasmids with cell specific promoters are solutions for reducing the ectopic expression. Using "gutless" viral vectors devoid of the immunogenic regions of viral plasmid is an attractive option to reduce the immunologic response, but we have to wait for more *in vivo* data using these third-generation vectors to reach a conclusive result [160]. Non-viral methods have more barriers to overcome to successfully transfect the cell; however, with the advent of innovative technologies like nanobots [170], stimuli responsive polymers [171], novel erythrocyte based carriers [172], magnetically targeted delivery [173] and focused *in vivo* plasmid DNA delivery to the vascular wall via intravascular ultrasound destruction of microbubbles [174]; we expect enhanced transgene expression in vascular cells in future studies. This will also be a possible solution to tackle with the immune response associated with the viral vectors. Site specific biodegradable stent based gene delivery approach [175] and modified percutaneous gene delivery systems offer new opportunities for enhanced gene delivery to vascular cells.

Acknowledgements

This work was supported by research grants from the National Institute of Health, R01 HL104516, R01 HL112597 and R01 HL116042 to DKA. The content is solely the responsibility of the authors and does not necessarily represent the official views of the National Heart, Lung, and Blood Institute or the National Institutes of Health. Both authors declare no conflict of any sort with the content in this paper.

Author details

Divya Pankajakshan* and Devendra K. Agrawal

*Address all correspondence to: DivyaPankajakshan@creighton.edu and dkagr@creighton.edu

Department of Biomedical Sciences and Center for Clinical & Translational Science Creighton University School of Medicine, Omaha, NE, USA

References

[1] Roger VL, Go AS, Lloyd-Jones DM, Benjamin EJ, Berry JD, Borden WB, Bravata DM, Dai S, Ford ES, Fox CS, Fullerton HJ, Gillespie C, Hailpern SM, Heit JA, Howard VJ, Kissela BM, Kittner SJ, Lackland DT, Lichtman JH, Lisabeth LD, Makuc DM, Marcus GM, Marelli A, Matchar DB, Moy CS, Mozaffarian D, Mussolino ME, Nichol G, Paynter NP, Soliman EZ, Sorlie PD, Sotoodehnia N, Turan TN, Virani SS, Wong ND, Woo D, Turner MB. Heart disease and stroke statistics--2012 update: a report from the American Heart Association. Circulation. 2012;125(1) e2-e220.

[2] Brewster LP, Brey EM, Greisler HP. Cardiovascular gene delivery: The good road is awaiting. Adv Drug Deliv Rev. 2006;58(4) 604-629.

[3] Yla-Herttuala S, Martin JF. Cardiovascular gene therapy. Lancet. 2000;355(9199) 213-222.

[4] Pankajakshan D, Agrawal DK. Scaffolds in tissue engineering of blood vessels. Can J Physiol Pharmacol. 2010;88(9) 855-873.

[5] Williams PD, Ranjzad P, Kakar SJ, Kingston PA. Development of viral vectors for use in cardiovascular gene therapy. Viruses. 2010;2(2) 334-371.

[6] Kahn ML, Lee SW, Dichek DA. Optimization of retroviral vector-mediated gene transfer into endothelial cells in vitro. Circ Res. 1992;71(6) 1508-1517.

[7] Inaba M, Toninelli E, Vanmeter G, Bender JR, Conte MS. Retroviral gene transfer: effects on endothelial cell phenotype. J Surg Res. 1998;78(1) 31-36.

[8] Zelenock JA, Welling TH, Sarkar R, Gordon DG, Messina LM. Improved retroviral transduction efficiency of vascular cells in vitro and in vivo during clinically relevant incubation periods using centrifugation to increase viral titers. J Vasc Surg. 1997;26(1) 119-127.

[9] Yu H, Eton D, Wang Y, Kumar SR, Tang L, Terramani TT, Benedict C, Hung G, Anderson WF. High efficiency in vitro gene transfer into vascular tissues using a pseudotyped retroviral vector without pseudotransduction. Gene Ther. 1999;6(11) 1876-1883.

[10] Dishart KL, Denby L, George SJ, Nicklin SA, Yendluri S, Tuerk MJ, Kelley MP, Dona-hue BA, Newby AC, Harding T, Baker AH. Third-generation lentivirus vectors effi-ciently transduce and phenotypically modify vascular cells: implications for gene therapy. J Mol Cell Cardiol. 2003;35(7) 739-748.

[11] Cefai D, Simeoni E, Ludunge KM, Driscoll R, von Segesser LK, Kappenberger L, Vas-salli G. Multiply attenuated, self-inactivating lentiviral vectors efficiently transduce human coronary artery cells in vitro and rat arteries in vivo. J Mol Cell Cardiol. 2005;38(2) 333-344.

[12] Bonci D, Cittadini A, Latronico MV, Borello U, Aycock JK, Drusco A, Innocenzi A, Follenzi A, Lavitrano M, Monti MG, Ross J, Jr., Naldini L, Peschle C, Cossu G, Con-dorelli G. 'Advanced' generation lentiviruses as efficient vectors for cardiomyocyte gene transduction in vitro and in vivo. Gene Ther. 2003;10(8) 630-636.

[13] Harvey BG, Hackett NR, El-Sawy T, Rosengart TK, Hirschowitz EA, Lieberman MD, Lesser ML, Crystal RG. Variability of human systemic humoral immune responses to adenovirus gene transfer vectors administered to different organs. J Virol. 1999;73(8) 6729-6742.

[14] Mastrangeli A, Harvey BG, Yao J, Wolff G, Kovesdi I, Crystal RG, Falck-Pedersen E. "Sero-switch" adenovirus-mediated in vivo gene transfer: circumvention of anti-ade-novirus humoral immune defenses against repeat adenovirus vector administration by changing the adenovirus serotype. Hum Gene Ther. 1996;7(1) 79-87.

[15] Wen S, Driscoll RM, Schneider DB, Dichek DA. Inclusion of the E3 region in an ade-noviral vector decreases inflammation and neointima formation after arterial gene transfer. Arterioscler Thromb Vasc Biol. 2001;21(11) 1777-1782.

[16] Sasano T, Kikuchi K, McDonald AD, Lai S, Donahue JK. Targeted high-efficiency, ho-mogeneous myocardial gene transfer. J Mol Cell Cardiol. 2007;42(5) 954-961.

[17] Pankajakshan D, Makinde TO, Gaurav R, Del Core M, Hatzoudis G, Pipinos I, Agrawal DK. Successful transfection of genes using AAV-2/9 vector in swine coro-nary and peripheral arteries. J Surg Res. 2012;175(1) 169-175.

[18] Choi VW, McCarty DM, Samulski RJ. AAV hybrid serotypes: improved vectors for gene delivery. Curr Gene Ther. 2005;5(3) 299-310.

[19] Kwon I, Schaffer DV. Designer gene delivery vectors: molecular engineering and evolution of adeno-associated viral vectors for enhanced gene transfer. Pharm Res. 2008;25(3) 489-499.

[20] Morris VB, Sharma CP. Folate mediated in vitro targeting of depolymerised trime-thylated chitosan having arginine functionality. J Colloid Interface Sci. 2010;348(2) 360-368.

[21] Shim MS, Kwon YJ. Stimuli-responsive polymers and nanomaterials for gene deliv-ery and imaging applications. Adv Drug Deliv Rev. 2012;64(11) 1046-1059.

[22] Al-Dosari MS, Gao X. Nonviral gene delivery: principle, limitations, and recent progress. Aaps J. 2009;11(4) 671-681.

[23] Asahara T, Chen D, Tsurumi Y, Kearney M, Rossow S, Passeri J, Symes JF, Isner JM. Accelerated restitution of endothelial integrity and endothelium-dependent function after phVEGF165 gene transfer. Circulation. 1996;94(12) 3291-3302.

[24] Lawrie A, Brisken AF, Francis SE, Cumberland DC, Crossman DC, Newman CM. Microbubble-enhanced ultrasound for vascular gene delivery. Gene Ther. 2000;7(23) 2023-2027.

[25] Nishi T, Yoshizato K, Yamashiro S, Takeshima H, Sato K, Hamada K, Kitamura I, Yoshimura T, Saya H, Kuratsu J, Ushio Y. High-efficiency in vivo gene transfer using intraarterial plasmid DNA injection following in vivo electroporation. Cancer Res. 1996;56(5) 1050-1055.

[26] Williams PD, Kingston PA. Plasmid-mediated gene therapy for cardiovascular disease. Cardiovasc Res. 2011;91(4) 565-576.

[27] Parkes R, Meng QH, Siapati KE, McEwan JR, Hart SL. High efficiency transfection of porcine vascular cells in vitro with a synthetic vector system. J Gene Med. 2002;4(3) 292-299.

[28] Kader KN, Sweany JM, Bellamkonda RV. Cationic lipid-mediated transfection of bovine aortic endothelial cells inhibits their attachment. J Biomed Mater Res. 2002;60(3) 405-410.

[29] Wang T, Upponi JR, Torchilin VP. Design of multifunctional non-viral gene vectors to overcome physiological barriers: dilemmas and strategies. Int J Pharm. 2012;427(1) 3-20.

[30] Zaric V, Weltin D, Erbacher P, Remy JS, Behr JP, Stephan D. Effective polyethylenimine-mediated gene transfer into human endothelial cells. J Gene Med. 2004;6(2) 176-184.

[31] Godbey WT, Wu KK, Mikos AG. Poly(ethylenimine)-mediated gene delivery affects endothelial cell function and viability. Biomaterials. 2001;22(5) 471-480.

[32] Turunen MP, Hiltunen MO, Ruponen M, Virkamaki L, Szoka FC, Jr., Urtti A, Yla-Herttuala S. Efficient adventitial gene delivery to rabbit carotid artery with cationic polymer-plasmid complexes. Gene Ther. 1999;6(1) 6-11.

[33] Brito L, Little S, Langer R, Amiji M. Poly(beta-amino ester) and cationic phospholipid-based lipopolyplexes for gene delivery and transfection in human aortic endothelial and smooth muscle cells. Biomacromolecules. 2008;9(4) 1179-1187.

[34] Chen SL, Zhu CC, Liu YQ, Tang LJ, Yi L, Yu BJ, Wang DJ. Mesenchymal stem cells genetically modified with the angiopoietin-1 gene enhanced arteriogenesis in a porcine model of chronic myocardial ischaemia. J Int Med Res. 2009;37(1) 68-78.

[35] Das H, George JC, Joseph M, Das M, Abdulhameed N, Blitz A, Khan M, Sakthivel R, Mao HQ, Hoit BD, Kuppusamy P, Pompili VJ. Stem cell therapy with overexpressed VEGF and PDGF genes improves cardiac function in a rat infarct model. PLoS One. 2009;4(10) e7325.

[36] Behrendt D, Ganz P. Endothelial function. From vascular biology to clinical applications. Am J Cardiol. 2002;90(10C) 40L-48L.

[37] Griese DP, Achatz S, Batzlsperger CA, Strauch UG, Grumbeck B, Weil J, Riegger GA. Vascular gene delivery of anticoagulants by transplantation of retrovirally-transduced endothelial progenitor cells. Cardiovasc Res. 2003;58(2) 469-477.

[38] Chen L, Wu F, Xia WH, Zhang YY, Xu SY, Cheng F, Liu X, Zhang XY, Wang SM, Tao J. CXCR4 gene transfer contributes to in vivo reendothelialization capacity of endothelial progenitor cells. Cardiovasc Res. 2010;88(3) 462-470.

[39] Ohno N, Itoh H, Ikeda T, Ueyama K, Yamahara K, Doi K, Yamashita J, Inoue M, Masatsugu K, Sawada N, Fukunaga Y, Sakaguchi S, Sone M, Yurugi T, Kook H, Komeda M, Nakao K. Accelerated reendothelialization with suppressed thrombogenic property and neointimal hyperplasia of rabbit jugular vein grafts by adenovirus-mediated gene transfer of C-type natriuretic peptide. Circulation. 2002;105(14) 1623-1626.

[40] Kong D, Melo LG, Mangi AA, Zhang L, Lopez-Ilasaca M, Perrella MA, Liew CC, Pratt RE, Dzau VJ. Enhanced inhibition of neointimal hyperplasia by genetically engineered endothelial progenitor cells. Circulation. 2004;109(14) 1769-1775.

[41] Laitinen M, Hartikainen J, Hiltunen MO, Eranen J, Kiviniemi M, Narvanen O, Makinen K, Manninen H, Syvanne M, Martin JF, Laakso M, Yla-Herttuala S. Catheter-mediated vascular endothelial growth factor gene transfer to human coronary arteries after angioplasty. Hum Gene Ther. 2000;11(2) 263-270.

[42] Channon KM, Annex BH. Antithrombotic strategies in gene therapy. Curr Cardiol Rep. 2000;2(1) 34-38.

[43] Waugh JM, Yuksel E, Li J, Kuo MD, Kattash M, Saxena R, Geske R, Thung SN, Shenaq SM, Woo SL. Local overexpression of thrombomodulin for in vivo prevention of arterial thrombosis in a rabbit model. Circ Res. 1999;84(1) 84-92.

[44] Yin X, Yutani C, Ikeda Y, Enjyoji K, Ishibashi-Ueda H, Yasuda S, Tsukamoto Y, Nonogi H, Kaneda Y, Kato H. Tissue factor pathway inhibitor gene delivery using HVJ-AVE liposomes markedly reduces restenosis in atherosclerotic arteries. Cardiovasc Res. 2002;56(3) 454-463.

[45] Rade JJ, Schulick AH, Virmani R, Dichek DA. Local adenoviral-mediated expression of recombinant hirudin reduces neointima formation after arterial injury. Nat Med. 1996;2(3) 293-298.

[46] Zoldhelyi P, McNatt J, Xu XM, Loose-Mitchell D, Meidell RS, Clubb FJ, Jr., Buja LM, Willerson JT, Wu KK. Prevention of arterial thrombosis by adenovirus-mediated transfer of cyclooxygenase gene. Circulation. 1996;93(1) 10-17.

[47] Levonen AL, Inkala M, Heikura T, Jauhiainen S, Jyrkkanen HK, Kansanen E, Maatta K, Romppanen E, Turunen P, Rutanen J, Yla-Herttuala S. Nrf2 gene transfer induces antioxidant enzymes and suppresses smooth muscle cell growth in vitro and reduces oxidative stress in rabbit aorta in vivo. Arterioscler Thromb Vasc Biol. 2007;27(4) 741-747.

[48] Levonen AL, Vahakangas E, Koponen JK, Yla-Herttuala S. Antioxidant gene therapy for cardiovascular disease: current status and future perspectives. Circulation. 2008;117(16) 2142-2150.

[49] Li Q, Bolli R, Qiu Y, Tang XL, Guo Y, French BA. Gene therapy with extracellular superoxide dismutase protects conscious rabbits against myocardial infarction. Circulation. 2001;103(14) 1893-1898.

[50] Laukkanen MO, Kivela A, Rissanen T, Rutanen J, Karkkainen MK, Leppanen O, Brasen JH, Yla-Herttuala S. Adenovirus-mediated extracellular superoxide dismutase gene therapy reduces neointima formation in balloon-denuded rabbit aorta. Circulation. 2002;106(15) 1999-2003.

[51] Woo YJ, Zhang JC, Vijayasarathy C, Zwacka RM, Englehardt JF, Gardner TJ, Sweeney HL. Recombinant adenovirus-mediated cardiac gene transfer of superoxide dismutase and catalase attenuates postischemic contractile dysfunction. Circulation. 1998;98(19 Suppl) II255-260; discussion II260-251.

[52] Duckers HJ, Boehm M, True AL, Yet SF, San H, Park JL, Clinton Webb R, Lee ME, Nabel GJ, Nabel EG. Heme oxygenase-1 protects against vascular constriction and proliferation. Nat Med. 2001;7(6) 693-698.

[53] Kashyap VS, Santamarina-Fojo S, Brown DR, Parrott CL, Applebaum-Bowden D, Meyn S, Talley G, Paigen B, Maeda N, Brewer HB, Jr. Apolipoprotein E deficiency in mice: gene replacement and prevention of atherosclerosis using adenovirus vectors. J Clin Invest. 1995;96(3) 1612-1620.

[54] Tsukamoto K, Tangirala R, Chun SH, Pure E, Rader DJ. Rapid regression of atherosclerosis induced by liver-directed gene transfer of ApoE in ApoE-deficient mice. Arterioscler Thromb Vasc Biol. 1999;19(9) 2162-2170.

[55] Greeve J, Jona VK, Chowdhury NR, Horwitz MS, Chowdhury JR. Hepatic gene transfer of the catalytic subunit of the apolipoprotein B mRNA editing enzyme results in a reduction of plasma LDL levels in normal and watanabe heritable hyperlipidemic rabbits. J Lipid Res. 1996;37(9) 2001-2017.

[56] Khurana R, Martin JF, Zachary I. Gene therapy for cardiovascular disease: a case for cautious optimism. Hypertension. 2001;38(5) 1210-1216.

[57] Granada JF, Ensenat D, Keswani AN, Kaluza GL, Raizner AE, Liu XM, Peyton KJ, Azam MA, Wang H, Durante W. Single perivascular delivery of mitomycin C stimulates p21 expression and inhibits neointima formation in rat arteries. Arterioscler Thromb Vasc Biol. 2005;25(11) 2343-2348.

[58] Chang MW, Barr E, Lu MM, Barton K, Leiden JM. Adenovirus-mediated over-expression of the cyclin/cyclin-dependent kinase inhibitor, p21 inhibits vascular smooth muscle cell proliferation and neointima formation in the rat carotid artery model of balloon angioplasty. J Clin Invest. 1995;96(5) 2260-2268.

[59] McArthur JG, Qian H, Citron D, Banik GG, Lamphere L, Gyuris J, Tsui L, George SE. p27-p16 Chimera: a superior antiproliferative for the prevention of neointimal hyperplasia. Mol Ther. 2001;3(1) 8-13.

[60] Tsui LV, Camrud A, Mondesire J, Carlson P, Zayek N, Camrud L, Donahue B, Bauer S, Lin A, Frey D, Rivkin M, Subramanian A, Falotico R, Gyuris J, Schwartz R, McArthur JG. p27-p16 fusion gene inhibits angioplasty-induced neointimal hyperplasia and coronary artery occlusion. Circ Res. 2001;89(4) 323-328.

[61] Takagi Y. Adenovirus-mediated overexpression of a cyclin-dependent kinase inhibitor, p57Kip2, suppressed vascular smooth muscle cell proliferation. Hokkaido Igaku Zasshi. 2002;77(3) 221-230.

[62] Maillard L, Van Belle E, Smith RC, Le Roux A, Denefle P, Steg G, Barry JJ, Branellec D, Isner JM, Walsh K. Percutaneous delivery of the gax gene inhibits vessel stenosis in a rabbit model of balloon angioplasty. Cardiovasc Res. 1997;35(3) 536-546.

[63] Chen L, Daum G, Forough R, Clowes M, Walter U, Clowes AW. Overexpression of human endothelial nitric oxide synthase in rat vascular smooth muscle cells and in balloon-injured carotid artery. Circ Res. 1998;82(8) 862-870.

[64] Kopp CW, de Martin R. Gene therapy approaches for the prevention of restenosis. Curr Vasc Pharmacol. 2004;2(2) 183-189.

[65] Yukawa H, Miyatake SI, Saiki M, Takahashi JC, Mima T, Ueno H, Nagata I, Kikuchi H, Hashimoto N. In vitro growth suppression of vascular smooth muscle cells using adenovirus-mediated gene transfer of a truncated form of fibroblast growth factor receptor. Atherosclerosis. 1998;141(1) 125-132.

[66] Kotani M, Fukuda N, Ando H, Hu WY, Kunimoto S, Saito S, Kanmatsuse K. Chimeric DNA-RNA hammerhead ribozyme targeting PDGF A-chain mRNA specifically inhibits neointima formation in rat carotid artery after balloon injury. Cardiovasc Res. 2003;57(1) 265-276.

[67] Ando H, Fukuda N, Kotani M, Yokoyama S, Kunimoto S, Matsumoto K, Saito S, Kanmatsuse K, Mugishima H. Chimeric DNA-RNA hammerhead ribozyme targeting transforming growth factor-beta 1 mRNA inhibits neointima formation in rat carotid artery after balloon injury. Eur J Pharmacol. 2004;483(2-3) 207-214.

[68] Ahn JD, Morishita R, Kaneda Y, Lee SJ, Kwon KY, Choi SY, Lee KU, Park JY, Moon IJ, Park JG, Yoshizumi M, Ouchi Y, Lee IK. Inhibitory effects of novel AP-1 decoy oligodeoxynucleotides on vascular smooth muscle cell proliferation in vitro and neointimal formation in vivo. Circ Res. 2002;90(12) 1325-1332.

[69] Ehsan A, Mann MJ, Dell'Acqua G, Dzau VJ. Long-term stabilization of vein graft wall architecture and prolonged resistance to experimental atherosclerosis after E2F decoy oligonucleotide gene therapy. J Thorac Cardiovasc Surg. 2001;121(4) 714-722.

[70] Luo Z, Garron T, Palasis M, Lu H, Belanger AJ, Scaria A, Vincent KA, Date T, Akita GY, Cheng SH, Barry J, Gregory RJ, Jiang C. Enhancement of Fas ligand-induced inhibition of neointimal formation in rabbit femoral and iliac arteries by coexpression of p35. Hum Gene Ther. 2001;12(18) 2191-2202.

[71] Newby AC. Matrix metalloproteinases regulate migration, proliferation, and death of vascular smooth muscle cells by degrading matrix and non-matrix substrates. Cardiovasc Res. 2006;69(3) 614-624.

[72] Ramirez Correa GA, Zacchigna S, Arsic N, Zentilin L, Salvi A, Sinagra G, Giacca M. Potent inhibition of arterial intimal hyperplasia by TIMP1 gene transfer using AAV vectors. Mol Ther. 2004;9(6) 876-884.

[73] George SJ, Baker AH, Angelini GD, Newby AC. Gene transfer of tissue inhibitor of metalloproteinase-2 inhibits metalloproteinase activity and neointima formation in human saphenous veins. Gene Ther. 1998;5(11) 1552-1560.

[74] Johnson TW, Wu YX, Herdeg C, Baumbach A, Newby AC, Karsch KR, Oberhoff M. Stent-based delivery of tissue inhibitor of metalloproteinase-3 adenovirus inhibits neointimal formation in porcine coronary arteries. Arterioscler Thromb Vasc Biol. 2005;25(4) 754-759.

[75] Guo YH, Gao W, Li Q, Li PF, Yao PY, Chen K. Tissue inhibitor of metalloproteinases-4 suppresses vascular smooth muscle cell migration and induces cell apoptosis. Life Sci. 2004;75(20) 2483-2493.

[76] Gurjar MV, Sharma RV, Bhalla RC. eNOS gene transfer inhibits smooth muscle cell migration and MMP-2 and MMP-9 activity. Arterioscler Thromb Vasc Biol. 1999;19(12) 2871-2877.

[77] Eefting D, de Vries MR, Grimbergen JM, Karper JC, van Bockel JH, Quax PH. In vivo suppression of vein graft disease by nonviral, electroporation-mediated, gene transfer of tissue inhibitor of metalloproteinase-1 linked to the amino terminal fragment of urokinase (TIMP-1.ATF), a cell-surface directed matrix metalloproteinase inhibitor. J Vasc Surg. 2010;51(2) 429-437.

[78] Emanueli C, Madeddu P. Angiogenesis gene therapy to rescue ischaemic tissues: achievements and future directions. Br J Pharmacol. 2001;133(7) 951-958.

[79] Syed IS, Sanborn TA, Rosengart TK. Therapeutic angiogenesis: a biologic bypass. Cardiology. 2004;101(1-3) 131-143.

[80] Losordo DW, Vale PR, Isner JM. Gene therapy for myocardial angiogenesis. Am Heart J. 1999;138(2 Pt 2) S132-141.

[81] Rosengart TK, Lee LY, Patel SR, Kligfield PD, Okin PM, Hackett NR, Isom OW, Crystal RG. Six-month assessment of a phase I trial of angiogenic gene therapy for the

treatment of coronary artery disease using direct intramyocardial administration of an adenovirus vector expressing the VEGF121 cDNA. Ann Surg. 1999;230(4) 466-470; discussion 470-462.

[82] Grines C, Rubanyi GM, Kleiman NS, Marrott P, Watkins MW. Angiogenic gene therapy with adenovirus 5 fibroblast growth factor-4 (Ad5FGF-4): a new option for the treatment of coronary artery disease. Am J Cardiol. 2003;92(9B) 24N-31N.

[83] Safi J, Jr., DiPaula AF, Jr., Riccioni T, Kajstura J, Ambrosio G, Becker LC, Anversa P, Capogrossi MC. Adenovirus-mediated acidic fibroblast growth factor gene transfer induces angiogenesis in the nonischemic rabbit heart. Microvasc Res. 1999;58(3) 238-249.

[84] Nah JW, Yu L, Han SO, Ahn CH, Kim SW. Artery wall binding peptide-poly(ethylene glycol)-grafted-poly(L-lysine)-based gene delivery to artery wall cells. J Control Release. 2002;78(1-3) 273-284.

[85] Akagi D, Oba M, Koyama H, Nishiyama N, Fukushima S, Miyata T, Nagawa H, Kataoka K. Biocompatible micellar nanovectors achieve efficient gene transfer to vascular lesions without cytotoxicity and thrombus formation. Gene Ther. 2007;14(13) 1029-1038.

[86] Song C, Labhasetwar V, Cui X, Underwood T, Levy RJ. Arterial uptake of biodegradable nanoparticles for intravascular local drug delivery: results with an acute dog model. J Control Release. 1998;54(2) 201-211.

[87] Kagaya H, Oba M, Miura Y, Koyama H, Ishii T, Shimada T, Takato T, Kataoka K, Miyata T. Impact of polyplex micelles installed with cyclic RGD peptide as ligand on gene delivery to vascular lesions. Gene Ther. 2012;19(1) 61-69.

[88] Theoharis S, Krueger U, Tan PH, Haskard DO, Weber M, George AJ. Targeting gene delivery to activated vascular endothelium using anti E/P-Selectin antibody linked to PAMAM dendrimers. J Immunol Methods. 2009;343(2) 79-90.

[89] White SJ, Nicklin SA, Sawamura T, Baker AH. Identification of peptides that target the endothelial cell-specific LOX-1 receptor. Hypertension. 2001;37(2 Part 2) 449-455.

[90] Jarver P, Langel K, El-Andaloussi S, Langel U. Applications of cell-penetrating peptides in regulation of gene expression. Biochem Soc Trans. 2007;35(Pt 4) 770-774.

[91] Golda A, Pelisek J, Klocke R, Engelmann MG, Rolland PH, Mekkaoui C, Nikol S. Small poly-L-lysines improve cationic lipid-mediated gene transfer in vascular cells in vitro and in vivo. J Vasc Res. 2007;44(4) 273-282.

[92] Cartier R, Reszka R. Utilization of synthetic peptides containing nuclear localization signals for nonviral gene transfer systems. Gene Ther. 2002;9(3) 157-167.

[93] Hebert E. Improvement of exogenous DNA nuclear importation by nuclear localization signal-bearing vectors: a promising way for non-viral gene therapy? Biol Cell. 2003;95(2) 59-68.

[94] Young JL, Benoit JN, Dean DA. Effect of a DNA nuclear targeting sequence on gene transfer and expression of plasmids in the intact vasculature. Gene Ther. 2003;10(17) 1465-1470.

[95] Vasileva A, Jessberger R. Precise hit: adeno-associated virus in gene targeting. Nat Rev Microbiol. 2005;3(11) 837-847.

[96] Vasileva A, Linden RM, Jessberger R. Homologous recombination is required for AAV-mediated gene targeting. Nucleic Acids Res. 2006;34(11) 3345-3360.

[97] Russell DW, Hirata RK. Human gene targeting by viral vectors. Nat Genet. 1998;18(4) 325-330.

[98] Li L, Miano JM, Mercer B, Olson EN. Expression of the SM22alpha promoter in transgenic mice provides evidence for distinct transcriptional regulatory programs in vascular and visceral smooth muscle cells. J Cell Biol. 1996;132(5) 849-859.

[99] Mack CP, Owens GK. Regulation of smooth muscle alpha-actin expression in vivo is dependent on CArG elements within the 5' and first intron promoter regions. Circ Res. 1999;84(7) 852-861.

[100] Mack CP, Thompson MM, Lawrenz-Smith S, Owens GK. Smooth muscle alpha-actin CArG elements coordinate formation of a smooth muscle cell-selective, serum response factor-containing activation complex. Circ Res. 2000;86(2) 221-232.

[101] Hoggatt AM, Simon GM, Herring BP. Cell-specific regulatory modules control expression of genes in vascular and visceral smooth muscle tissues. Circ Res. 2002;91(12) 1151-1159.

[102] Madsen CS, Regan CP, Hungerford JE, White SL, Manabe I, Owens GK. Smooth muscle-specific expression of the smooth muscle myosin heavy chain gene in transgenic mice requires 5'-flanking and first intronic DNA sequence. Circ Res. 1998;82(8) 908-917.

[103] Qian J, Kumar A, Szucsik JC, Lessard JL. Tissue and developmental specific expression of murine smooth muscle gamma-actin fusion genes in transgenic mice. Dev Dyn. 1996;207(2) 135-144.

[104] Mericskay M, Parlakian A, Porteu A, Dandre F, Bonnet J, Paulin D, Li Z. An overlapping CArG/octamer element is required for regulation of desmin gene transcription in arterial smooth muscle cells. Dev Biol. 2000;226(2) 192-208.

[105] Su H, Yeghiazarians Y, Lee A, Huang Y, Arakawa-Hoyt J, Ye J, Orcino G, Grossman W, Kan YW. AAV serotype 1 mediates more efficient gene transfer to pig myocardium than AAV serotype 2 and plasmid. J Gene Med. 2008;10(1) 33-41.

[106] Ribault S, Neuville P, Mechine-Neuville A, Auge F, Parlakian A, Gabbiani G, Paulin D, Calenda V. Chimeric smooth muscle-specific enhancer/promoters: valuable tools for adenovirus-mediated cardiovascular gene therapy. Circ Res. 2001;88(5) 468-475.

[107] Young JL, Zimmer WE, Dean DA. Smooth muscle-specific gene delivery in the vasculature based on restriction of DNA nuclear import. Exp Biol Med (Maywood). 2008;233(7) 840-848.

[108] Morishita K, Johnson DE, Williams LT. A novel promoter for vascular endothelial growth factor receptor (flt-1) that confers endothelial-specific gene expression. J Biol Chem. 1995;270(46) 27948-27953.

[109] Cowan PJ, Shinkel TA, Witort EJ, Barlow H, Pearse MJ, d'Apice AJ. Targeting gene expression to endothelial cells in transgenic mice using the human intercellular adhesion molecule 2 promoter. Transplantation. 1996;62(2) 155-160.

[110] Hegen A, Koidl S, Weindel K, Marme D, Augustin HG, Fiedler U. Expression of angiopoietin-2 in endothelial cells is controlled by positive and negative regulatory promoter elements. Arterioscler Thromb Vasc Biol. 2004;24(10) 1803-1809.

[111] Karantzoulis-Fegaras F, Antoniou H, Lai SL, Kulkarni G, D'Abreo C, Wong GK, Miller TL, Chan Y, Atkins J, Wang Y, Marsden PA. Characterization of the human endothelial nitric-oxide synthase promoter. J Biol Chem. 1999;274(5) 3076-3093.

[112] Neish AS, Williams AJ, Palmer HJ, Whitley MZ, Collins T. Functional analysis of the human vascular cell adhesion molecule 1 promoter. J Exp Med. 1992;176(6) 1583-1593.

[113] Jahroudi N, Lynch DC. Endothelial-cell-specific regulation of von Willebrand factor gene expression. Mol Cell Biol. 1994;14(2) 999-1008.

[114] Korhonen J, Lahtinen I, Halmekyto M, Alhonen L, Janne J, Dumont D, Alitalo K. Endothelial-specific gene expression directed by the tie gene promoter in vivo. Blood. 1995;86(5) 1828-1835.

[115] Patterson C, Perrella MA, Hsieh CM, Yoshizumi M, Lee ME, Haber E. Cloning and functional analysis of the promoter for KDR/flk-1, a receptor for vascular endothelial growth factor. J Biol Chem. 1995;270(39) 23111-23118.

[116] Aoyama T, Sawamura T, Furutani Y, Matsuoka R, Yoshida MC, Fujiwara H, Masaki T. Structure and chromosomal assignment of the human lectin-like oxidized low-density-lipoprotein receptor-1 (LOX-1) gene. Biochem J. 1999;339 (Pt 1) 177-184.

[117] Hou J, Baichwal V, Cao Z. Regulatory elements and transcription factors controlling basal and cytokine-induced expression of the gene encoding intercellular adhesion molecule 1. Proc Natl Acad Sci U S A. 1994;91(24) 11641-11645.

[118] Tessitore A, Pastore L, Rispoli A, Cilenti L, Toniato E, Flati V, Farina AR, Frati L, Gulino A, Martinotti S. Two gamma-interferon-activation sites (GAS) on the promoter of the human intercellular adhesion molecule (ICAM-1) gene are required for induction of transcription by IFN-gamma. Eur J Biochem. 1998;258(3) 968-975.

[119] Minami T, Kuivenhoven JA, Evans V, Kodama T, Rosenberg RD, Aird WC. Ets motifs are necessary for endothelial cell-specific expression of a 723-bp Tie-2 promoter/

enhancer in Hprt targeted transgenic mice. Arterioscler Thromb Vasc Biol. 2003;23(11) 2041-2047.

[120]   White SJ, Papadakis ED, Rogers CA, Johnson JL, Biessen EA, Newby AC. In vitro and in vivo analysis of expression cassettes designed for vascular gene transfer. Gene Ther. 2008;15(5) 340-346.

[121]   Gigout L, Rebollo P, Clement N, Warrington KH, Jr., Muzyczka N, Linden RM, Weber T. Altering AAV tropism with mosaic viral capsids. Mol Ther. 2005;11(6) 856-865.

[122]   Nicklin SA, Baker AH. Tropism-modified adenoviral and adeno-associated viral vectors for gene therapy. Curr Gene Ther. 2002;2(3) 273-293.

[123]   Baker AH. Designing gene delivery vectors for cardiovascular gene therapy. Prog Biophys Mol Biol. 2004;84(2-3) 279-299.

[124]   White SJ, Nicklin SA, Buning H, Brosnan MJ, Leike K, Papadakis ED, Hallek M, Baker AH. Targeted gene delivery to vascular tissue in vivo by tropism-modified adeno-associated virus vectors. Circulation. 2004;109(4) 513-519.

[125]   Nicklin SA, Buening H, Dishart KL, de Alwis M, Girod A, Hacker U, Thrasher AJ, Ali RR, Hallek M, Baker AH. Efficient and selective AAV2-mediated gene transfer directed to human vascular endothelial cells. Mol Ther. 2001;4(3) 174-181.

[126]   Work LM, Nicklin SA, Brain NJ, Dishart KL, Von Seggern DJ, Hallek M, Buning H, Baker AH. Development of efficient viral vectors selective for vascular smooth muscle cells. Mol Ther. 2004;9(2) 198-208.

[127]   Takakura Y, Nishikawa M, Yamashita F, Hashida M. Influence of physicochemical properties on pharmacokinetics of non-viral vectors for gene delivery. J Drug Target. 2002;10(2) 99-104.

[128]   Mahato RI, Kawabata K, Takakura Y, Hashida M. In vivo disposition characteristics of plasmid DNA complexed with cationic liposomes. J Drug Target. 1995;3(2) 149-157.

[129]   Gonin P, Gaillard C. Gene transfer vector biodistribution: pivotal safety studies in clinical gene therapy development. Gene Ther. 2004;11 Suppl 1 S98-S108.

[130]   Ye X, Gao GP, Pabin C, Raper SE, Wilson JM. Evaluating the potential of germ line transmission after intravenous administration of recombinant adenovirus in the C3H mouse. Hum Gene Ther. 1998;9(14) 2135-2142.

[131]   Beck C, Uramoto H, Boren J, Akyurek LM. Tissue-specific targeting for cardiovascular gene transfer. Potential vectors and future challenges. Curr Gene Ther. 2004;4(4) 457-467.

[132]   Sharif F, Daly K, Crowley J, O'Brien T. Current status of catheter- and stent-based gene therapy. Cardiovasc Res. 2004;64(2) 208-216.

[133]   Fram DB, Aretz T, Azrin MA, Mitchel JF, Samady H, Gillam LD, Sahatjian R, Waters D, McKay RG. Localized intramural drug delivery during balloon angioplasty using

hydrogel-coated balloons and pressure-augmented diffusion. J Am Coll Cardiol. 1994;23(7) 1570-1577.

[134] Opie SR, Dib N. Local endovascular delivery, gene therapy, and cell transplantation for peripheral arterial disease. J Endovasc Ther. 2004;11 Suppl 2 II151-162.

[135] Barath P, Popov A, Dillehay GL, Matos G, McKiernan T. Infiltrator Angioplasty Balloon Catheter: a device for combined angioplasty and intramural site-specific treatment. Cathet Cardiovasc Diagn. 1997;41(3) 333-341.

[136] Fernandez-Ortiz A, Meyer BJ, Mailhac A, Falk E, Badimon L, Fallon JT, Fuster V, Chesebro JH, Badimon JJ. A new approach for local intravascular drug delivery. Iontophoretic balloon. Circulation. 1994;89(4) 1518-1522.

[137] Walter DH, Cejna M, Diaz-Sandoval L, Willis S, Kirkwood L, Stratford PW, Tietz AB, Kirchmair R, Silver M, Curry C, Wecker A, Yoon YS, Heidenreich R, Hanley A, Kearney M, Tio FO, Kuenzler P, Isner JM, Losordo DW. Local gene transfer of phVEGF-2 plasmid by gene-eluting stents: an alternative strategy for inhibition of restenosis. Circulation. 2004;110(1) 36-45.

[138] Sharif F, Hynes SO, McCullagh KJ, Ganley S, Greiser U, McHugh P, Crowley J, Barry F, O'Brien T. Gene-eluting stents: non-viral, liposome-based gene delivery of eNOS to the blood vessel wall in vivo results in enhanced endothelialization but does not reduce restenosis in a hypercholesterolemic model. Gene Ther. 2012;19(3) 321-328.

[139] Sharif F, Hynes SO, McMahon J, Cooney R, Conroy S, Dockery P, Duffy G, Daly K, Crowley J, Bartlett JS, O'Brien T. Gene-eluting stents: comparison of adenoviral and adeno- associated viral gene delivery to the blood vessel wall in vivo. Hum Gene Ther. 2006;17(7) 741-750.

[140] Klugherz BD, Song C, DeFelice S, Cui X, Lu Z, Connolly J, Hinson JT, Wilensky RL, Levy RJ. Gene delivery to pig coronary arteries from stents carrying antibody-tethered adenovirus. Hum Gene Ther. 2002;13(3) 443-454.

[141] Nishio S, Kosuga K, Igaki K, Okada M, Kyo E, Tsuji T, Takeuchi E, Inuzuka Y, Takeda S, Hata T, Takeuchi Y, Kawada Y, Harita T, Seki J, Akamatsu S, Hasegawa S, Bruining N, Brugaletta S, de Winter S, Muramatsu T, Onuma Y, Serruys PW, Ikeguchi S. Long-Term (>10 Years) clinical outcomes of first-in-human biodegradable poly-l-lactic acid coronary stents: Igaki-Tamai stents. Circulation. 2012;125(19) 2343-2353.

[142] George SJ, Baker AH. Gene transfer to the vasculature: historical perspective and implication for future research objectives. Mol Biotechnol. 2002;22(2) 153-164.

[143] Siow RC, Churchman AT. Adventitial growth factor signalling and vascular remodelling: potential of perivascular gene transfer from the outside-in. Cardiovasc Res. 2007;75(4) 659-668.

[144] Dourron HM, Jacobson GM, Park JL, Liu J, Reddy DJ, Scheel ML, Pagano PJ. Perivascular gene transfer of NADPH oxidase inhibitor suppresses angioplasty-induced ne-

ointimal proliferation of rat carotid artery. Am J Physiol Heart Circ Physiol. 2005;288(2) H946-953.

[145] Schneider DB, Sassani AB, Vassalli G, Driscoll RM, Dichek DA. Adventitial delivery minimizes the proinflammatory effects of adenoviral vectors. J Vasc Surg. 1999;29(3) 543-550.

[146] Laitinen M, Pakkanen T, Donetti E, Baetta R, Luoma J, Lehtolainen P, Viita H, Agrawal R, Miyanohara A, Friedmann T, Risau W, Martin JF, Soma M, Yla-Herttuala S. Gene transfer into the carotid artery using an adventitial collar: comparison of the effectiveness of the plasmid-liposome complexes, retroviruses, pseudotyped retroviruses, and adenoviruses. Hum Gene Ther. 1997;8(14) 1645-1650.

[147] March KL, Woody M, Mehdi K, Zipes DP, Brantly M, Trapnell BC. Efficient in vivo catheter-based pericardial gene transfer mediated by adenoviral vectors. Clin Cardiol. 1999;22(1 Suppl 1) I23-29.

[148] Baek S, March KL. Gene therapy for restenosis: getting nearer the heart of the matter. Circ Res. 1998;82(3) 295-305.

[149] Marshall E. Gene therapy death prompts review of adenovirus vector. Science. 1999;286(5448) 2244-2245.

[150] Manno CS, Pierce GF, Arruda VR, Glader B, Ragni M, Rasko JJ, Ozelo MC, Hoots K, Blatt P, Konkle B, Dake M, Kaye R, Razavi M, Zajko A, Zehnder J, Rustagi PK, Nakai H, Chew A, Leonard D, Wright JF, Lessard RR, Sommer JM, Tigges M, Sabatino D, Luk A, Jiang H, Mingozzi F, Couto L, Ertl HC, High KA, Kay MA. Successful transduction of liver in hemophilia by AAV-Factor IX and limitations imposed by the host immune response. Nat Med. 2006;12(3) 342-347.

[151] Bessis N, GarciaCozar FJ, Boissier MC. Immune responses to gene therapy vectors: influence on vector function and effector mechanisms. Gene Ther. 2004;11 Suppl 1 S10-17.

[152] Waters B, Lillicrap D. The molecular mechanisms of immunomodulation and tolerance induction to factor VIII. J Thromb Haemost. 2009;7(9) 1446-1456.

[153] Hartman ZC, Appledorn DM, Amalfitano A. Adenovirus vector induced innate immune responses: impact upon efficacy and toxicity in gene therapy and vaccine applications. Virus Res. 2008;132(1-2) 1-14.

[154] Seregin SS, Amalfitano A. Improving adenovirus based gene transfer: strategies to accomplish immune evasion. Viruses. 2010;2(9) 2013-2036.

[155] Kawai T, Akira S. Toll-like receptor and RIG-I-like receptor signaling. Ann N Y Acad Sci. 2008;1143 1-20.

[156] Varnavski AN, Calcedo R, Bove M, Gao G, Wilson JM. Evaluation of toxicity from high-dose systemic administration of recombinant adenovirus vector in vector-naive and pre-immunized mice. Gene Ther. 2005;12(5) 427-436.

[157] Rafii S, Dias S, Meeus S, Hattori K, Ramachandran R, Feuerback F, Worgall S, Hackett NR, Crystal RG. Infection of endothelium with E1(-)E4(+), but not E1(-)E4(-), adenovirus gene transfer vectors enhances leukocyte adhesion and migration by modulation of ICAM-1, VCAM-1, CD34, and chemokine expression. Circ Res. 2001;88(9) 903-910.

[158] Lieber A, He CY, Meuse L, Schowalter D, Kirillova I, Winther B, Kay MA. The role of Kupffer cell activation and viral gene expression in early liver toxicity after infusion of recombinant adenovirus vectors. J Virol. 1997;71(11) 8798-8807.

[159] Shayakhmetov DM, Gaggar A, Ni S, Li ZY, Lieber A. Adenovirus binding to blood factors results in liver cell infection and hepatotoxicity. J Virol. 2005;79(12) 7478-7491.

[160] Alba R, Bosch A, Chillon M. Gutless adenovirus: last-generation adenovirus for gene therapy. Gene Ther. 2005;12 Suppl 1 S18-27.

[161] Bangari DS, Mittal SK. Current strategies and future directions for eluding adenoviral vector immunity. Curr Gene Ther. 2006;6(2) 215-226.

[162] Miao CH. Advances in Overcoming Immune Responses following Hemophilia Gene Therapy. J Genet Syndr Gene Ther. 2011;S1.

[163] Coughlan L, Alba R, Parker AL, Bradshaw AC, McNeish IA, Nicklin SA, Baker AH. Tropism-modification strategies for targeted gene delivery using adenoviral vectors. Viruses. 2010;2(10) 2290-2355.

[164] Schulick AH, Vassalli G, Dunn PF, Dong G, Rade JJ, Zamarron C, Dichek DA. Established immunity precludes adenovirus-mediated gene transfer in rat carotid arteries. Potential for immunosuppression and vector engineering to overcome barriers of immunity. J Clin Invest. 1997;99(2) 209-219.

[165] Herzog RW, Dobrzynski E. Immune implications of gene therapy for hemophilia. Semin Thromb Hemost. 2004;30(2) 215-226.

[166] Jayandharan GR, Aslanidi G, Martino AT, Jahn SC, Perrin GQ, Herzog RW, Srivastava A. Activation of the NF-kappaB pathway by adeno-associated virus (AAV) vectors and its implications in immune response and gene therapy. Proc Natl Acad Sci U S A. 2011;108(9) 3743-3748.

[167] Moskalenko M, Chen L, van Roey M, Donahue BA, Snyder RO, McArthur JG, Patel SD. Epitope mapping of human anti-adeno-associated virus type 2 neutralizing antibodies: implications for gene therapy and virus structure. J Virol. 2000;74(4) 1761-1766.

[168] Wu TL, Ertl HC. Immune barriers to successful gene therapy. Trends Mol Med. 2009;15(1) 32-39.

[169] Verthelyi D. Adjuvant properties of CpG oligonucleotides in primates. Methods Mol Med. 2006;127 139-158.

[170] Jacob T, Hemavathy K, Jacob J, Hingorani A, Marks N, Ascher E. A nanotechnology-based delivery system: Nanobots. Novel vehicles for molecular medicine. J Cardiovasc Surg (Torino). 2011;52(2) 159-167.

[171] Piskin E. Stimuli-responsive polymers in gene delivery. Expert Rev Med Devices. 2005;2(4) 501-509.

[172] Lande C, Cecchettini A, Tedeschi L, Taranta M, Naldi I, Citti L, Trivella MG, Grimaldi S, Cinti C. Innovative Erythrocyte-based Carriers for Gene Delivery in Porcine Vascular Smooth Muscle Cells: Basis for Local Therapy to Prevent Restenosis. Cardiovasc Hematol Disord Drug Targets. 2012;12(1) 68-75.

[173] Chorny M, Fishbein I, Adamo RF, Forbes SP, Folchman-Wagner Z, Alferiev IS. Magnetically targeted delivery of therapeutic agents to injured blood vessels for prevention of in-stent stenosis. Methodist Debakey Cardiovasc J. 2012;8(1) 23-27.

[174] Phillips LC, Klibanov AL, Bowles DK, Ragosta M, Hossack JA, Wamhoff BR. Focused in vivo delivery of plasmid DNA to the porcine vascular wall via intravascular ultrasound destruction of microbubbles. J Vasc Res. 2010;47(3) 270-274.

[175] Fishbein I, Chorny M, Levy RJ. Site-specific gene therapy for cardiovascular disease. Curr Opin Drug Discov Devel. 2010;13(2) 203-213.

Feasibility of Gene Therapy for Tooth Regeneration by Stimulation of a Third Dentition

Katsu Takahashi, Honoka Kiso, Kazuyuki Saito,
Yumiko Togo, Hiroko Tsukamoto, Boyen Huang and
Kazuhisa Bessho

Additional information is available at the end of the chapter

1. Introduction

The tooth is a complex biological organ that consists of multiple tissues, including enamel, dentin, cementum, and pulp. Missing teeth is a common and frequently occurring problem in aging populations. To treat these defects, the current approach involves fixed or removable prostheses, autotransplantation, and dental implants. The exploration of new strategies for tooth replacement has become a hot topic. Using the foundations of experimental embryology, developmental and molecular biology, and the principles of biomimetics, tooth regeneration is becoming a realistic possibility. Several different methods have been proposed to achieve biological tooth replacement[1-8]. These include scaffold-based tooth regeneration, cell pellet engineering, chimeric tooth engineering, stimulation of the formation of a third dentition, and gene-manipulated tooth regeneration. The idea that a third dentition might be locally induced to replace missing teeth is an attractive concept[5,8,9]. This approach is generally presented in terms of adding molecules to induce de novo tooth initiation in the mouth. It might be combined with gene-manipulated tooth regeneration; that is, endogenous dental cells in situ can be activated or repressed by a gene-delivery technique to produce a tooth. Tooth development is the result of reciprocal and reiterative signaling between oral ectoderm-derived dental epithelium and cranial neural crest cell-derived dental mesenchyme under genetic control [10-12]. More than 200 genes are known to be expressed during tooth development (http://bite-it.helsinki.fi/). A number of mouse mutants are now starting to provide some insights into the mechanisms of supernumerary tooth formation. Multiple supernumerary teeth may have genetic components in their etiology and partially represent the third dentition in humans. Such candidate molecules or genes might be those that are involved in embryonic tooth induction, in successional tooth formation, or in the control of the number of teeth. This means that it may be possible to induce *de novo* tooth formation by the in situ repression or activation of a single candidate gene. In this review, we present an overview of the collective knowledge of tooth regeneration, especially regarding the control of the number of teeth for gene therapy by the stimulation of a third dentition.

2. The third dentition

It has been suggested that, in humans, a "third dentition" with one or more supernumerary teeth can occur in addition to the permanent dentition, and supernumerary teeth are sometimes thought to represent a partial post-permanent dentition [13-15]. The basic dentition pattern observed in mammals is diphyodont, and consists of three incisors, one canine, four premolars, and three molars, while Human teeth are diphyodont excepting the permanent molars [16]. The deciduous teeth are, ontogenetically, the first generation of teeth. The permanent teeth (except molar) belong to the second dentition. The term "third dentition" refers to the opinion that one more set of teeth can occur in addition to the permanent teeth (Figure 1). Human teeth are diphyodont excepting the permanent molars. The normal mouse dentition is monophyodont and composed of one incisor and three molars in each quadrant. The number of teeth is usually strictly determined. It was initially reported that there is an anlage of the third dentition in some mammals [17]. The presence of an epithelial anlage of the third dentition was also noticed in humans [18,19]. The teeth and anlagen that appear in third dentition in serial sections of infant jaws and some fetuses have been analyzed. The epithelium which is considered as the anlagen of the third dentition develops lingual to all permanent tooth germs [15]. Furthermore, when it appears, the predecessor (permanent tooth germ) is in the bell-shaped stage [15]. The timing of appearance of the third dentition seems to be after birth (Table 1). This means that we have a chance to access the formation of the third dentition in the mouth.

Teeth	The time of appearance of the third dentition	
	Maxilla	Mandible
central incisors	∼ 3 months after birth	2 ∼ 3 months after birth
lateral incisors	8 ∼ 9 months after birth	2 ∼ 3 months after birth
canines	2 ∼ 7 months after birth	2 ∼ 3 months after birth
the first premolar	1 year 1 month ∼ 5 years 4 months after birth	1 year 1 month ∼ 5 years 4 months after birth
the second premolar	1 year 1 month ∼ 5 years 4 months after birth	2 years ∼ 5 years 4 months after birth

Table 1. Timing of appearance of the third dentition

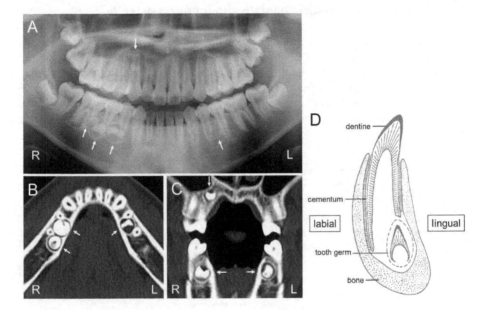

Figure 1. Multiple impacted supernumerary teeth in a 13-year-old non-syndromic patient. The third dentition develops lingual to the permanent tooth germ (D). All impacted supernumerary teeth in this patient are located to the lingual side of the permanent teeth (white arrow) (A-C). These multiple supernumerary teeth seem to be post-permanent dentition ("third dentition").

Analysis of other model systems with continuous tooth replacement or secondary tooth formation, such as in the fish, snake, lizard, and ferret, is providing insights into the molecular and cellular mechanisms underlying successional tooth development, and will assist in studies on supernumerary tooth formation in humans. While some nonmammalian species have multi rowed dentition and replace their teeth regularly throughout life, mammalian vertebrates have one row of teeth and only renew their teeth once, or, in some rodents, show no replacement [20-23]. Detailed histological analysis of the tooth replacement in these models indicates that the successional teeth are initiated from the dental lamina epithelium, which grows from the lingual side of the deciduous tooth enamel organ, and it later elongates and buds into the jaw mesenchyme, forming successional teeth. Jarvien et al. showed that, in the ferret, Sostdc1 (also known as USAG-1, ectodin, and Wise) is expressed in the elongating successional dental lamina at the interface between the lamina and deciduous tooth, as well as the buccal side of the dental lamina, suggesting that Sostdc1 plays a role in defining the identity of the dental lamina [20]. Handrigan et al. analyzed successional tooth formation in the snake and in lizard, and proposed that dental epithelium stem cells are responsible for the formation of successional lamina, and Wnt signaling may regulate the stem cell fate in these cells [24]. Maintenance or reactivation of component dental lamina is thus pivotal for the replacement tooth and supernumerary formation.

3. Human syndromes associated with supernumerary teeth

Supernumerary teeth can be associated with a syndrome (Table 2) or they can be found in non-syndromic patients [25-28]. Only 1% of non-syndromic cases have multiple supernumerary teeth, which occur most frequently in the mandibular premolar area, followed by the molar and anterior regions, respectively [29-34]. There are special cases exhibiting permanent supernumerary teeth developing as supplementary teeth forming after the permanent teeth. These are thought to represent a third dentition, best known as manifestations of cleidocranial dysplasia (CCD).

Syndrome	Gene	Genetics	References
Cleidocranial Dysplasia; CCD (Dental anomalies, isolated dental phenotype) (MIM 119600)	Runx2 (MIM 600211)	Chromosome 6p21, autosomal dominant	Lee et al., 1997; Mundlos et al., 1997.
Familial adenomatous polyposis 1; FAP1 (including Gardner syndrome) (MIM 175100)	APC (MIM 611731)	Chromosome 5q21-22, autosomal dominant	Fader et al., 1962; Ida et al., 1981; Shafer et al.,1983; Jensen and Kreiborg, 1990.
Nance–Horan syndrome (Cataract-Dental syndrome) (MIM 302350)	NHS (MIM 300457)	Chromosome Xp22.13, X-linked dominant	Bixler et al., 1984; Van Dorp and Delleman, 1979; Walpole et al., 1990; Burdon et al., 2003.
Trichorhinophalangeal syndrome, Type III (TRPS3) (MIM 190351)	TRPS1 (MIM 604386)	Chromosome 8q23.3, autosomal dominant	Giedion., 1966; Momeni et al., 2000; Kantaputra et al., 2008.
Robinow syndrome (MIM 180700)	WNT5A (MIM 164975)	Chromosome 3p14.3, autosomal dominant	Mazzeu et al., 2007.
Hallermann-Streiff syndrome; HSS (MIM 234100)	GJA1 (MIM 121014)	Chromosome 6q22.31, Isolated cases	da Fonseca and Mueller, 1994; Robotta and Schafer, 2011.
Rothmund–Thomson Syndrome; RTS (MIM 268400)	RECQL4 (MIM 603780)	Chromosome 8q24.3, autosomal recessive	Kitao et al., 1999.
Orofaciodigital Syndrome I ; OFD1 (Papillon-Leage and Psaume syndrome) (MIM 311200)	OFD1 (MIM 300170)	Chromosome Xp22.2, X-linked dominant	Ferrante et al., 2001.
Uncombable Hair,Retinal Pigmentary Dystrophy,Dental Anomalies,and Brachydactyly (Bork Syndrome) (MIM 191482)	Unknown	autosomal dominant	Silengo et al., 1993.

Table 2. Human syndromes associated with supernumerary teeth

Genetic mutations have been associated with the presence or absence of individual types of teeth. Supernumerary teeth are associated with more than 20 syndromes and developmental abnormalities like CCD, and Gardner syndrome [35]. The percentage occurrence in CCD is 22% in the maxillary incisor region and 5% in the molar region[36-38]. CCD is a dominantly inherited skeletal dysplasia caused by mutations in *Runx2* [39-40]. It is characterized by persistently open sutures or the delayed closure of sutures, hypoplastic or aplastic clavicles, a short stature, delayed eruption of permanent dentition, supernumerary teeth, and other skeletal anomalies. There is a wide spectrum of phenotypic variability ranging from the full-blown phenotype to an isolated dental phenotype characterized by supernumerary tooth formation and/or the delayed eruption of permanent teeth in CCD (Figure 1) [41-44]. A dose-related effect seems to be present, as the milder case of CCD, and those exhibiting primary dental anomalies, are related to mutations that reduce, but do not abolish, protein stability, DNA binding, and transactivation [41,43-45]. Runx2-deficient mice were found to exhibit lingualbuds in front of the upper molars, and these were much more prominent than in wild-type mice[46,47].These buds presumably represent the mouse secondary dentition, and it is likely that Runx2 acts to prevent the formation of these buds. Runx2 usually functions as a cell growth inhibitor[43]. Runx2 regulates the proliferation of cells and may exert specific control on the dental lamina and formation of successive dentitions. Runx2 heterozygous mutant mice mostly phenocopied the skeletal defects of CCD in humans, but with no supernumerary tooth formation [48] (Otto, 1997). Notably, in Runx2 homozygous and heterozygous mouse upper molars, a prominent epithelial bud regularly presents. This epithelial bud protrudes lingually with active Shh signaling, and it may represent the extension of the dental lamina for successional tooth formation in mice. Hence, although Runx2 is required for primary tooth development, it prevents the growth of the dental lamina and successional tooth formation [47].

Familial adenomatous polyposis (FAP), also named adenomatous polyposis of the colon (APC), is an autosomal dominant hereditary disorder characterized by the development of many precancerous colorectal adenomatous polyps, some of which will inevitably develop into cancer. In addition to colorectal neoplasm, individuals can develop variable extracolonic lesions, including upper gastrointestinal polyposis, osteomas, congenital hypertrophy of the retinal pigment epithelium, soft tissue tumors, desmoid tumors, and dental anomalies [49-53]. Dental abnormalities include impacted teeth, congenital absence of one or more teeth, supernumerary teeth, dentigerous cysts associated with the crown of an unerupted tooth, and odontomas[50,52]. Gardner syndrome is a variant of FAP characterized by multiple adenomas of the colon and rectum typical of FAP together with osteomas and soft tissue tumors[49,51]. Supernumerary teeth and osteomas were originally described as a part of Gardner syndrome, but they can also occur in FAP patients with or without other extracolonic lesions [51,52]. FAP and Gardner syndrome are caused by a large number of germinal mutations in the APC gene [52,53]. APC is a tumor suppressor gene involved in the down-regulation of free intracellular ß-catenin, the major signal transducer of the canonical Wnt signaling pathway, as well as a central component of the E-cadherin adhesion complex [54,55]. In addition, the APC protein may also play roles in chromosomal stability, the regulation of cell migration up the colonic crypt and cell adhesion through association with GSK3ß, and other functions associated with microtubule bundles [55,56]. Inactivation of APC would lead to the stabilization and accumulation of the proto-oncogene ß-catenin, dysregulation of the cell cycle, and chromosomal instability [52]. Approximately 11-27% of patients have supernumerary teeth, but, so far, no specific codon mutation of the APC gene has been found to correlate with supernumerary teeth. Correlations seem to exist between dental abnormalities and the number and type of osteomas, with the highest incidence of supernumerary teeth and odontomas being found in FAP patients with three or more osteomas[52]. Conditional knockout of the Apc-gene resulted in supernumerary teeth in mice [57-59]. Notably, adult oral tissues, especially young adult tissues, are still responsive to the loss of Apc[60]. In old adult mice, supernumerary teeth can be induced on both labial and lingual sides of the incisors, which contain adult stem cells supporting the continuous growth of mouse incisors [60,61]. In young mice, supernumerary tooth germs were induced in multiple regions of the jaw in both incisor and molar regions. They can form directly from the oral epithelium, in the dental lamina connecting the developing molar or incisor tooth germ to the oral epithelium, in the crown region, as well as in the elongating and furcation area of the developing root [60].

The identification of mutations in RUNX2 causing an isolated dental phenotype in CCD and in APC causing FAP has attracted attention as a possible route towards inducing de novo tooth formation.

4. Supernumerary tooth formation in a mouse model

The number of teeth is usually strictly determined. Whereas evidence supporting a genetic etiology for tooth agenesis is well established, the etiology of supernumerary tooth formation is only partially understood in the mouse model (Table 3). Unlike humans, mice have only molars and incisors separated by a toothless region called the diastema. In addition, mice only have a single primary dentition and their teeth are not replaced. Therefore, mice may not be an optimal model for studying tooth replacement and supernumerary tooth formation [62]. Most of the reported mouse supernumerary teeth are located in the diastema region. This is not a *de novo* tooth formation but the rescue of vestigial tooth rudiments. During the early stages of tooth development, many transient vestigial dental buds develop in the diastema area. Some of them can develop into the bud stage, but later regress and disappear by apoptosis, or merge with the mesial crown of the first molar tooth [63-68]. Major signaling pathways regulating tooth development are also expressed in these vestigial dental buds. Modulation of these signals can rescue these vestigial tooth rudiments to develop into supernumerary diastema teeth [23]. A number of mutant mouse strains have been reported exhibiting supernumerary diastema teeth. Although the rudimentary tooth buds form in the embryonic diastema, they regress apoptically [69]. Transgenic mice in which the keratin 14 promoter directs Ectodysplasin (Eda), a member of the tumor necrosis factor (TNF) family of signaling molecules, or Eda receptor expression to the epithelium had supernumerary teeth mesial to the first molar as a result of diastema tooth development [70-72]. It has also been reported that Sprouty2 (Spry2) or Spry4 (which encode negative feedback regulators of fibroblast growth factor (FGF)) deficient mice showed supernumerary tooth formation as a result of diastema tooth development[73]. Hypomorphic Polaris mice and *Wnt-Cre* (Polaris conditional mutant mice with affected Shh signaling) [73-74], Pax6 mutant mice [75] and Gas1 null mutants [73] were also included. Uterine sensitization associated gene-1 (USAG-1) is a BMP antagonist, and also modulates Wnt signaling. We reported that USAG-1-deficient mice have supernumerary teeth (Figure 2).

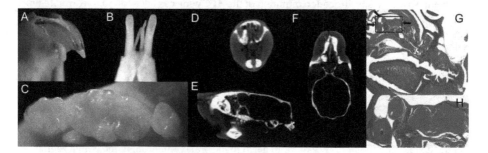

Figure 2. Supernumerary teeth formation in Sostdc 1 (USAG-1) (A-C) and CEBPB (D-H) adult mutant mice. A: Oblique view of the maxillary incisors. B: Occlusal view of the mandibular incisors. C: Occlusal view of the mandibular molars. Micro-CT images (D-F) and HE-staining (G,H) of the murine head. A frontal view (D), a sagittal view (E) and a horizontal view (F) showed supernumerary tooth (red arrow). Two supernumerary teeth and an odontoma were seen in a low (G) and a high (H) magnification.

Mutant mouse	Tooth phenotype	references
Sostdc1−/− (USAG-1, ectodin, Wise)	Supernumerary incisors in the maxilla and mandible Premolar mesial to first molar, peg-shaped tooth lingual to first molar	Munne et al., 2009; Ohazama et al., 2008; Yanagita et al., 2006; Murashima-Suginami et al., 2007, 2008.
CEBPB−/−	Supernumerary teeth and/or odontomas in the diastema between the incisor and the first molar	Huang et al., 2012.
Gas1−/−	Premolar mesial to first molar, both jaws (100% penetrance)	Ohazama et al., 2009.
Gas1−/−; Shh+/−	Mandibular molar (associated with jaw duplication)	Seppala et al., 2007.
Tg737orpk hypomorph	Premolar mesial to first molar, both jaws (100% penetrance)	Zhang et al., 2003; Ohazama et al., 2009,.
Wnt1-Cre; Polarisflox/flox	Premolar mesial to first molar, both jaws (100% penetrance)	Ohazama et al., 2009.
Spry2−/−	Premolar mesial to first molar; maxilla (>5%), mandible (97%: 92% bilateral; 5% unilateral)	Klein et al., 2006; Peterkova et al., 2009.
Spry4−/−	Both jaws? 16% penetrance (most unilateral)	Klein et al., 2006.
Lrp4−/− (Megf7) hypomorph	Supernumerary incisors in the maxilla and mandible Premolar mesial to first molar (varying penetrance in both jaws) Lingual peg-shaped tooth (maxilla, variable penetrance)	Ohazama et al., 2008.
Osr2−/−	Lingual molars	Zhang et al., 2009.
Epiprofin−/−	Multiple incisors and molars in both jaws	Nakamura et al., 2008.
K14-Cre; Apccko/cko	Multiple incisor and molar tooth buds	Kuraguchi et al., 2006.
K14-CreΔBm; Apccko/cko	Numerous labial and lingual incisor and molar teeth (↑ with age)	Wang et al., 2009.
K14-Cre1Amc; Apccko/cko	Numerous epithelial buds from E14.5	Wang et al., 2009.
K14-CreERTM; Apccko/cko	Numerous labial and lingual incisors (age P5–10/12)	Wang et al., 2009.
K14-CreERTM; Ctnb1(ex3)fl/+	Numerous labial and lingual incisors (age P5–6/12) P5 molar supernumeraries	Wang et al., 2009.
K14-Cre/+; β-cateninex3fl/+	Multiple incisor and molar epithelial invaginations in both jaws	Jarvinen et al., 2006.
K14-Cre; Ctnnb1(ex3)fl/+	Multiple molar epithelial invaginations	Liu et al., 2008.
K14-Lef1	Rudimentary teeth at inappropriate sites	Zhou et. Al., 1995.
Pax6Sey	Incisor supernumeraries: 35% unilateral; 45% bilateral incisors	Kaufman et al., 1995.
K14-Eda	Premolar mesial to first molar; incomplete penetrance	Kangas et al., 2004; Mustonen et al., 2003.
K14-Edar	Premolar mesial to first molar; incomplete penetrance	Tucker et al., 2004.
Tabby+/−	Molar (2.5%; mandible > maxilla)	Gruneberg et al., 1966; Sofaer et al., 1969.
B6CBACa-Aw−J/A-EdaTa/0	Molar (1%; mandible >maxilla)	Peterkova et al., 2005.
di	Mandibular incisors (right > left)	Danforth et al., 1958.
β-catΔex3K14/+	Supernumerary molars in the maxilla and mandible	Järvinen, E., 2006

Table 3. Mutant mouse associated with supernumerary teeth

The supernumerary maxillary incisor appears to form as a result of the successive development of the rudimentary upper incisor. USAG-1 abrogation rescued apoptotic elimination of odontogenic mesenchymal cells [14]. BMP signaling in the rudimentary maxillary incisor, assessed by expressions of Msx1 and Dlx2 and the phosphorylation of Smad protein, was significantly enhanced. Wnt signaling, as demonstrated by the nuclear localization of β-catenin, was also up-regulated. The inhibition of BMP signaling rescues supernumerary tooth formation in E15 incisor explant culture. Based upon these results, we conclude that enhanced BMP signaling results in supernumerary teeth and BMP signaling was modulated by Wnt signaling in the USAG-1-deficient mouse model (Figure 3) [76]. Canonical Wnt/β-catenin signaling and its down-stream molecule Lef-1 are essential for tooth development [77].

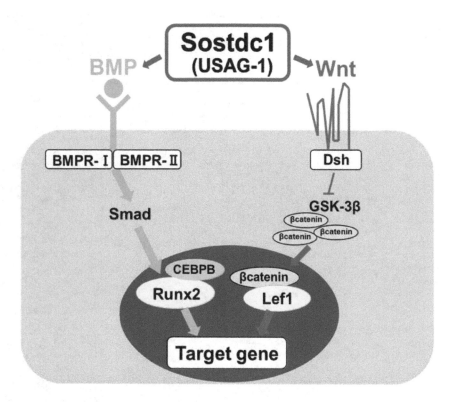

Figure 3. Diagrammatic representation of the Sostdc (USAG-1) pathway during development

Overexpression of Lef-1 under the control of the K14 promoter in transgenic mice leads to the development abnormal invaginations of the dental epithelium in the mesenchyme and formation of a tooth-like structure [78]. *De novo* supernumerary teeth arising directly from the primary tooth germ or dental lamina have been reported in *Apc* loss-of-function (as discussed in the previous section) or β-catenin gain-of-function mice, and *Sp6* (*Epiprofin*)-deficient mice. It was demonstrated that mouse tooth buds expressing stabilized β-catenin give rise to extra teeth[58] (Jarvinen et al., 2006). More recently, Epiprofin (Epfn) (a zinc finger transcription factor belonging to the Sp transcription factor superfamily)-deficient mice developed an excess number of teeth[79]. Mammals only have one row of teeth in each jaw. Interestingly, in the *Osr2* null mutant mouse embryo, supernumerary tooth germs were found developing directly from the oral epithelium lingual to their molar tooth germs [80]. More recently, we also demonstrated that CEBPB deficiency was related to the formation of supernumerary teeth[81]. A total of 66.7% of CEBPB$^{-/-}$ 12-month-olds sustained supernumerary teeth and/or odontomas in the diastema between the incisor and the first molar. Two supernumerary teeth accompanied with a complex odontoma near the root of the upper right incisor were identified in a CEBPB$^{-/-}$ adult (Figure 2), whilst two other CEBPB-/- mice simply showed a supernumerary tooth in the upper left quadrant. Another CEBPB$^{-/-}$ adult mouse did not display any supernumerary teeth in either jaw, but an odontoma in the lower-right quadrant. All of the CEBPB$^{-/-}$ adults appeared with a normal number of erupted incisors and molars. Nevertheless, 20%of the CEBPB$^{+/-}$ 12-month-olds hada missing lower third molar. Dental anomalies such as supernumerary teeth, odontomas, or hypodontia were not found in mice of any other genotypes and/or age[81].

These mouse models clearly demonstrated that it was possible to induce *de novo* tooth formation by the in situ repression or activation of single candidate gene such as USAG-1.

5. Gene therapy approaches

Gene therapy provides a unique tool for the delivery of previously identified signaling molecules in both time and space that may significantly augment our progress toward clinical tooth regeneration. Stimulation of the formation of a third dentition and gene-manipulated tooth regeneration comprise an attractive concept (Figure 4). This approach is generally presented in terms of adding molecules to induce *de novo* tooth initiation in the mouth. It might be combined with gene-manipulated tooth regeneration; that is, endogenous dental cells *in situ* can be activated or repressed by a gene-delivery technique to make a tooth. We have a chance to access the formation of the third dentition in the mouth, because the time of appearance of the third dentition seems to be after birth. As the half-life of targeted proteins in vivo is transient, tooth regeneration is not a common outcome following conventional therapy. Typically, high concentrations are required to promote regeneration [82]). Therefore, supplemental local production via gene transfer could be superior to bolus delivery methods.

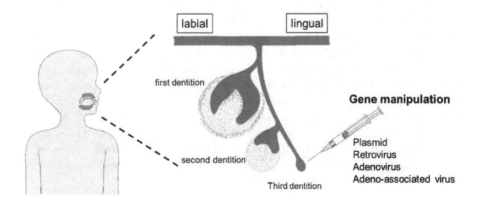

Figure 4. *In vivo* gene delivery approach for the tooth regeneration by stimulation of a third dentition.

Simply stated, gene therapy consists of the insertion of genes into an individual's cells directly or indirectly with a matrix to promote a specific biological effect. Gene therapy can be used to induce a more favorable host response. Targeting cells for gene therapy requires the use of vectors or direct delivery methods to transfect them. To overcome the short half-lives of peptides in vivo, gene therapy that uses a vector that encodes the candidate genes is utilized to stimulate the formation of the third dentition. The two main strategies of gene vector delivery have been applied. Gene vectors can be introduced directly to the target site (*in vivo* gene delivery) [83] or selected cells can be harvested, expanded, genetically transduced, and then reimplanted (*ex vivo* gene delivery). *In vivo* gene transfer involves the insertion of the gene of interest directly into the body, anticipating the genetic modification of the target cells. *Ex vivo* gene transfer includes the incorporation of genetic material into cells exposed from a tissue biopsy with subsequent reimplantation into the recipient. So far, *in vivo* gene delivery has been a suitable gene therapy approach in tooth regeneration by stimulation of the third dentition, but *ex vivo* gene delivery is not realistic because of the poor availability of ideal cells.

Gene transfer is accomplished through the use of viral and nonviral vectors. The three main classes of virus used for gene therapy are the retrovirus, adenovirus, and adenoassociated viruses. Retroviruses are ideal for long-term gene therapy since, once introduced, their DNA integrates and becomes part of the genome of the host cells. Indeed, the current human genome contains up to 5 to 8% of endogenous retroviral sequences that have been acquired over the course of evolution [84]. Adenoviruses are more commonly suited for short-term gene delivery and are highly targeted for tissue engineering strategies that desire protein production over the course of several weeks. Efficient adenovirus-directed gene delivery to odontogenic mesenchymal cells derived from cranial neural crest cells was reported [85,86]. In addition, because the adenovirus is well-known as the "virus of the common cold," infection is generally nontoxic and self-limiting. However, determination of the genotoxicity for each specific application is necessary to keep the safety profile within acceptable parameters. Adenoassociated viruses have become the focus of much research in recent years because of their complete inability to replicate without a helper virus, potential for tissue-specific targeting, and gene expression in the order of months to years. The ability to specifically target one tissue type without adverse effects on neighboring tissues is highly desired in fields such as tooth regeneration. On the other hand, nonviral methods are safe and do not require immunosuppression for successful gene delivery, but suffer from lower transfection efficiencies. DNA injection followed by application of electric fields (electroporation) has been more effective for introducing DNA than the use of simple DNA injection [87]. However, this method involves the concern that the electric pulse causes tissue damage. Recently, we reported that gene transfer using an ultra-fine needle [88], in addition to microbubbles enhanced transcutaneous sonoporation [87].

In vivo gene delivery seems to be a suitable gene therapy approach in tooth regeneration by stimulation of the third dentition.

6. Conclusion

We have a chance to access the formation of the third dentition in the mouth, because the timing of the appearance of the third dentition seems to be after birth. The identification of mutations in *RUNX2* causing an isolated dental phenotype in CCD and supernumerary tooth formation in the mouse model clearly demonstrated that it was possible to induce *de novo* tooth formation by the in situ repression or activation of a single candidate gene. These results support the idea that the *de novo* repression or activation of candidate genes such as RUNX2 or USAG-1 might be used to stimulate the third dentition in order to induce new tooth formation in the mouse (Figure 4). *In vivo* gene delivery seems to be a suitable gene therapy approach in tooth regeneration by stimulation of the third dentition.

Acknowledgement

This work was supported by Grant-in-Aid for Scientific Research(C):22592213 and Grant-in-Aid for JSPS Fellows:02109741.

Author details

Katsu Takahashi[1], Honoka Kiso[1], Kazuyuki Saito[1], Yumiko Togo[1], Hiroko Tsukamoto[1], Boyen Huang[2] and Kazuhisa Bessho[1]

1 Department of Oral and Maxillofacial Surgery, Graduate School of Medicine, Kyoto University, Sakyo-ku, Kyoto, Japan

2 Department of Paediatric Dentistry, School of Medicine and Dentistry, James Cook University, Cairns, Australia

References

[1] Ohazama A, Modino SA, Miletich I, Sharpe PT. Stem-cell-based tissue engineering of murine teeth. J Dent Res 2004;83(7):518-522.

[2] Duailibi MT, Duailibi SE, Young CS, Bartlett JD, Vacanti JP, Yelick PC. Bioengineered teeth from cultured rat tooth bud cells. J Dent Res 2004;83(7):523-528.

[3] Young CS, Abukawa H, Asrican R, Ravens M, Troulis MJ, Kaban LB, Vacanti JP, Yelick PC. Tissue-engineered hybrid tooth and bone. Tissue Eng 2005;11(9-10): 1599-1610.

[4] Edwards PC, Mason JM. Gene-enhanced tissue engineering for dental hard tissue re-generation: (1) overview and practical considerations. Head Face Med2006;2:12.

[5] Sartaj R, Sharpe P. Biological tooth replacement. J Anat2006;209(4):503-509.

[6] Nakao K, Morita R, Saji Y, Ishida K, Tomita Y, Ogawa M, Saitoh M, Tomooka Y, Tsuji T. The development of a bioengineered organ germ method. Nat Methods.2007;4(3): 227-230.

[7] Ferreira CF, Magini RS, Sharpe PT. Biological tooth replacement and repair. J Oral Rehabil2007;34(12):933-939.

[8] Yu J, Shi J, Jin Y. Current Approaches and Challenges in Making a Bio-Tooth. Tissue Eng Part B Rev2008;14(3):307-319.

[9] Takahashi, K., Sakata, T., Murashima-Suginami, A., Tsukamoto, H., Kiso, H. and Bes-sho, K. Tooth regeneration: Potential for stimulation of the formation of a third denti-tion by one gene. Current Topics in Genetics 2008;3: 77-82.

[10] Thesleff I, Sharpe P. Signalling networks regulating dental development. MechDev 1997;67(2):111-123.

[11] Chai Y, Slavkin HC. Prospects for tooth regeneration in the 21st century: a perspec-tive. Microsc Res Tech2003;60(5):469-479.

[12] ThesleffI. The genetic basis of tooth development and dental defects. Am J Med Gen-et A2006;140(23):2530-2535.

[13] Jensen BL, Kreiborg S. Development of the dentition in cleidocranial dysplasia. J Oral Pathol Med 1990;19(2):89-93.

[14] Murashima-Suginami A, Takahashi K, Kawabata T, Sakata T, Tsukamoto H, Sugai M, Yanagita M, Shimizu A, Sakurai T, Slavkin HC, Bessho K. Rudiment incisors sur-vive and erupt as supernumerary teeth as a result of USAG-1 abrogation. Biochem. Biophys. Res. Commun 2007;359(3):549-555.

[15] Ooë T. Epithelial anlagen of human third dentition and their migrations in the man-dible and maxilla. OkajimasFolAnatJap 1969; 46(5):243-251.

[16] Hillson S. Teeth. Cambridge:Cambridge University Press; 1986.

[17] Leche W. Studienuber die Entwicklung des Zahnsstemsbei den Saugetieren. Morph Jb 1893;19: 502-574.

[18] Rose C. Uberesteeinervorzeitigenpralaktealen und einerviertenZahnreihebeim Men-schen. Oester-ungarViertjschrZhik 1895;11:45-50.

[19] Ahrens H. Entwicklung der menschlichenZahne. AnatHefte 1913;48:169-267

[20] Järvinen E, Tummers M, Thesleff I. The role of the dental lamina in mammalian tooth replacement. J ExpZool B MolDevEvol2009 ;312B(4):281-291.

[21] Koussoulakou DS, Margaritis LH, Koussoulakos SL. A curriculum vitae of teeth: evolution, generation, regeneration.Int J BiolSci2009;5(3):226-243.

[22] Mikkola ML. Controlling the number of tooth rows. Sci Signal2009;2(85):pe53.

[23] Tummers M, Thesleff I. The importance of signal pathway modulation in all aspects of tooth development. J ExpZool B MolDevEvol2009;312B(4):309-319

[24] Handrigan GR, Leung KJ, Richman JM. Identification of putative dental epithelial stem cells in a lizard with life-long tooth replacement. Development2010;137(21): 3545-3549.

[25] Garvey MT, Barry HJ, Blake M. Supernumerary teeth--an overview of classification, diagnosis and management. J Can Dent Assoc1999;65(11):612-616

[26] Liu DG, Zhang WL, Zhang ZY, Wu YT, Ma XC. Three-dimensional evaluations of supernumerary teeth using cone-beam computed tomography for 487 cases. Oral Surg Oral Med Oral Pathol Oral RadiolEndod2007;103(3):403-11.

[27] Díaz A, Orozco J, Fonseca M. Multiple hyperodontia: report of a case with 17 supernumerary teeth with non syndromic association. Med Oral Patol Oral Cir Bucal2009;14(5):E229-31.

[28] Ferrés-Padró E, Prats-Armengol J, Ferrés-Amat E. A descriptive study of 113 unerupted supernumerary teeth in 79 pediatric patients in Barcelona. Med Oral Patol Oral Cir Bucal2009;14(3):E146-52

[29] Yusof WZ. Non-syndrome multiple supernumerary teeth: literature review. J Can Dent Assoc1990;56(2):147-149.

[30] Batra P, Duggal R, Parkash H. Non-syndromic multiple supernumerary teeth transmitted as an autosomal dominant trait. J Oral Pathol Med2005;34(10):621-625.

[31] Orhan AI, Ozer L, Orhan K. Familial occurrence of nonsyndromal multiple supernumerary teeth. A rare condition. Angle Orthod 2006;76(5):891-897.

[32] Hyun HK, Lee SJ, Ahn BD, Lee ZH, Heo MS, Seo BM, Kim JW. Nonsyndromic multiple mandibular supernumerary premolars. J Oral MaxillofacSurg2008;66(7): 1366-1369.

[33] Yagüe-García J, Berini-Aytés L, Gay-Escoda C. Multiple supernumerary teeth not associated with complex syndromes: a retrospective study.Med Oral Patol Oral Cir Bucal 2009;14(7):E331-336

[34] Inchingolo F, Tatullo M, Abenavoli FM, Marrelli M, Inchingolo AD, Gentile M, Inchingolo AM, Dipalma G. Non-syndromic multiple supernumerary teeth in a family unit with a normal karyotype: case report.Int J Med Sci 2010;7(6):378-384.

[35] Zhu JF, Marcushamer M, King DL, Henry RJ. Supernumerary and congenitally absent teeth: a literature review. J ClinPediatr Dent1996;20(2):87-95.

[36] Ida, M., Nakamura, T., and Utsunomiya, J. Osteomatous changes and tooth abnormalities found in the jaw of patients with adenomatosis coli. Oral Surg. Oral Med. Oral Pathol 1981;52(1), 2-11.

[37] Shafer, W. G., Hine, M. K., and Levi, B. M.Textbook of oral pathology 4th Ed. Philadelphia:WB Saunders Co;1983.

[38] Jensen, B. L., and Kreiborg, S. Craniofacial growth in cleidocranial dysplasia--a roentgencephalometric study. J Craniofac Genet DeveBiol 1995;15(1): 35-43.

[39] Lee B, Thirunavukkarasu K, Zhou L, Pastore L, Baldini A, Hecht J, Geoffroy V, Ducy P, Karsenty G. Misense mutations abolishing DNA binding of the osteoblast-specific transcription factor OSF2/CBFA1 in cleidocranial dysplasia, Nature Genetics 1997 ; 16(3): 307-310.

[40] Mundlos S, Otto F, Mundlos C, Mulliken JB, Aylsworth AS, Albright S, Lindhout D, Cole WG, Henn W, Knoll JH, Owen MJ, Mertelsmann R, Zabel BU, Olsen BR. Mutations involving the transcription factor CBFA1 cause cleidocranial dysplasia. Cell 1997; 89(5): 773-779.

[41] Zhou G, Chen Y, Zhou L, Thirunavukkarasu K, Hecht J, Chitayat D, Gelb BD, Pirinen S, Berry SA, Greenberg CR, Karsenty G, Lee B. CBFA1 mutation analysis and functional correlation with phenotypic variability in cleidocranial dysplasia, Hum Mol Genet 1999; 8(12): 2311-2316.

[42] Quack I, Vonderstrass B, Stock M, Aylsworth AS, Becker A, Brueton L, Lee PJ, Majewski F, Mulliken JB, Suri M, Zenker M, Mundlos S, Otto F. Mutation analysis of core biding factor A1 in patients with cleidocranial dysplasia. Am J hum Genet 1999; 65(5): 1268-1278.

[43] Yoshida T, Kanegane H, Osato M, Yanagida M, Miyawaki T, Ito Y, Shigesada K. Functional analysis of RUNX2 mutations in Japanese patients with cleidocranial dysplasia demonstrates novel genotype-phenotype correlations. Am J Hum Genet2002;71(4):724-738.

[44] Baumert U, Golan I, Redlich M, Aknin JJ, Muessig D. Cleidocranial dysplasia: molecular genetic analysis and phenotypic-based description of a Middle European patient group. Am J Med Genet A2005;139A(2):78-85.

[45] Yoshida T, Kanegane H, Osato M, Yanagida M, Miyawaki T, Ito Y, Shigesada K. Functional analysis of RUNX2 mutations in cleidocranial dysplasia: novel insights into genotype-phenotype correlations. Blood Cells Mol Dis 2003;30(2):184-193.

[46] [46] Aberg T, Cavender A, Gaikwad JS, Bronckers AL, Wang X, Waltimo-Sirén J, Thesleff I, D'Souza RN. Phenotypic changes in dentition of Runx2 homozygote-null mutant mice. J HistochemCytochem2004;52(1):131-139.

[47] Wang XP, Aberg T, James MJ, Levanon D, Groner Y, Thesleff I. Runx2 (Cbfa1) inhibits Shh signaling in the lower but not upper molars of mouse embryos and prevents the budding of putative successional teeth. J Dent Res2005;84(2):138-143.

[48] Otto F, Thornell AP, Crompton T, Denzel A, Gilmour KC, Rosewell IR, Stamp GW, Beddington RS, Mundlos S, Olsen BR, Selby PB, Owen MJ. Cbfa1, a candidate gene for cleidocranial dysplasia syndrome, is essential for osteoblast differentiation and bone development. Cell1997;89(5):765-771.

[49] Gardner EJ, Richards RC. Multiple cutaneous and subcutaneous lesions occurring simultaneously with hereditary polyposis and osteomatosis. Am J Hum Genet1953;5(2):139-147.

[50] Chimenos-Küstner E, Pascual M, Blanco I, Finestres F. Hereditary familial polyposis and Gardner's syndrome: contribution of the odonto-stomatology examination in its diagnosis and a case description. Med Oral Patol Oral Cir Bucal2005;10(5):402-409.

[51] Ramaglia L, Morgese F, Filippella M, Colao A. Oral and maxillofacial manifestations of Gardner's syndrome associated with growth hormone deficiency: case report and literature review. Oral Surg Oral Med Oral Pathol Oral RadiolEndod2007;103(6):e30-34.

[52] Wijn MA, Keller JJ, Giardiello FM, Brand HS. Oral and maxillofacial manifestations of familial adenomatous polyposis. Oral Dis2007;13(4):360-365.

[53] Okamoto M, Sato C, Kohno Y, Mori T, Iwama T, Tonomura A, Miki Y, Utsunomiya J, Nakamura Y, White R, et al. Molecular nature of chromosome 5q loss in colorectal tumors and desmoids from patients with familial adenomatous polyposis. Hum Genet1990;85(6):595-599.

[54] Groden J, Thliveris A, Samowitz W, Carlson M, Gelbert L, Albertsen H, Joslyn G, Stevens J, Spirio L, Robertson M, et al. Identification and characterization of the familial adenomatous polyposis coli gene. Cell 1991;66(3):589-600.

[55] Heinen CD. Genotype to phenotype: analyzing the effects of inherited mutations in colorectal cancer families. Mutat Res2010;693(1-2):32-45.

[56] Phelps RA, Broadbent TJ, Stafforini DM, Jones DA. New perspectives on APC control of cell fate and proliferation in colorectal cancer. Cell Cycle2009;8(16):2549-2556

[57] Kuraguchi M, Wang XP, Bronson RT, Rothenberg R, Ohene-Baah NY, Lund JJ, Kucherlapati M, Maas RL, Kucherlapati R. Adenomatous polyposis coli (APC) is required for normal development of skin and thymus. PLoS Genet2006;2(9):e146.

[58] Järvinen E, Salazar-Ciudad I, Birchmeier W, Taketo MM, Jernvall J, Thesleff I. Continuous tooth generation in mouse is induced by activated epithelial Wnt/beta-catenin signaling. ProcNatlAcadSci U S A 2006;103(49):18627-18632.

[59] Liu F, Chu EY, Watt B, Zhang Y, Gallant NM, Andl T, Yang SH, Lu MM, Piccolo S, Schmidt-Ullrich R, Taketo MM, Morrisey EE, Atit R, Dlugosz AA, Millar SE. Wnt/beta-catenin signaling directs multiple stages of tooth morphogenesis. DevBiol2008;313(1):210-224.

[60] Wang XP, O'Connell DJ, Lund JJ, Saadi I, Kuraguchi M, Turbe-Doan A, Cavallesco R, Kim H, Park PJ, Harada H, Kucherlapati R, Maas RL. Apc inhibition of Wnt signaling

regulates supernumerary tooth formation during embryogenesis and throughout adulthood. Development2009;136(11):1939-1949.

[61] Liu F, Dangaria S, Andl T, Zhang Y, Wright AC, Damek-Poprawa M, Piccolo S, Nagy A, Taketo MM, Diekwisch TG, Akintoye SO, Millar SE beta-Catenin initiates tooth neogenesis in adult rodent incisors. J Dent Res2010;89(9):909-914.

[62] Huysseune A, Thesleff I. Continuous tooth replacement: the possible involvement of epithelial stem cells. Bioessays2004;26(6):665-671.

[63] Peterková R, Peterka M, Viriot L, Lesot H. Development of the vestigial tooth primordia as part of mouse odontogenesis. Connect Tissue Res2002;43(2-3):120-128.

[64] Peterková R, Lesot H, Viriot L, Peterka M. The supernumerary cheek tooth in tabby/EDA mice-a reminiscence of the premolar in mouse ancestors. Arch Oral Biol 2005;50(2):219-225.

[65] Peterkova R, Churava S, Lesot H, Rothova M, Prochazka J, Peterka M, Klein OD. Revitalization of a diastemal tooth primordium in Spry2 null mice results from increased proliferation and decreased apoptosis. J ExpZool B MolDevEvol2009;312B(4): 292-308.

[66] Prochazka J, Pantalacci S, Churava S, Rothova M, Lambert A, Lesot H, Klein O, Peterka M, Laudet V, Peterkova R. Patterning by heritage in mouse molar row development. ProcNatlAcadSci U S A2010;107(35):15497-15502

[67] Viriot L, Peterková R, Peterka M, Lesot H. Evolutionary implications of the occurrence of two vestigial tooth germs during early odontogenesis in the mouse lower jaw. Connect Tissue Res 2002;43(2-3):129-133.

[68] Witter K, Lesot H, Peterka M, Vonesch JL, Mísek I, Peterková R Origin and developmental fate of vestigial tooth primordia in the upper diastema of the field vole (Microtusagrestis, Rodentia). Arch Oral Biol2005;50(4):401-409.

[69] Keranen SV, Kettunen P, Aberg T,Thesleff T,Jernvall T. Gene expression patterns associated with suppression of odontogenesis in mouse and vole diastema region, Dev. Genes Evol 1999;209(8): 495-506.

[70] Mustonen T, Pispa J, Mikkola ML, Pummila M, Kangas AT, Pakkasjärvi L, Jaatinen R, Thesleff I. Stimulation of ectodermal organ development by Ectodysplasin-A1. DevBiol2003;259(1):123-136.

[71] Pispa J, Mustonen T, Mikkola ML, Kangas AT, Koppinen P, Lukinmaa PL, Jernvall J, Thesleff I. Tooth patterning and enamel formation can be manipulated by misexpression of TNF receptor Edar. DevDyn2004;231(2):432-440.

[72] Tucker AS, Headon DJ, Courtney JM, Overbeek P, Sharpe PT. The activation level of the TNF family receptor, Edar, determines cusp number and tooth number during tooth development. DevBiol2004;268(1):185-194.

[73] OD. Klein, G. Minowada, R. Peterkova, A. Kangas, BD. Yu, H. Lesot , M. Peterka, J. Jernvall, GR. Martin, Sprouty genes control diastema tooth development via bidirevtional antagonism of epithelial-messenchymal FGF signaling,Dev.Cell 2006;11(2): 181-190.

[74] Ohazama A, Haycraft CJ, Seppala M, Blackburn J, Ghafoor S, Cobourne M, Martinelli DC, Fan CM, Peterkova R, Lesot H, Yoder BK, Sharpe PT. Primary cilia regulate Shh activity in the control of molar tooth number. Development2009;136(6):897-903.

[75] Zhang Q, Murcia NS, Chittenden LR, Richards WG, Michaud EJ, Woychik RP, Yoder BK. Loss of the Tg737 protein results in skeletal patterning defects.DevDyn2003 ; 227(1):78-90.

[76] Kaufman MH, Chang HH, Shaw JP. Craniofacial abnormalities in homozygous Small eye (Sey/Sey) embryos and newborn mice. JAnat1995;186 (Pt 3):607-617.

[77] Murashima-Suginami A, Takahashi K, Sakata T, Tsukamoto H, Sugai M, Yanagita M, Shimizu A, Sakurai T, Slavkin HC, Bessho K. Enhanced BMP signaling results in supernumerary tooth formation in USAG-1 deficient mouse. BiochemBiophys Res Commun2008;369(4):1012-1016.

[78] Kratochwil K, Dull M, Farinas I, Galceran J, Grosschedl R. Lef1 expression is activated by BMP-4 and regulates inductive tissue interactions in tooth and hair development. Genes Dev1996;10(11):1382-1394.

[79] Zhou P, Byrne C, Jacobs J, Fuchs E. Lymphoid enhancer factor 1 directs hair follicle patterning and epithelial cell fate. Genes Dev1995;9(6):700-713.

[80] Nakamura T, de Vega S, Fukumoto S, Jimenez L, Unda F, Yamada Y. Transcription factor epiprofin is essential for tooth morphogenesis by regulating epithelial cell fate and tooth number. J Biolchem2008;283(8):4825-4833.

[81] Zhang Z, Lan Y, Chai Y, Jiang R. Antagonistic actions of Msx1 and Osr2 pattern mammalian teeth into a single row. Science2009;323(5918):1232-1234.

[82] Huang B, Takahashi K, Sakata-Goto T, Kiso H, Togo Y, Saito K, Tsukamoto H, Sugai M, Akira A, Shimizu A, Bessho K. Phenotypes of CEBPB Deficiency: Supernumerary Teeth and Elongated Coronoid Process. Oral Dis 2012; in press,

[83] Fang J, Zhu YY, Smiley E, Bonadio J, Rouleau JP, Goldstein SA, McCauley LK, Davidson BL, Roessler BJ. Stimulation of new bone formation by direct transfer of osteogenic plasmid genes. ProcNatlAcadSci USA 1996;93(12):5753-5758.

[84] Jin Q, Anusaksathien O, Webb SA, Printz MA, Giannobile WV. Engineering of tooth-supporting structures by delivery of PDGF gene therapy vectors. MolTher2004 ;9(4): 519-526.

[85] Lander ES, Linton LM, Birren B, Nusbaum C, Zody MC, Baldwin J, Devon K, Dewar K, Doyle M, FitzHugh W, Funke R, Gage D, Harris K, Heaford A, et al. Initial sequencing and analysis of the human genome. Nature2001;409(6822):860-921.

[86] Takahashi, K., Nuckolls, G.H., Tanaka, O., Semba, I., Takahashi, I., Dashner,R., Shum, L. Slavkin, H.C. Adenovirus mediated ectopic expression of Msx2 in even-numbered rhombomeres cause apoptotic elimination of cranial neural crest cells en ovo. Development 1998;125(9), 1627-1635.

[87] Takahashi K, Nuckolls GH, Takahashi I, Nonaka K, Nagata M, Ikura T, Slavkin HC and Shum L. Msx2 is a repressor of chondrogenic differentiation in migratory crainal neural crest cells. DevDyn 2001, 222(2), 252-262.

[88] Aihara H, Miyazaki J. Gene transfer into muscle by electroporation in vivo. Nat Biotechnol 1998;16(9):867-870.

[89] Osawa K, Okubo Y, Nakao K, Koyama N, Bessho K. Osteoinduction by microbubble-enhanced transcutaneous sonoporation of human bone morphogenetic protein-2. J Gene Med2009;11(7):633-641.

[90] Osawa K, Okubo Y, Nakao K, Koyama N, Bessho K. Feasibility of BMP-2 gene therapy using an ultra-fine needle. In: You Y. (ed.) Targets in Gene Therapy. Rijeka:InTech; 2011.p159-166

Chapter 13

Gene Therapy Perspectives Against Diseases of the Respiratory System

Dimosthenis Lykouras, Kiriakos Karkoulias,
Christos Tourmousoglou, Efstratios Koletsis,
Kostas Spiropoulos and Dimitrios Dougenis

Additional information is available at the end of the chapter

1. Introduction

Gene therapy uses a variety of techniques as the introduction of a normal allele of a gene in cases where the cell does not express the gene or in other cases where the gene is under-expressed. In order to achieve effective gene therapy for a specific gene in a certain type of cells a lot of work is needed. More specifically the following steps are essential: 1. Isolation of target gene, 2. Development of a specific gene vector, 3. Specification of the target cell, 4. Definition of route of administration, and 5. Identification of other potential uses of the gene.

The value of gene of gene therapy is often discussed, especially in some diseases who have a known protein defect and the protein itself can be produced in a large scale and could then be administered to the patient. Genetic engineering could be beneficial in the production of the target protein. Nevertheless, the infusion of the protein is not curative, because of the half-life of the protein itself and the growth factors that are essential.

In order to isolate a specific gene, it is essential to produce a cDNA library that contains the total number of unique genes expressed in a specific tissue. The DNA contained in a cDNA library is not genomic, therefore it contains only the encoding sequences of the DNA.

The standard procedure of the construction of a cDNA library includes 1) isolation of the total amount of mRNA that is produced in the target cells, 2) Hybridization using a multi-T promoter, 3) Synthesis of complementary DNA (cDNA) to the mRNA prototype using the enzyme reverse transcriptase, 4) Degradation of the mRNA by the means of an alkali, 5) Synthesis of the second DNA strand using nucleotides and the enzyme DNA polymerase.

The cDNA library contains only the exons of the genes that are expressed in the specific tissue; therefore the cDNA can show the activity of the studied tissue.

As soon as the isolation of the gene that is to be administered to the patient is achieved, an appropriate vector is needed in order to deliver the gene to the target cells. The most important vectors that are generally used in gene therapy applications in order to perform transfection of the targeted cellular population are:

1. Plasmids which are well-tolerated and safe, but transfer towards the nucleus is not so easy

2. Adeno-virus which may transfect differentiating as well as stale cells and have a very good percentage of transfection, but is not inserted in the nucleus and there is a possibility of reaction against the adeno-virus

3. Retro-virus which are inserted in the genome and are stable during transport, but they can only used in transfection of multiplying cells

4. Lenti-virus which is a subtype of retro-virus that may be inserted in stable cells and it is quite stable during the procedure

5. AAV (adeno-associated-based vector) which is inserted in the genome, is quite stable during the procedure and stable cells can be transfected as well, but only 4,7 kb can be inserted and there is a possibility of mutations

6. Liposomes – Oligonucleotides (ODN-based) which are very easy to use, selective for the endothelium, special alterations can improve the availability and reduce toxicity

The target cell has to be defined carefully in order to achieve the best curative result. In the case of gene therapy in the lung, the airway epithelia or even the lung vasculature may be efficient cellular targets.

The route of administration has to be defined so as the target gene is transported to the target cells in order to perform the transfection of the target tissue cells.

The use of a target gene in the therapy of a certain condition of the lung does not exclude a possible use of the gene in another therapeutic strategy, where there is a similar pathophysiology (e.g. inflammation). Therefore, the identification of other potential uses of the target gene is always important.

2. Gene therapy in cystic fibrosis

Gene therapy is still far from becoming a curative treatment for cystic fibrosis (CF). Despite the outstanding technological and medical progress there is still number of interesting genetic, biological, pharmaceutical and ethical problems. Only when these issues are to be solved will gene therapy become an option for the treatment of CF.

As for the biology of CF, the cystic fibrosis transmembrane conductance regulator (CFTR) is expressed in airway epithelia, on the luminal side of the plasma membrane, where it plays an important role as a phosphorylation-regulated Cl– channel and a regulator of channels and transporters [1, 2]. More specifically, the activation of CFTR results in a parallel inhibition of the epithelial Na+ channel (ENaC), which is lost when CFTR is absent or not functioning. There is a so called "low volume" hypothesis, which suggests that a loss of Cl– secretion and an increase in Na+ absorption reduce the thickness of the airway surface liquid (ASL), thus impairing mucociliary clearance [3]. Moreover, a reduction in the secretion of bicarbonates (mediated by the CFTR) might affect the hydration of the secreted mucus, thus altering its physical properties [4]. CFTR is also expressed in submucosal glands in the airways, which mainly participate in host defence. A loss of CFTR function in duct-lining serous cells prevents the secretion of mucus and anti-microbial factors by submucosal glands [5].

Since the discovery of the cystic fibrosis transmembrane conductance regulator (CFTR) gene in 1989, it was thought that scientists could prevent or delay the onset or even the progression of lung disease by using gene transfer. Although loss of CFTR function may affect a great number of different cells and tissues, progressive lung disease is responsible for the rates of morbidity and mortality. Therefore, the efforts of gene therapy have focused so far on gene transfer to the airways. CFTR is expressed in various epithelial cells in the lumen and in submucosal glands of the airways, where the mRNA is expressed [6, 7].

The fact that CF is an autosomal recessive disease lead to the idea that the delivery of a CFTR cDNA to the airway epithelium with a viral or non-viral vector could have beneficial effect. The delivery method could be either direct instillation or aerosol delivery. Furthermore, early studies indicated that the transfection of 6–10% of CF epithelia generated wild-type levels of chloride transport in vitro [8].

The selection of targets cells for gene therapy in CF is still controversial. The available strategies suggest correcting cells of the surface epithelium, the submucosal glands, or both [9, 10, 11]. The CFTR is expressed in the airways, including ciliated cells within the surface epithelium and a subpopulation of cells in submucosal gland ducts and acini. There are several epithelial cell types in the lung that seem to have progenitor functions, thus allowing long-term correction if these cells are targeted with selected vectors [12]. Experiments from several species and model systems have revealed potential progenitor populations, including: basal cells [13] and non-ciliated columnar cells of the airways [14, 15], submucosal gland epithelia [16], Clara cells [17] and alveolar type II cells in the distal lung.

Many viral and nonviral vectors have been tested for their usefulness in CF gene therapy. Adenoviral (AV) vectors have as a great disadvantage their low transduction efficiency of human airway epithelia and by their induction of strong immune responses [18]. In contrast adeno-associated viral (AAV) vectors may lead to long-term gene transfer and expression in bronchial epithelia of rabbits and nonhuman primates.

In addition to the DNA viruses, AV and AAV, various RNA viruses have been investigated for uses in airway gene transfer. Murine parainfluenza virus type 1, human respiratory syncytial virus (RSV) and human parainfluenza virus type 3 (PIV3) can effectively transfect airway epithelial cells by attaching to sialic acid and cholesterol [19], which are found on the apical surface of these cells. These viruses replicate in the cytoplasm and do not seem to cause mutagenesis during the insertion in DNA. Although RSV and PIV3 are human pathogens, SeV, the only RNA virus for which efficiency has been assessed in vivo, is not. However, gene expression mediated by recombinant SeV-based vectors needs repeated administration, which does not seem feasible because of the development of neutralizing antibodies against the vector itself [20].

Lentiviral (LV) vectors derived from human immunodeficiency virus type 1 (HIV-1) and feline immunodeficiency virus (FIV) are integrating retroviruses which can be adequately utilized to achieve efficient transfection of airway epithelia [21].

Among the many nonviral gene therapy vectors investigated so far, GL67 ([Cholest-5-en-3-ol(3b)- 3-[(3-aminopropyl)[4-[(3-aminopropyl)amino]butyl] carbamate]) has emerged as a promising lipid for efficient lung transfection [22].

Finally, mRNA-based nonviral gene transfer is a new strategy in order to express the CFTR in target cells [23]. By the use of mRNA instead of plasmid DNA as the transgene, transfection efficacy depends on the cytoplasmic expression machinery. However, when compared to DNA, much less is known about immune responses to RNA, although responses to both seem to be mediated by Toll-like receptors (TLRs).

As a chronic, lifelong disease, CF will be best treated with a continuous level of CFTR expression. This could be achieved either by repeated application or with a long-duration expression system. Viral vectors, which are mainly used in gene therapy appear difficult to administer repeatedly [24], in contrast to synthetic approaches [25].

The use of genomic DNA that contains all the control elements that allow gene expression at physiological levels has been utilized [26]. Extensive knowledge of the critical regulatory elements in the CFTR locus is required.

The CFTR gene maps at 7q31.2 and the expression is regulated during development and in different tissues. The CFTR locus is in connection with genes with different tissue-specific expression profiles, suggesting the presence of specific control promoters and insulators. Nuclear localization studies of CFTR and its adjacent gene loci in humans and mice demonstrate that different chromatin regions behave independently, depending on their expression profiles [27].

2.1. Applications of RNA interference to treat CF

The recent knowledge in the field of small interfering RNAs has led to the development of applications in relevance to CF. The RNAi technology has been used in order to identify gene products that contribute to steps in wild-type and mutant CFTR production and action [28]. Therefore, there is a possibility that RNAi-based strategies could be developed to increase the expression of ΔF508 CFTR, to rescue ΔF508 CFTR from proteosomal degradation or prolong its action on cell membrane. Similarly, targeting other cellular pathways, such as the inflammatory process, might lead to the reduction of symptoms. A significant obstacle to overcome is the identification of methods to efficiently deliver RNAi to differentiated airway epithelia.

2.2. Lung tissue engineering

Lung transplantation is currently the only definitive treatment for end-stage CF lung disease. However, the availability of donors is limited and the survival of transplantation is hardly 10–20% at 10 years [29]. Recently, two groups independently used similar tissue-engineering strategies to develop an autologous bioartificial lung that may begin to help overcome the limited availability of donor tissues [30, 31]. Evidence for gas exchange within the resulting grafts was demonstrated. Following the development of this technology, the ex vivo correction of patient-derived cells and the transplantation of these cells could lead to the cure of the disease. Although these initial results are very exciting, several steps need to be further optimized before long-term tissue-engineered lung function can be used in patient applications [32].

3. Gene therapy in Chronic Obstructive Pulmonary Disease (COPD)

Chronic obstructive pulmonary disease is a disease characterised by the presence of airflow obstruction generally progressive due to chronic bronchitis or emphysema and may be partially reversible. COPD is the 4th leading cause of death in the United States. In 2000, the WHO estimated 2.74 million deaths worldwide from COPD. In-patient hospitalization and emergency department care accounts for >73% of this cost COPD costs $1,522 per person per year (3 times asthma costs) [GOLD 2008].

Tobacco smoke is by far the most important risk factor for COPD worldwide. Other important risk factors are occupational exposure, socioeconomic status and genetic predisposition [33]. Thus, investigating into copd and into management possibilities is of high importance in order to provide the essential help to the patients. The currently used drugs can manage effectively the main symptoms of copd and may control the symptoms of this condition.

To date, there are no effective treatments for emphysema, nor are there efficient clinical management strategies. Novel approaches using gene therapy and stem cell technologies may offer new opportunities. However, this will remain almost entirely dependent on a more thorough understanding of the pathogenesis of COPD [34]. Currently, the most accepted theory for the development of COPD is protease/ antiprotease imbalance similar to emphysema due to hereditary 1-antitrypsin deficiency [35]. Newer studies [36] have shown that the pathogenesis of COPD involves not only elastases, but also collagenases and gelatinases. Experimental models [37] have suggested a role for 1-antitrypsin and secretory leukoprotease inhibitor in the treatment of this disorder. However, there is still need for a convincing study proving the concept of antiprotease treatment for COPD and emphysema [38] Neutrophils are a major source of proteases and reactive oxygen, so gene therapy could also target adhesion molecules for neutrophils to reduce their accumulation into the lung parenchyma.

3.1. A1-antitrypsin deficiency

A1-antitrypsin (AAT), is a major anti-protease serum protein, counteracting the effects of neutrophil elastase and other pro-inflammatory molecules released at sites of lung inflammation [39]. There are not effective treatments using protein therapy so gene therapy is being evaluated as an alternative approach.

Early studies in cotton rats using first-generation Ad vectors resulted in detection of AAT in bronchoalveolar fluid for only 1 week post-administration [40]. Cationic liposomes have also been used to express human AAT in the rabbit lung following aerosolisation [41]. Recombinant AAV vectors are being evaluated for more persistent expression of therapeutic serum levels of human AAT in murine and non-human primate models following intramuscular injection [42]. A1-antitrypsin deficiency is a pulmonary disease with an underlying single gene defect and a target for gene therapy. One specific treatment for AAT deficiency available is the administration of AAT intravenously, but only 2–3% of the infused AAT actually reach the lungs. Another method of administration is the inhalation of nebulized AAT powder or aerosolized AAT solution [43]. However, the treatment by the means of an alternative therapy, namely gene therapy, provides long term solution [44]. Several vectors containing cDNA of AAT have been constructed for treating AAT deficiency diseases. These vectors are retroviral [45], adenoviral [46] and adeno-associated viral [47]. Besides this, AAT gene can also be transferred by liposomal vectors [48]. First clinical trial has demonstrated that AAT gene could be transferred in humans [49]. Patients with AAT deficiency received a single dose of non-viral cationic liposome. Protein Gene Therapy for Alpha-1-Antitrypsin Deficiency Diseases was detected in nasal lavage fluid, with maximum levels on fifth day, which is approximately one third of the normal levels. The retroviral vector containing cDNA of human AAT with constitutive promoter have also been used as a delivery system. The disadvantage of retroviral vector system is that transgene expression is low. The adenoviral vectors containing human AAT cDNA have been delivered to different organs and cells [50]. Results in vitro demonstrated that human alpha-1-antitrypsin was synthesized as well as secreted. The adenoviruses are pathogenic in nature as well as immunogenic, therefore they have limited applications in treating AAT deficiency diseases. Recombinant adeno-associated viral vectors have been most successful delivery system so far, as they are capable of achieving therapeutic levels of AAT [51], and are less likely to induce an inflammatory response than adenoviral vectors. These viral and non-viral vectors showed advantages as well as disadvantages in curing AAT deficiency diseases. Among tested rAAV serotypes, the rAAV8 was found to be more powerful gene therapy vector for treating lungs and liver diseases [52]. Newly developed AAV vector looks promising for treating AAT deficiency diseases.

4. Gene therapy in asthma

Asthma is a disorder defined by certain clinical, physiological and pathological characteristics. Asthma is a chronic inflammatory disorder of the airways associated with airway hyper-responsiveness that leads to recurrent episodes of wheezing, breathlessness, chest tightness, and coughing, usually associated with widespread, but variable, airflow obstruction that is often reversible either spontaneously or with treatment [GINA 2000]. Since its pathogenesis is not clear, this definition is descriptive and inclusive of different phenotypes that are being increasingly recognized. Worldwide, 300 million people are supposed to be affected by asthma [53]. It appears that the global prevalence of asthma ranges 1–18% of the population in different countries. The WHO has estimated that 15 million disability-adjusted life-yrs are lost annually due to asthma, representing 1% of the total global disease burden [54]. Annual worldwide deaths from asthma have been estimated at 250,000 and mortality does not appear to correlate well with prevalence.

The best treatment of asthma is inhaled corticosteroids and bronchodilators, for the majority of asthmatic patients [55]. Gene therapy could bring some benefit for asthmatic patients with uncontrolled asthma who require high doses of corticosteroids and for patients with corticosteroid- resistant asthma. The target of gene therapy in bronchial asthma could be the overexpression of T-helper (Th) type 1 cytokines that influence the Th2 cytokine reactions [56]. Moreover the overexpression of IL-12 also restored local antiviral immunity, which is impaired in a Th2-dominated environment particulary during exacerbations of bronchial asthma due to viral infections [57]. Another study [58],examined the gene transfer of IFN that is a very interesting mediator in the airway hyper-responsiveness. Furthermore, another newer study [59] has shown that the transfer of the glucocorticoid receptor gene in vitro mediated the inhibition of nuclear factor-B activities even in absence of exogenous corticosteroids, and the authors suggested that this approach could restore corticosteroid sensitivity in patients.

5. Gene therapy in lung cancer

Lung cancer is the most common cancer worldwide, it is responsible for 12.4% of new cases of cancer in 2002. The overall mortality is 87% and 5-year survival is estimated to range from 15% in USA to 8.9% in developing countries [60]. It ranks first as the cause of death and it is responsible for 1.18 million deaths in 2002 and it is accounted by the World Health Organization for 18.4% of all cancer deaths by 2015. Non-small cell cancer (NSCLC) accounts for approximately 85% of lung cancers [61].

Even if there have been a lot of advances in surgery, radiation and chemotherapy, the 5-year survival for lung cancer remains poor. There is now great interest in gene therapy approaches for thoracic malignancies. Lung cancer is usually metastatic at the time of diagnosis and systemic therapy is needed rather than local therapy.

Gene therapy for thoracic malignancies represents a therapeutic approach that has been evaluated in clinical trials for the last two decades. Using viral vectors or antisense RNA, strategies have included induction of apoptosis, suicide gene expression,cytokine based therapy, various vaccinations and adoptive transfer of modified immune cells.

5.1. Clinical trials

5.1.1. Replacement of tumor suppressors

The goal of this strategy is to use a gene vector in order to encode a tumor-suppressor protein in tumor cells that is mutated or absent in the majority of lung cancers.

Tumor-based p53 therapy: It has been shown that the replacement of the normal p53 tumor suppressor gene in tumor cells induces rapid cell death by studies in cellular and animal models. In several early-phase clinical studies the strategy of the restoring the wild-type p53 expression in lung tumor cells was studied. The first study to demonstrate the feasibility of tumor suppressor gene replacement mediating tumor regression was a phase I study in which a retrovirus vector carrying wild-type p53 was administered to 7 patients with lung cancer with direct intra-tumoral injection. There was evidence of increased apoptosis in 6 patients and tumor regression in 3 patients [62]. Other phase I studies of p53 replacement with adenoviral vectors resulted in few partial responses and several patients with stabilization of disease[63, 64, 65]. Weill et al. delivered Ad.p53 to obstructive lesions endobronchially and they had several partial responses [66]. In another large phase I study of Ad.p53 gene transfer that was delivered intra-tumoraly in combination with chemotherapy, it was shown that there was increased apoptosis in transduced tumors when examined histologically [67]. A single-arm phase II study of intratumoral Ad.p53 in combination with radiation showed tumor regression in 63% (12 of 19) and was well tolerated [68]. But in another phase II study there was no difference in response rates for Ad.p53/chemotherapy-treated lesions for primary tumor lesions versus lesions treated with chemotherapy alone and this showed that Ad.p53 provided little local benefit over chemotherapy [69]. Keedy et al. delivered repeatedly Ad.p53 by bronchoalveolar lavage (BAL) to patients with bronchoalveolar carcinoma. It was shown that this delivery resulted in transient expression of p53 in 19% (3 of 16) of patients,2 of the 3 patients achieved stable disease. It was suggested that BAL could be used for adenoviral delivery, but toxicity was a serious issue with this approach [70]. Guan et al. delivered Ad.p53 alone or in combination with bronchial artery instillation (BIA) of chemotherapy (fluorouracil, navelbine or cisplatin). The delivery of Ad.p53 was performed via direct percutaneous delivery or via BIA. There was 47% response rate in the combination group and an improvement in time to progression when compared with BAI alone [71]. The Adp53 has been approved for usage in neck and head cancers in China, but there are not any trials using Ad.p53 in lung cancer in USA. Vanchani et al. believed that there is a strong issue with the application of this method in lung cancer (especially treating endobronchial lesions) as there is no bystander effect in combination with low transfection efficiency of adenoviral vectors [72].

FUS1 Replacement: FUS1 is a novel tumor suppressor gene that was identified in human chromosome 3p21.3 region where allele losses and genetic alterations occur for some human cancers. In most premalignant lung lesions and lung cancers the expression of FUS1 protein is absent. It was shown that wt-FUS1 function was restored in 3p21.3-deficient non-small cell lung carcinoma cells and this function inhibited tumor cell growth by induction of apoptosis and alteration of cell cycle kinetics [73].

Gene-Modified Dentritic Cell-Based Vaccination: Dentritic cells (DC) are the most potent antigen presenting cells in the immune system and they have been used for vaccination as vaccine vehicles. They have been used in two ways. The first one is to modify DC ex vivo with chemokines or cytokines and inject them directly into tumors and then they take antigen and induce immune response. The second one is to load immature, phagocytic DC with antigen with the aid of purified protein, cell extracts, mRNA and gene vectors and after that they inject these DC subcutaneously.

Ad.p53: p53 protein: It is proposed as a tumor antigen for vaccines as mutant p53 exists in very high levels in tumor cells and has more prolonged half-time than normal cells. p53-based gene therapy (p53 transduced DC) with standard chemotherapy showed promising results [74]. In a phase I trial, 29 patients with small cell lung cancer were vaccinated with DC transduced with Ad.p53 and the result was 1 patient with partial response and 7 cases with stable disease. Besides, out of the 21 patients that received a second line of chemotherapy, there was 62% response rate much higher from the rate that it is known for the second line therapy in small cell lung cancer. There was also a better survival (12.1 months instead of 9.6 months) in patients that showed an immune response to vaccination.

CCL21: CCL21 is a CC chemokine which is expressed in high levels in high endothelial venules and T cell zones of spleen and lymph nodes and also it attracts mature DC, naive T cells and induces T-cell activation [75]. Preclinical data showed that there was potent activity against lung cancers when DC transduced with CCL1 were injected into tumors.

Gene-Modified Tumor Cell-Based Vaccination: Killed tumor cells (usually irradiated) have been injected into patients as vaccines against recurrent cancers for many years with partial successful results.

Transforming growth factor β2 antisense vector modified cells: It is known that increased levels of transforming growth factor (TGF-β2) are associated with greater immunosuppression and poorer prognosis in patients with NSCLC. Preclinical studies showed that the delivery of an antisense gene to TGF-β2 to ex vivo tumor cells inhibited cellular TGF-β2 expression and resulted in increased immunogenicity when these tumor cells were administered as a vaccine. In a phase II trial this method of vaccination with irradiated tumor cells modified with a TGF-β2 antisense vector (belagenpumatucel-L) was evaluated. There was better survival (dose-related) with minimal toxicity. Besides there were different immunologic end points such as increased levels of cytokines (INF-γ, interleukin-6, interleukin-4) and increased levels of antibody production to vaccine HLAs. In a trial, 21 patients received belagenpumatucel-L at a single dose [76]. It was shown that 70% of cases were stable, but there was no complete or partial response. There is an ongoing phase III trial in which this vaccination is evaluated.

Tumor cells modified to secrete granulocyte-monocyte colony stimulating factor(GVAX): Granulocyte-monocyte colony stimulating factor (GM-CSF) is a cytokine that is involved in the maturation and proliferation of myeloid progenitor cells and stimulates proliferation, maturation and migration of DC and that leads to induction of T-cell immune responses against cancer. There are preclinical studies in which the transfection of tumor cells with the

GM-CSF gene has led these cells to induce antitumor immune responses. The clinical trials in lung cancer started using a vaccine platform with intradermal vaccination of irradiated autologous tumor cells that were virally enginnered to secrete GM-CSF [77, 78]. In the first trial of cases of metastatic NSCLC, GM-CSF was transduced into autologous tumor cells with the aid of adenoviral vector before irradiation and vaccination. There were a few clinical responses with a strong immune response. A delayed hypersensitivity reaction to irradiated, autologous nontransfected tumor cells was observed in patients. Nemunaitis J,et al. used a similar strategy in early-stage and late-stage patients and they showed that there were several clinical responses with similar immunologic outcomes [79]. In another trial, Nemunaitis J,et al. used a vaccine of unmodified, irradiated autologous tumor cells mixed with a GM-CSF-secreting bystander cell line. The vaccine GM-CSF secretion was higher than with the autologous vaccine, but the frequency of vaccine site reactions, tumor responses and survival were less favorable with the bystander vaccine [80]. Finally, the GVAX approach was not used more in lung cancer because the results were not satisfied and now only studies in pancreatic cancer are going on.

a(1,3)Galactosyltransferase: The gene that encodes a(1,3) Galactosyltransferase is not active in humans and it is functional in other mammalian cells. The major mechanism of hyperacute rejection of xenotransplants is the production of anti-a Gal antibodies in humans. Morris J et al. used allogeneic NSCLC tumor cells that were retrovirally modified to express aGT. It was shown that 6 of 17 patients, that received intradermal treatments, had prolonged stable disease [81].

B7.1/HLA vaccination: B7.1 is the one that costimulates T cells during priming by an antigen-priming cell. In a phase I trial of 19 patients with advanced NSCLC, treatment with an allogeneic lung cancer cell line vaccine transfected with B7.1,HLA-A1 and HLA-A2 was done. There was one partial response and 5 cases with stable disease. In the 6 responders, the CD8 T cell titers to tumor cell stimulations were elevated steadily till 150 weeks after therapy [82].A phase II trial is ongoing in patients with stage IIIB/IV who fail after the first line chemotherapy.

5.1.2. Vaccines

MUC-1 vaccination: MUC-1 is a tumor-associated mucin-type surface antigen normally found on epithelial cells in many tissues. In cases of lung cancer the targeting of MUC-1 has been used in a lot of ways with gene and non-gene therapy approaches. Ramlau R et al. in their 2 arm phase II trial with 65 patients with IIIB/IV NSCLC used a vaccinia virus containing the coding sequences for MUC1 and IL-2 (TG4010).The patients that participated in the trial had MUC-1 antigen expression on the primary tumor or metastases. In the 1ST arm (44 patients), combination therapy with TG4010 and cisplatin/vinorelbine was given, and in the 2nd arm TG4010 monotherapy was given followed by combination therapy at progression. In the 1st arm there was partial response in 29.5% and survival rate of 53% for the 1st year. In the 2nd arm, two of the 21 patients had stable disease for more than 6 months with monotherapy of TG4010 and this arm was terminated early as the results were not satisfied. There were MUC1-specific responses for 12 of 21 patients with stable disease or partial response.

Disease control was observed for 4 of 5 patients. The existence of MUC1 specific responses was translated to longer time to progression and better overall survival [83].

L523S vaccination: L523S is an immunogetic lung antigen that is expressed in 80% of lung cancer cells. Nemunaitis et al. in a phase I study, they gave two doses of intramuscular recombinant DNA followed by two doses of Ad.L523S (given 4 weeks apart) to 13 patients with early stage NSCLC(stage 1B,IIA and IIB). The authors found that only 1 patient showed a L523S-specific antibody response [84].

5.2. Antisense therapy

This technology is able to downregulate a lot of molecules that promote lung cancer tumor growth. There are 3 trials with antisense therapy. In the first trial aprinocarsen was used. Aprinocarsen is an oligonucleotide that binds to mRNA for protein kinase C-a and inhibits its expression. It was demonstrated that this molecule was safe in patients with lung cancer and it was characterized by modest activity in combination with chemotherapy [85]. In another trial with chemotherapy with or without aprinocarsen as first line therapy, it was shown that there was no better survival but with some toxicity as well [86]. In phase I studies it was shown that few patients had prolonged stable disease and 1 patient had response with the administration of Raf antisense molecules [87]. In patients with lung cancer in two phase II studies, these molecules did not show any antitumor activity [88]. Next, in other trials, the authors used Bcl-2, an apoptotic inhibitor which is overexpressed by many tumors and especially by 80-90% of SCLCs; the existence of this inhibitor means increased resistance to chemotherapy. In two trials there were encouraging results [89, 90], but in another trial of standard chemotherapy with or without a bcl-2 antisense oligonucleotide (oblimersen) more hematologic toxicity and worse overall survival was observed in the experimental arm [91].

5.3. New directions

The trials that have been made about gene therapy in lung cancer, preclinically and clinically, have demonstrated intermittent efficacy. The technology of gene transfer is promising but it is not easy to transduce more than a small number of tumor cells. This is a very important issue especially with approaches that they do not have bystander effects. It is very important to create vectors that they are able to induce long term in vivo expression as lentiviruses and AAVs.

Another interesting strategy is the immune-gene therapy, which requires gene transduction for stimulating an endogenous immune response and in this way a bystander effect is generated. There are some engouraging approaches with gene therapy to stimulate anti-tumor responses by delivering immunostimulatory cytokines or by administering a vaccine.

There is another important field of creating adoptive transfer of gene-modified autologous lymphocytes that are modified ex vivo by using lentiviruses or retroviruses. This approach is directed against mesothelioma and lung cancer cells.

6. Conclusion

Gene therapy is a very promising tool for the respiratory clinician and a few clinical trials have been performed. All these trials have shown safety but intermittent efficacy. Gene therapy for pulmonary diseases has not yet reached the point of clinical practice. But we can say that this tool will find a very interesting role in our efforts for treating respiratory diseases in the future.

Author details

Dimosthenis Lykouras[1], Kiriakos Karkoulias[1], Christos Tourmousoglou[2], Efstratios Koletsis[2], Kostas Spiropoulos[1] and Dimitrios Dougenis[2]

1 Department of Pulmonary Medicine, University Hospital of Patras, Greece

2 Department of Cardiothoracic Surgery, University Hospital of Patras, Greece

References

[1] Mall M, Bleich M, Greger R, Schreiber R, Kunzelmann K. The amiloride-inhibitable Na+ conductance is reduced by the cystic fibrosis transmembrane conductance regulator in normal but not in cystic fibrosis airways. J Clin Invest 1998;102:15–21

[2] Stutts MJ, Canessa CM, Olsen JC, et al. CFTR as a cAMP-dependent regulator of sodium channel. Science 1995;269:847–50. 1–3

[3] Matsui H, Grubb BR, Tarran R, et al. Evidence for periciliary liquid layer depletion, not abnormal ion composition, in the pathogenesis of cystic fibrosis airway disease. Cell 1998;95:1005–15

[4] Quinton PM. Cystic fibrosis: impaired bicarbonate secretion and mucoviscidosis. Lancet 2008;372:415–7

[5] Wine JJ, Joo NS. Submucosal glands and airway defense. Proc Am Thorac Soc 2004;1:47–53

[6] Devidas, S. and Guggino, W.B. (1997) CFTR: domains, structure, and function. J. Bioenerg. Biomembr., 29, 443–451

[7] Riordan, J.R. (2008) CFTR function and prospects for therapy. Annu. Rev. Biochem., 77, 701–726

[8] Johnson, L.G., Olsen, J.C., Sarkadi, B., Moore, K.L., Swanstrom, R. and Boucher, R.C. (1992) Efficiency of gene transfer for restoration of normal airway epithelial function in cystic fibrosis. Nat. Genet., 2, 21–25

[9]   Engelhardt, J.F., Yankaskas, J.R., Ernst, S.A., Yang, Y., Marino, C.R., Boucher, R.C., Cohn, J.A. and Wilson, J.M. (1992) Submucosal glands are the predominant site of CFTR expression in the human bronchus. Nat. Genet., 2, 240–248

[10] Zhou, L., Dey, C.R., Wert, S.E., DuVall, M.D., Frizzell, R.A. and Whitsett, J.A. (1994) Correction of lethal intestinal defect in a mouse model of cystic fibrosis by human CFTR. Science, 266, 1705–1708

[11] Joo, N.S., Cho, H.J., Khansaheb, M. and Wine, J.J. (2010) Hyposecretion of fluid from tracheal submucosal glands of CFTR-deficient pigs. J. Clin. Invest., 120, 3161–3166

[12] Liu, X., Luo, M., Guo, C., Yan, Z., Wang, Y., Lei-Butters, D.C. and Engelhardt, J.F. (2009) Analysis of adeno-associated virus progenitor cell transduction in mouse lung. Mol. Ther., 17, 285–293

[13] Rock, J.R., Onaitis, M.W., Rawlins, E.L., Lu, Y., Clark, C.P., Xue, Y., Randell, S.H. and Hogan, B.L. (2009) Basal cells as stem cells of the mouse trachea and human airway epithelium. Proc. Natl Acad. Sci. USA, 106, 12771–12775

[14] Randell, S.H. (1992) Progenitor-progeny relationships in airway epithelium. Chest, 101, 11S–16S

[15] Ford, J.R. and Terzaghi-Howe, M. (1992) Basal cells are the progenitors of primary tracheal epithelial cell cultures. Exp. Cell Res., 198, 69–77

[16] Borthwick, D.W., Shahbazian, M., Krantz, Q.T., Dorin, J.R. and Randell, S.H. (2001) Evidence for stem-cell niches in the tracheal epithelium. Am. J. Respir. Cell Mol. Biol., 24, 662–670

[17] Hong, K.U., Reynolds, S.D., Giangreco, A., Hurley, C.M. and Stripp, B.R. (2001) Clara cell secretory protein-expressing cells of the airway neuroepithelial body microenvironment include a label-retaining subset and are critical for epithelial renewal after progenitor cell depletion. Am. J. Respir. Cell Mol. Biol., 24, 671–681

[18] Flotte TR, Ng P, Dylla DE, et al. Viral vector-mediated and cell-based therapies for treatment of cystic fibrosis. Mol Ther 2007;15:229–41

[19] Zhang L, Bukreyev A, Thompson CI, et al. Infection of ciliated cells by human para-influenza virus type 3 in an in vitro model of human airway epithelium. J Virol 2005;79:1113–24

[20] Griesenbach U, Boyton RJ, Somerton L, et al. Effect of tolerance induction to immunodominant T-cell epitopes of Sendai virus on gene expression following repeat administration. Gene Ther 2006;13:449–56

[21] Copreni E, Penzo M, Carrabino S, Conese M. Lentiviral-mediated gene transfer to the respiratory epithelium: a promising approach to gene therapy of Cystic Fibrosis. Gene Ther 2004;11:S67–75

[22] Lee ER, Marshall J, Siegel CS, et al. Detailed analysis of structures and formulations of cationic lipids for efficient gene transfer to the lung. Hum Gene Ther 1996;7:1701–17

[23] Yamamoto A, Kormann M, Rosenecker J, Rudolph C. Current prospects for mRNA gene delivery. Eur J Pharm Biopharm 2009;71:484–9

[24] Moss, R. B.,Milla, C., Colombo, J., Accurso, F., Zeitlin, P. L., Clancy, J. P., et al. (2007) Repeated aerosolized AAV-CFTR for treatment of cystic fibrosis: a randomized placebocontrolled phase 2B trial. Hum. Gene Ther. 18, 726–732

[25] Hyde, S. C., Southern, K. W., Gileadi, U., Fitzjohn, E. M., Mofford, K. A., Waddell, B. E., et al. (2000) Repeat administration of DNA/liposomes to the nasal epithelium of patients with cystic fibrosis. Gene Ther. 7, 1156–1165

[26] Conese M, Boyd AC, Di Gioia S, Auriche C, Ascenzioni F. Genomic context vectors and artificial chromosomes for cystic fibrosis gene therapy. Curr Gene Ther 2007;7:175–87

[27] Zink D, Amaral MD, Englmann A, et al. Transcription-dependent spatial arrangements of CFTR and adjacent genes in human cell nuclei. J Cell Biol 2004;166:815–25

[28] Wang, X., Venable, J., LaPointe, P., Hutt, D.M., Koulov, A.V., Coppinger, J., Gurkan, C., Kellner, W., Matteson, J., Plutner, H. et al. (2006) Hsp90 cochaperone Aha1 downregulation rescues misfolding of CFTR in cystic fibrosis. Cell, 127, 803–815

[29] Orens, J.B. and Garrity, E.R. Jr (2009) General overview of lung transplantation and review of organ allocation. Proc. Am. Thorac. Soc., 6, 13–19

[30] Petersen, T.H., Calle, E.A., Zhao, L., Lee, E.J., Gui, L., Raredon, M.B., Gavrilov, K., Yi, T., Zhuang, Z.W., Breuer, C. et al. (2010) Tissue-engineered lungs for in vivo implantation. Science, 329, 538–541

[31] Ott, H.C., Clippinger, B., Conrad, C., Schuetz, C., Pomerantseva, I., Ikonomou, L., Kotton, D. and Vacanti, J.P. (2010) Regeneration and orthotopic transplantation of a bioartificial lung. Nat. Med., 16, 927–933

[32] de Perrot, M., Fischer, S., Liu, M., Imai, Y., Martins, S., Sakiyama, S., Tabata, T., Bai, X.H., Waddell, T.K., Davidson, B.L. et al. (2003) Impact of human interleukin-10 on vector-induced inflammation and early graft function in rat lung transplantation. Am. J. Respir. Cell Mol. Biol., 28, 616–625

[33] Menzies D, Nair A, Williamson PA, Schembri S, Al-Khairalla MZ, Barnes M, et al. Respiratory symptoms, pulmonary function, and markers of inflammation among bar workers before and after a legislative ban on smoking in public places. JAMA 2006;296(14):1742-8

[34] Eisner MD, Balmes J, Katz BP, Trupin L, Yelin E, Blanc P. Lifetime environmental tobacco smoke exposure and the risk of chronic obstructive pulmonary disease. Environ Health Perspect 2005;4:7-15

[35] Barnes, P. J. Mediators of chronic obstructive pulmonary disease. Pharm. Rev. 56, 515–548 (2004)

[36] Segura-Valdez L, Pardo A, Gaxiola M, et al. Upregulation of gelatinases A and B, collagenases 1 and 2, and increased parenchymal cell death in COPD. Chest 2000; 117:684–694

[37] Tomee JF, Koeter GH, Hiemstra PS, et al. Secretory leukoprotease inhibitor: a native antimicrobial protein presenting a new therapeutic option? Thorax 1998; 53:114–116

[38] Rogers DF, Laurent GJ. New ideas on the pathophysiology and treatment of lung disease. Thorax 1998; 53:200–203

[39] Carrell R. W. (1986) alpha 1-Antitrypsin: molecular pathology, leukocytes, and tissue damage. J Clin Invest 78: 1427–1431

[40] Rosenfeld M. A., Siegfried W., Yoshimura K., Yoneyama K., Fukayama M., Stier L. E. et al. (1991) Adenovirus-mediated transfer of a recombinant alpha 1-antitrypsin gene to the lung epithelium in vivo. Science 252: 431–434

[41] Canonico A. E., Conary J. T., Meyrick B. O. and Brigham K. L. (1994) Aerosol and intravenous transfection of human alpha- 1-antitrypsin gene to lungs of rabbits. Am J Respir Cell Mol. Biol. 10: 24–29

[42] Song S., Scott-Jorgensen M., Wang J., Poirier A., Crawford J. and Campbell-Thompson M. et al. (2002) Intramuscular administration of recombinant adeno-associated virus 2 alpha- 1 antitrypsin (rAAV-SERPINA1) vectors in a nonhuman primate model: safety and immunologic aspects. Mol. Ther. 6: 329–335

[43] Crystal, R. G.(1992). Gene therapy strategies for pulmonary diseases. American Journal of Medicine, Vol 92, No. 6A, pp.44S-52S, ISSN 1175-6365]. [Hubbard, R. C. & Crystal, R. G. (1990). Strategies for aerosol therapy of alpha l-antitrypsin deficiency by the aerosol route. Lung, Vol 168, Supplement, pp.565-578, ISSN 0341- 2040

[44] Flotte, T. (March 2011).Alpha-1-antitrypsin Deficiency, In:Project, 20.3.2011, Available from http://www.gtc.ufl.edu/research/gtc-rppulm.htm#aa

[45] Kay, M. A.; Baley, P.; Rothenberg, S.; Leland, F.; Fleming, L.; Ponder, K. P.; Liu, T.; Finegold, M.; Darlington, G.; Pokorny, W, et al. (1992). Expression of human α- 1- antitrypsin in dogs after autologous transplantation of retroviral transduced hepatocytes. Proceeding of the National Academy of Science of the United State of America, Vol 89, No. 1, pp. 89–93, ISSN 0027-8424

[46] Jaffe, H. A.; Danel, C.; Longenecker, G.; Metzger, M.; Setoguchi,Y.; Rosenfeld, M. A.; Gant, T.W.; Thorgeirsson, S. S.; Stratford-Perricaudet, L. D.; Perricaudet, M, et al. (1992). Adenovirus-mediated in vivo gene transfer and expression in normal rat liver. Nature Genetics, Vol 1, No.5, pp. 372–378, ISSN 1061-4036

[47] Song, S.; Morgan, M.; Ellis, T.; Poirier, A.; Chesnut, K.; Wang, J.; Brantley, M.; Muzyczka, N.; Byrne, B. J.; Atkinson, M. & Flotte, T. R. (1998). Sustained secretion of hu-

man α -1-antitrypsin from murine muscle transduced with adeno-associated virus vectors. Proceeding of the National Academy of Science of the United State of America, Vol 95, No.24, pp.14384–14388, ISSN 0027-8424

[48] Canonico, A. E.; Conary, J. T.; Meyrick, B.O. & Brigham, K.L.(1994).Aerosol and intravenous transfection of human -1 antitrypsin gene to lungs of rabbits. American Journal of Respiratory Cell and Molecular Biology, Vol 10, No.1, pp. 24–29, ISSN 1044-1549]

[49] Brigham, K. L.; Lane, K. B.; Meyrick, B.; Stecenko, A. A.; Strack, S.; Cannon, D. R.; Caudill, M. & Canonico, A. E. (2000).Transfection of nasal mucosa with a normal alpha-1 antitrypsin (AAT) gene in AAT deficient subjects: comparison with protein therapy. Human Gene Therapy, Vol 11, No.7, pp. 1023–1032, ISSN 1043-0342

[50] Rosenfeld, M. A.; Siegfried, W.; Yoshimura, K.; Yoneyama, K.; Fukayama, M.; Stier, L. E.; Paakko, P. K.; Gilardi, P.; Stratford-Perricaudet, L. D.; Perricaudet, M, et al. (1991).Adenovirus-mediated transfer of a recombinant α-1-antitrypsin gene to the lung epithelium in vivo. Science, Vol 252, No.5004, pp. 431–434

[51] Song, S.; Morgan, M.; Ellis, T.; Poirier, A.; Chesnut, K.; Wang, J.; Brantley, M.; Muzyczka, N.; Byrne, B. J.; Atkinson, M. & Flotte, T. R. (1998). Sustained secretion of human α -1-antitrypsin from murine muscle transduced with adeno-associated virus vectors. Proceeding of the National Academy of Science of the United State of America, Vol 95, No.24, pp.14384–14388, ISSN 0027-8424

[52] Sifers, R. N.; Brashears-Macatee, S.; Kidd, V. J.; Muensch, H. & Woo, S.L. (1988). A frameshift mutation results in a truncated α-1-antitrypsin that is retained within the rough endoplasmic reticulum. Journal of Biological Chemistry, Vol 263, No.15, pp. 7330–7335, ISSN 0021-9258

[53] Global Strategy for Asthma Management and Prevention. Global Initiative for Asthma (GINA), 2006. Available from www.ginasthma.org Date last updated, 2006

[54] Masoli M, Fabian D, Holt S, Beasley R. The global burden of asthma: executive summary of the GINA Dissemination Committee report. Allergy 2004; 59: 469 478

[55] Alton EW, Griesenbach U, Geddes DM. Gene therapy for asthma: inspired research or unnecessary effort? Gene Ther 1999; 6:155–156

[56] Mathieu M, Gougat C, Jaffuel D, et al. The glucocorticoid receptor gene as a candidate for gene therapy in asthma. Gene Ther 1999; 6:245–252

[57] Hogan SP, Foster PS, Tan X, et al. Mucosal IL-12 gene delivery inhibits allergic airways disease and restores local antiviral immunity. Eur J Immunol 1998; 28:413–423

[58] Dow SW, Schwarze J, Heath TD, et al. Systemic and local interferon gamma gene delivery to the lungs for treatment of allergen-induced airway hyperresponsiveness in mice. Hum Gene Ther 1999; 10:1905–1914.29

[59] Mathieu M, Gougat C, Jaffuel D, et al. The glucocorticoid receptor gene as a candidate for gene therapy in asthma. Gene Ther 1999; 6:245–252.30

[60] Parkin DM, Bray F, Ferlay J, et al. Global cancer statistics, 2002. CA Cancer J Clin 2005; 55:74-108

[61] Sher T, Dy GK, Adjei AA. Small cell lung cancer. Mayo Clin Proc 2008; 83:355-67

[62] Roth JA, Nguyen D, Lawrence DD, et al. Retrovirusmediated wild-type p53 gene transfer to tumors of patients with lung cancer. Nat Med 1996;2(9): 985–91

[63] Schuler M, Rochlitz C, Horowitz JA, et al. A phase I study of adenovirus-mediated wild-type p53 gene transfer in patients with advanced non-small cell lung cancer. Hum Gene Ther 1998;9(14):2075–82

[64] Swisher SG, Roth JA, Nemunaitis J, et al. Adenovirus- mediated p53 gene transfer in advanced non-small-cell lung cancer. J Natl Cancer Inst1999;91(9):763–71

[65] Fujiwara T, Tanaka N, Kanazawa S, et al. Multicenter phase I study of repeated intratumoral delivery of adenoviral p53 in patients with advanced nonsmall- cell lung cancer. J Clin Oncol 2006;24(11): 1689–99

[66] Weill D,Mack M,Roth J,et al. Adenoviral-mediated p53 gene transfer to non-small cell lung cancer through endobronchial injection.Chest 2000,118:966-970

[67] Nemunaitis J, Swisher SG, Timmons T, et al. Adenovirus-mediated p53 gene transfer in sequence with cisplatin to tumors of patients with non-small-cell lung cancer. J Clin Oncol 2000;18(3):609–22

[68] Swisher SG, Roth JA, Komaki R, et al. Induction of p53-regulated genes and tumor regression in lung cancer patients after intratumoral delivery of adenoviral p53 (INGN 201) and radiation therapy. Clin Cancer Res 2003;9(1):93–101

[69] Schuler M, Herrmann R, De Greve JL, et al. Adenovirus-mediated wild-type p53 gene transfer in patients receiving chemotherapy for advanced non-small-cell lung cancer: results of a multicenter phase II study. J Clin Oncol 2001;19(6):1750–8

[70] Keedy V, Wang W, Schiller J, et al. Phase I study of adenovirus p53 administered by bronchoalveolarlavage in patients with bronchioloalveolar cell lung carcinoma: ECOG 6597. J Clin Oncol 2008;26(25):4166–71

[71] Guan YS,Liu Y, Zou Q,et al.Adenovirus-mediated wild type p53 gene transfer in combination with bronchial arterial infusion for treatment of advanced non-small cell lung cancer,one year follow up.J Zhejiang Univ Sci B 2009; 10,5: 331-40

[72] Vanchani A,Moon E,Wakeam E, et al.Gene therapy for mesothelioma and lung cancer.Am J Respir Cell Mol Biol, 2010,42,385-393

[73] Ji L, Roth JA. Tumor suppressor FUS1 signaling pathway. J Thorac Oncol 2008;3(4): 327–30

[74] Antonia SJ, Mirza N, Fricke I, et al. Combination of p53 cancer vaccine with chemotherapy in patients with extensive stage small cell lung cancer. Clin Cancer Res 2006;12(3 Pt 1):878–87

[75] Baratelli F, Takedatsu H, Hazra S, et al. Pre-clinical characterization of GMP grade CCL21-gene modified dendritic cells for application in a phase I trial in non-small cell lung cancer. J Transl Med 2008;6:38

[76] Nemunaitis J, Dillman RO, Schwarzenberger PO, et al. Phase II study of belagenpumatucel-L, a transforming growth factor beta-2 antisense gene modified allogeneic tumor cell vaccine in nonsmall-cell lung cancer. J Clin Oncol 2006;24(29): 4721–30

[77] Nemunaitis J, Nemunaitis M, Senzer N, et al. Phase II trial of belagenpumatucel-L, a TGF-beta2 antisense gene modified allogeneic tumor vaccine in advanced non small cell lung cancer (NSCLC) patients. Cancer Gene Ther 2009;16(8):620–4

[78] Salgia R, Lynch T, Skarin A, et al. Vaccination with irradiated autologous tumor cells engineered to secrete granulocyte-macrophage colony-stimulating factor augments antitumor immunity in some patients with metastatic non-small-cell lung carcinoma. J Clin Oncol 2003;21(4):624–30

[79] Nemunaitis J, Sterman D, Jablons D, et al. Granulocyte- macrophage colony-stimulating factor genemodified autologous tumor vaccines in non-small-cell lung cancer. J Natl Cancer Inst 2004;96(4):326–31

[80] Nemunaitis J, Jahan T, Ross H, et al. Phase 1/2 trial of autologous tumor mixed with an allogeneic GVAX vaccine in advanced-stage non-small-cell lung cancer. Cancer Gene Ther 2006;13(6):555–62

[81] Morris JC, Vahanian N, Janik JE, et al. Phase I study of an antitumor vaccination using alpha(1,3)galactosyltransferase expressing allogeneic tumor cells in patients with refractory or recurrent non-small cell lung cancer (NSCLC). J Clin Oncol 2005;23(16S): 2586

[82] Raez LE, Cassileth PA, Schlesselman JJ, et al. Allogeneic vaccination with a B7.1 HLA-A gene-modified adenocarcinoma cell line in patients with advanced non-small-cell lung cancer. J Clin Oncol 2004;22(14):2800–7

[83] Ramlau R, Quoix E, Rolski J, et al. A phase II study of Tg4010 (mva-Muc1-Il2) in association with chemotherapy in patients with stage III/IV non-small cell lung cancer. J Thorac Oncol 2008;3(7):735–44

[84] Nemunaitis J, Meyers T, Senzer N, et al. Phase I trial of sequential administration of recombinant DNA and adenovirus expressing L523S protein in early stage non-small-cell lung cancer. Mol Ther 200613(6):1185–91

[85] Ritch P, Rudin CM, Bitran JD, et al. Phase II study ofnPKC-alpha antisense oligonucleotide aprinocarsen in combination with gemcitabine and carboplatin in patients with advanced non-small cell lung cancer.Lung Cancer 2006;52(2):173–80

[86] Paz-Ares L, Douillard JY, Koralewski P, et al. Phase III study of gemcitabine and cisplatin with or without aprinocarsen, a protein kinase C-alpha antisense oligonucleotide, in patients with advanced-stage non-small-cell lung cancer. J Clin Oncol 2006; 24(9):1428–34

[87] Rudin CM, Holmlund J, Fleming GF, et al. Phase I trial of ISIS 5132, an antisense oligonucleotide inhibitor of c-Raf-1, administered by 24-hour weekly infusion to patients with advanced cancer. Clin Cancer Res 2001;7(5):1214–20

[88] Coudert B, Anthoney A, Fiedler W, et al. Phase II trial with ISIS 5132 in patients with small-cell (SCLC) and non-small cell (NSCLC) lung cancer. A European Organization for Research and Treatment of Cancer (EORTC) early clinical studies group report. Eur J Cancer 2001;37 (17):2194–8

[89] Rudin CM, Otterson GA, Mauer AM, et al. A pilot trial of G3139, a bcl-2 antisense oligonucleotide, and paclitaxel in patients with chemorefractory smallcell lung cancer. Ann Oncol 2002;13(4):539–45

[90] Rudin CM, Kozloff M, Hoffman PC, et al. Phase I study of G3139, a bcl-2 antisense oligonucleotide, combined with carboplatin and etoposide in patients with small-cell lung cancer. J Clin Oncol 2004;22(6): 1110–7

[91] Rudin CM, Salgia R, Wang X, et al. Randomized phase II study of carboplatin and etoposide with or without the bcl-2 antisense oligonucleotide oblimersen for extensive-stage small-cell lung cancer: CALGB 30103. J Clin Oncol 2008;26(6):870–6

Permissions

The contributors of this book come from diverse backgrounds, making this book a truly international effort. This book will bring forth new frontiers with its revolutionizing research information and detailed analysis of the nascent developments around the world.

We would like to thank Francisco Martín Molina, for lending his expertise to make the book truly unique. He has played a crucial role in the development of this book. Without his invaluable contribution this book wouldn't have been possible. He has made vital efforts to compile up to date information on the varied aspects of this subject to make this book a valuable addition to the collection of many professionals and students.

This book was conceptualized with the vision of imparting up-to-date information and advanced data in this field. To ensure the same, a matchless editorial board was set up. Every individual on the board went through rigorous rounds of assessment to prove their worth. After which they invested a large part of their time researching and compiling the most relevant data for our readers. Conferences and sessions were held from time to time between the editorial board and the contributing authors to present the data in the most comprehensible form. The editorial team has worked tirelessly to provide valuable and valid information to help people across the globe.

Every chapter published in this book has been scrutinized by our experts. Their significance has been extensively debated. The topics covered herein carry significant findings which will fuel the growth of the discipline. They may even be implemented as practical applications or may be referred to as a beginning point for another development. Chapters in this book were first published by InTech; hereby published with permission under the Creative Commons Attribution License or equivalent.

The editorial board has been involved in producing this book since its inception. They have spent rigorous hours researching and exploring the diverse topics which have resulted in the successful publishing of this book. They have passed on their knowledge of decades through this book. To expedite this challenging task, the publisher supported the team at every step. A small team of assistant editors was also appointed to further simplify the editing procedure and attain best results for the readers.

Our editorial team has been hand-picked from every corner of the world. Their multi-ethnicity adds dynamic inputs to the discussions which result in innovative outcomes. These outcomes are then further discussed with the researchers and contributors who give their valuable feedback and opinion regarding the same. The feedback is then collaborated with the researches and they are edited in a comprehensive manner to aid the understanding of the subject.

Apart from the editorial board, the designing team has also invested a significant amount of their time in understanding the subject and creating the most relevant covers. They scrutinized every image to scout for the most suitable representation of the subject and create an appropriate cover for the book.

The publishing team has been involved in this book since its early stages. They were actively engaged in every process, be it collecting the data, connecting with the contributors or procuring relevant information. The team has been an ardent support to the editorial, designing and production team. Their endless efforts to recruit the best for this project, has resulted in the accomplishment of this book. They are a veteran in the field of academics and their pool of knowledge is as vast as their experience in printing. Their expertise and guidance has proved useful at every step. Their uncompromising quality standards have made this book an exceptional effort. Their encouragement from time to time has been an inspiration for everyone.

The publisher and the editorial board hope that this book will prove to be a valuable piece of knowledge for researchers, students, practitioners and scholars across the globe.

List of Contributors

Hiroshi Tomitaand
Department of Chemistry and Bioengineering, Iwate University, Morioka, Iwate, Japan
Tohoku University Hospital, Sendai, Miyagi, Japan

Eriko Sugano, Hitomi Isago and Namie Murayama
Department of Chemistry and Bioengineering, Iwate University, Morioka, Iwate, Japan

Makoto Tamai
Tohoku University Hospital, Sendai, Miyagi, Japan

Francisco Martin, Alejandra Gutierrez-Guerrero and Karim Benabdellah
Gene and Cell Therapy Group, Human DNA variability department, GENYO, Centre for Genomics and Oncological Research: Pfizer, University of Granada, Andalusian Regional Government. Parque Tecnológico Ciencias de la Salud (PTCS), Granada, Spain

Qiuhong Li, Amrisha Verma, Ping Zhu, Bo Lei and William W Hauswirth
Departments of Ophthalmology, University of Florida, Gainesville, FL, USA

Yiguo Qiu
Departments of Ophthalmology, University of Florida, Gainesville, FL, USA
The First Affiliated Hospital of Chongqing Medical University, Chongqing Key Laboratory of Ophthalmology, Chongqing Eye Institute, China

Takahiko Nakagawa
Division of Renal Disease and Hypertension, University of Colorado Denver, Aurora, CO, USA

Mohan K Raizada
Department of Physiology & Functional Genomics, University of Florida, Gainesville, FL, USA

E. Mayr, U. Koller and J.W. Bauer
EB House Austria, Dept. Dermatol, Paracelsus Med Univ., Salzburg, Austria

Maria Garcia-Gomez, Oscar Quintana-Bustamante, Maria Garcia-Bravo, S. Navarro, Zita Garate and Jose C. Segovia
Differentiation and Cytometry Unit, Hematopoiesis and Gene Therapy Division, Centro de Investigaciones Energéticas, Medioambientales y Tecnológicas (CIEMAT) and Centro de Investigación Biomédica en Red de Enfermedades Raras (CIBER-ER), Madrid, Spain

George Kotzamanis, Athanassios Kotsinas and Vassilis G. Gorgoulis
University of Athens, Medical School, Greece

Apostolos Papalois
Experimental Research Center ELPEN SA, Greece

Daisuke Tsuji and Kohji Itoh
Department of Medicinal Biotechnology, Graduate School of Pharmaceutical Sciences, Institute for Medicinal Research, The University of Tokushima, Tokushima, Japan
NIBIO, Ibaraki, Osaka, Japan

Gabriel J. Moreno-González
Intensive Care Unit, Hospital Universitari de Bellvitge, L'Hospitalet Llobregat, Barcelona, Spain

Angel Zarain-Herzberg
Biochemistry Department, School of Medicine, Universidad Nacional Autónoma de México, Mexico City, México

Isaura Tavares and Isabel Martins
Department of Experimental Biology, Faculty of Medicine of Porto, University of Porto, Portugal
IBMC - Instituto de Biologia Molecular e Celular, University of Porto, Portugal

Ann M. Simpson, Chang Tao, Bronwyn A O'Brien, Edwin Ch'ng, Leticia M. Castro, Julia Ting, Zehra Elgundi, Donald K. Martin and Graham M. Nicholson
School of Medical & Molecular Biosciences, University of Technology Sydney, Sydney, Australia

Tony An and M. Anne Swan
School of Medical Sciences (Anatomy & Histology) and Bosch Institute, University of Sydney, Australia

Guo Jun Liu
Brain and Mind Research Institute, Faculty of Health Sciences, University of Sydney and Life Sciences, Australian Nuclear Science and Technology Organization, Sydney, Australia

Mark Lutherborrow
Australian Foundation for Diabetes Research & Diabetes Transplant Unit, Sydney, Australia

Fraser Torpy
School of the Environment, University of Technology Sydney, Sydney, Australia

Bernard E. Tuch
Australian Foundation for Diabetes Research & Diabetes Transplant Unit, Prince of Wales Hospital, and CSIRO, Division of Materials Science and Engineering, Sydney, Australia

Divya Pankajakshan and Devendra K. Agrawal
Department of Biomedical Sciences and Center for Clinical & Translational Science
Creighton University School of Medicine, Omaha, NE, USA

Katsu Takahashi, Honoka Kiso, Kazuyuki Saito, Yumiko Togo, Hiroko Tsukamoto and Kazuhisa Bessho
Department of Oral and Maxillofacial Surgery, Graduate School of Medicine, Kyoto University, Sakyo-ku, Kyoto, Japan

Boyen Huang
Department of Paediatric Dentistry, School of Medicine and Dentistry, James Cook University, Cairns, Australia

Dimosthenis Lykouras, Kiriakos Karkoulias and Kostas Spiropoulos
Department of Pulmonary Medicine, University Hospital of Patras, Greece

Christos Tourmousoglou, Efstratios Koletsis and Dimitrios Dougenis
Department of Cardiothoracic Surgery, University Hospital of Patras, Greece

Printed in the USA
CPSIA information can be obtained
at www.ICGtesting.com
JSHW011501221024
72173JS00005B/1165